Journal of Semitic Studies Supplement 27

Novel Medical and General Hebrew Terminology from the 13th Century

Translations by Hillel Ben Samuel of Verona, Moses Ben Samuel Ibn Tibbon, Shem Tov Ben Isaac of Tortosa, Zeraḥyah Ben Isaac Ben She'altiel Ḥen

by

Gerrit Bos

Published by Oxford University Press
on behalf of the University of Manchester
2011

OXFORD
UNIVERSITY PRESS

Great Clarendon Street, Oxford OX2 6DP

Oxford University Press is a department of the University of Oxford.
It furthers the University's objective of excellence in research, scholarship,
and education by publishing worldwide in

Oxford New York

Athens Auckland Bangkok Bogotá Buenos Aires Cape Town
Chennai Dar es Salaam Delhi Florence Hong Kong Istanbul Karachi
Kolkata Kuala Lumpur Madrid Melbourne Mexico City Mumbai Nairobi
Paris São Paulo Shanghai Singapore Taipei Tokyo Toronto Warsaw

with associated companies in Berlin Ibadan

Oxford is a registered trade mark of Oxford University Press
in the UK and in certain other countries

Published in the United Kingdom
by Oxford University Press, Oxford

First published 2011

A catalogue for this book is available from the British Library

Library of Congress Cataloguing in Publication Data
(Data available)

ISSN 0022-4480
ISBN 978-0-19-969749-6

Subscription information for the *Journal of Semitic Studies* is available at the journal website:
jss.oupjournals.org

Printed in Great Britain by Bell & Bain Ltd, Glasgow

Table of Contents

Introduction. Novel Medical and General Hebrew Terminology from the 13th Century 1

1. Hillel Ben Samuel of Verona, *Sefer Keritut* 9

    Introduction 9

    Bruno Longobucco (Longoburgensis) *Cyrurgia magna* and the Hebrew Translation by Hillel 11

    Hillel's Poem on a Doctor's Fees 14

    Study of the technical terminology employed by Hillel in his translation of Bruno's *Cyrurgia* 16

    List of Terms 16

    I. Hebrew terms 16

    II. Hebrew transcriptions of Latin terms 43

    III. Mixed terms 45

2. Moses Ibn Tibbon, *Sefer Ẓedat ha-Derakhim* 47

    Introduction 47

    A. Dated Translations 49

    B. Undated Translations 50

    Study of the technical terminology employed by Moses Ibn Tibbon in his translation of Ibn al-Jazzār, *Zād al-musāfir*, Bk. 7, Chs 7–30 53

    List of Terms 53

3. Shem Tov Ben Isaac, Sefer *ha-Shimmush* 73

    Introduction 73

    List of Terms 76

4. Zeraḥyah Ben Isaac Ben She'altiel Ḥen, Hebrew translation of Maimonides' *Medical Aphorisms* (*Fuṣūl Mūsā fī l-Ṭibb*) 121

    Introduction 121

Zeraḥyah as a Translator 122

Study of the Terminology Employed by Zeraḥyah in his Translation of Maimonides' *Medical Aphorisms* 127

List of Terms 128

Abbreviations 196

Index 201

The cover illustration features in Shem Tov Ben Isaac's *Sefer ha-Shimmush*; i.e. the Hebrew translation of al-Zahrāwī's *Kitāb al-taṣrīf*, MS Paris, heb. 1163, which was copied in a sephardic script in the fourteenth century. The illustration is part of Bk 30 which deals with the subject of surgery.

Novel Medical and General Hebrew Terminology from the 13th Century Translations by Hillel Ben Samuel of Verona, Moses Ben Samuel Ibn Tibbon, Shem Tov Ben Isaac of Tortosa, and Zeraḥyah Ben Isaac Ben She'altiel Ḥen

The current collective volume has two major objectives: 1) to map the medical terminology featuring in medieval Hebrew medical works translated in the thirteenth century, especially those terms that do not feature in the current dictionaries at all or in an insufficient[1] way and thus facilitating consultation of these medical works; 2) to specify the medical terminology used by specific authors/translators and thus facilitating the identification of anonymous medical material. Unfortunately, the terminology in medieval Hebrew medical literature, both original works and translations, has been sorely neglected by modern research.[2] Moreover, it is virtually lacking in the standard dictionaries for the Hebrew language, such as *Ha-Millon he-ḥadash* composed by Abraham Even-Shoshan.[3] The only medieval medical work to which Even-Shoshan refers is the Hebrew translation of Ibn Sīnā's *K. al-Qānūn* by Nathan ha-Me'ati;[4] and even those references are indirect, having been borrowed from the dictionary composed by Ben Yehuda. Ben Yehuda's dictionary is indeed the only one containing a certain number of medical terms.[5] However, it needs to be revised since it does not make a consequent use of the limited sources registered in the introduction. The only dictionary exclusively devoted to medical terms, both medieval and modern, is that by Masie, entitled 'Dictionary of Medicine and Allied Sciences'.[6] However, just like the

1 With insufficient I mean that these terms do not feature in the dictionaries in the sense given to them by the translator, or they do feature in the dictionaries but not for the period in question. The introduction to this volume is a slightly revised version of the introduction to the article: 'Medical Terminology in the Hebrew Tradition: Shem Tov Ben Isaac, *Sefer ha-Shimmush*, book 30', JSS LV/1 (2010), 53–101.

2 The following survey does not take into consideration the field of the medieval plant names and remedies, with the exception of some characteristic examples.

3 The edition I consulted is that in five volumes (Jerusalem 2000).

4 Ibid., vol. 1, p. 16.

5 E. Ben Yehuda, *Millon ha-Lashon ha-Ivrit. Thesaurus Totius Hebraitatis et Veteris et Recentioris*. 17 vols (Berlin-Tel Aviv 1910–59. Repr. Tel Aviv 1948–59).

6 A.M. Masie, *Dictionary of Medicine and Allied Sciences. Latin-English-Hebrew*. Edited by S. Tchernichowski. (Jerusalem 1934).

dictionary by Ben Yehuda it only makes an occasional use of the sources registered in the introduction and only rarely differentiates between the various medieval translators. Further, since Masie's work is alphabetised according to the Latin or English term, it cannot be consulted for Hebrew terms. The *Historical Dictionary of the Hebrew Language* which is currently being composed by the Academy of the Hebrew Language is not taken into consideration consistently as it is not a dictionary in the proper sense of the word.[7] Moreover, its consultation in the past made it clear that the medieval medical terminology is virtually completely lacking in it.[8] The Bar Ilan Responsa Project has also not been consulted throughout since it is not a dictionary, although it does contain a larger number of medieval medical terms than the *Historical Dictionary*.

Apart from these general dictionaries, the secondary literature dealing with the subject of the medieval Hebrew medical terminology is extremely limited and generally only deals with a small number of medical terms.[9] An early study is Joseph Hyrtl's 'Das Arabische und Hebräische in der Anatomie', which was published in 1879.[10] Although it was a pioneering work, it is of little use for scholars today for the following reasons: 1) It only deals with a small number of terms; 2) Most of these terms are derived from one source only, namely a printed edition of the Hebrew translation of Ibn Sīnā's *K. al-Qānūn fī al-ṭibb* by Nathan ha-Me'ati, which was published in Naples in 1491–2.[11] 3) It does not specify particular translators. Thus, Hyrtl states about the *almagabani* (fauces), i.e. larynx, that it was translated in the Hebrew Avicenna as לֹוֶעַ from לוע (to devour). He fails to specify to which of the different

7 Cf. the definition of the term 'dictionary' in *The New Oxford Dictionary of English* (Oxford 1998), p. 512: 'A book that lists the words of a language in alphabetical order and gives their meaning, or that gives the equivalent words in a different language'.

8 Cf. G. Bos, 'Medical terminology in the Hebrew tradition: Shem Tov Ben Isaac, Sefer ha-Shimmush, book 30', *JSS* LV/1 (2010): 53–101.

9 The following survey does not pretend to be complete or exhaustive.

10 J. Hyrtl, *Das Arabische und Hebräische in der Anatomie* (Vienna 1879).

11 For the Hebrew translations of the *K. al-Qānūn fī al-ṭibb* by Nathan ha-Me'ati, Zeraḥyah Ben Isaac Ben She'altiel Ḥen, Joshua Lorki and an anonymous translator, and the manuscripts of these translations see Ch. Rabin, 'Toledot Targum Sefer ha-Qanun le-Ivrit', *Melilah* III–IV (Manchester 1950), 132–46. B. Richler, 'Manuscripts of Avicenna's Kanon in Hebrew translation; a revised and up-to-date list', *Koroth* 30, vol. 8 (1982), 145–68; L. Ferre, 'Avicena Hebraico: La traducción del Canon de Medicina. The Hebrew translation of Avicenna's Canon', *BIBLID* (2003) 52: 163–82.

translations of Avicenna he refers. Shortly after Hyrtl, David Kaufmann's monograph on the five senses, entitled 'Die Sinne: Beiträge zur Geschichte der Physiologie und Psychologie im Mittelalter aus hebräischen und arabischen Quellen' was published in Budapest 1884.[12] The work is admittedly very useful even today; however, the medical terminology he discusses is limited to that of the physiology of the five senses.

A more general study dealing with medieval medical terminology was undertaken by Hermann Kroner, a Rabbi practicing in Bopfingen, southern Germany, and published in 1921 under the title 'Zur Terminologie der arabischen Medizin und zu ihrem zeitgenössischen hebräischen Ausdrucke'.[13] However, it only discusses a relatively small number of terms since it is based primarily on the Hebrew translations of some of Maimonides' minor works, and only distinguishes between two translators, Zeraḥyah Ben Isaac Ben She'altiel Ḥen and Moses Ben Samuel Ibn Tibbon. It also suffers from several mistakes, sometimes resulting from the fact that Kroner only had access to corrupt manuscripts. Thus the term منهرم featuring on p. 55 and translated as 'Apathischer (Lässiger)' should be corrected into منهزم meaning 'defeated, vanquished'. And ibidem تسجيع (Rhythmus (des Herzens) geben) should be read as تشجيع meaning 'strengthening' which was translated by Ibn Tibbon as לתת גבורה.

In 1945 Asher Goldstein published an article entitled *Ha-Refu'ah we-ha-Lashon ha-Ivrit* (Medicine and the Hebrew Language) in which he discusses different ways in which a novel medieval Hebrew medical terminology was created. However, he only discusses a few terms. Moreover, he seems to have had a certain bias against the Arabic medical terminology as he denies the important role it played in the formation of the medieval medical terminology in general, as he states explicitly:

I allow myself to remind [the reader] of my warning published in 'Ha-Rofe ha-Ivri', I (1927), p. 18, about the danger of using the Arabic [for the

12 It was published as part of the *Jahresbericht der Landes-Rabbinerschule in Budapest für das Schuljahr 1883–84* and reprinted in: David Kaufmann, *Die Spuren al-Baṭaljûsi's*, Budapest 1880, and *Studien über Salomon Ibn Gabirol* (Budapest 1899). With an introduction by L. Jacobs (Farnborough 1972).

13 H. Kroner, *Zur Terminologie der arabischen Medizin und zu ihrem zeitgenössischen hebräischen Ausdrucke. An der Hand dreier medizinischer Abhandlungen des Maimonides.* (Berlin 1921).

innovation of Hebrew medical terms], for it does not have any scientific value in our days. And also in the Golden Age of the Arabic medical science, in the Middle Ages, when it left its mark on medicine world-wide, [Hebrew] authors, doctors and translators of Arabic medical works were careful not to use Arabic medical terms. Only a few medical terms in Arabic infiltrated the Hebrew language.[14]

Accordingly when discussing the term חולי הפיל (elephantiasis) as it features in the *Sefer Ẓori ha-Guf* by Nathan Ben Jo'el Falaquera,[15] Goldstein simply states that it is a translation of Latin *elephantiasis*.[16] However, since the work is based on Arabic sources it would have been more appropriate to suggest that it is a loan translation from the Arabic داء الفيل. Again, in an article entitled 'Munaḥim refu'iyyim be-Ivrit mi-beḥinah historit' (Medical nomenclature in Hebrew from historical point of view), which was published in 1967, Goldstein's discussion of some medical terms, like hernia, duodenum, cirrhosis, and their Hebrew counterparts, is primarily based on the Hebrew translation of Ibn Sīnā's *K. al-Qānūn fī al-ṭibb* and some of Maimonides' medical writings, such as the *Pirkei Moshe* (= Medical Aphorisms).[17] However, he does not specify which of the Hebrew translations he used. For instance, when discussing the disease called 'Hemorrhagia' (i.e. bleeding) he mentions as Hebrew equivalents from Maimonides' writings and Ibn Sīnā's *K. al-Qānūn*; שטף דם, תשפוכת דם, רעף דם[18] without providing sources.

Following Goldstein, the research into medieval Hebrew medical terminology was generally limited to a study of the anatomical terms featuring in Vesalius' *Tabulae Anatomicae Sex*, which was published in 1538, and his *De Humani Corporis Fabrica Libri Septem*, commonly known as *Fabrica* and published in 1543. As Vesalius himself knew no Hebrew, the Hebrew (and Arabic) equivalents and their transliterations for the *Tabulae* hail from an anonymous friend; for the *Fabrica*, book one on osteology, he consulted his friend Lazarus de Frigeis of Venice who relied, in turn, on the Naples edition

14 A. Goldstein, 'Ha-Refu'ah we-ha-Lashon ha-Ivrit', *Harofé haivri. The Hebrew Medical Journal* 2 (1945), 88–96, p. 95 (transl. from the Hebrew by Gerrit Bos).

15 See G. Bos and R. Fontaine, 'Medico-philosophical controversies in Nathan b. Jo'el Falaquera, Sefer Zori ha-Guf', *Jewish Quarterly Review* XC (July-October 1999), 27–60.

16 Goldstein (ibid., p. 91) actually reads: אלשופנאנטטיאזים.

17 A. Goldstein, 'Munaḥim refu'iyyim be-Ivrit mi-beḥinah historit', *Koroth* vol. 4: 5–7 (1967), 452–62; vol. 4: 8–10 (1968), 625–36, and vol. 4: 11–12 (1968), 773–86.

18 Ibid., vol. 4: 5–7 (1967), 459.

of Ibn Sīnā's *K. al-Qānūn fī al-ṭibb* mentioned above. However, the Hebrew terminology in the Fabrica edition of 1543 is very corrupt. De Frigeis' knowledge of Hebrew and Arabic may have been sketchy; the transcriber and the typesetter, who were evidently unfamiliar with Hebrew, introduced many typographical errors.[19]

Mordecai Etziony studied the Hebrew material in two articles, published in 1945 and 1946. The first article deals with the Hebrew anatomical terminology featuring in Vesalius' *Tabulae*,[20] while the second article covers the Hebrew terms featuring in the *Fabrica*.[21] The value of both articles lies primarily in their elucidation of the Hebrew terminology; the author does not analyse the medieval source(s), but only refers to Rabbinic parallels on the basis of Jastrow's dictionary,[22] as in the case of the term שלבים (see below). In addition to Etzioni, Charles Singer and C. Rabin studied the Hebrew material in Vesalius' *Tabulae* in their monograph entitled: 'Prelude to Modern Science: Being a Discussion of the History Sources and Circumstances of the "Tabulae Anatomicae Sex" of Vesalius' which was published in 1946 as well.[23] The authors trace the Semitic terminology in the *Tabulae* to contemporary oral usage in Arabic, Hebrew and Romance.[24] They state explicitly that this work was not influenced by the printed Hebrew Avicenna.[25] The study is valuable insofar as the authors extensively discuss these Hebrew terms, compare them with the terminology in the *Fabrica* and that of the different medieval Hebrew

19 See Andreas Vesalius, *De humani corporis fabrica*, translation and annotation by D. Garrison and M. Hast (Vesalius.northwestern.edu), bk. 1, ch. 40, p. 166, esp. n. 5. See as well: B.L. Gordon, review of 'Charles Singer and C. Rabin, *Prelude to Modern Science: Being a Discussion of the History Sources and Circumstances of the "Tabulae Anatomicae Sex" of Vesalius'*, Cambridge 1946', The *Jewish Quarterly Review*, New Ser., Vol. 38, No. 2 (Oct. 1947), 201–3, p. 201.

20 M. Etziony, 'The Hebrew-Aramaic element in Vesalius' Tabulae Anatomicae Sex. A Critical Analysis', *Bulletin of the History of Medicine* 18 (1945), 413–24.

21 M. Etziony, 'The Hebrew-Aramaic element', 36–57.

22 Cf. the author's statement in 'The Hebrew-Aramaic element in Vesalius', p. 38: 'References are given only in the case of some Hebrew terms. The occurrence of those equivalents which are common use in old and modern Hebrew has not been traced to any particular place in literature. Practically all references quoted are those found in Jastrow'.

23 C. Singer and C. Rabin, *Prelude to Modern Science: Being a Discussion of the History Sources and Circumstances of the 'Tabulae Anatomicae Sex' of Vesalius* (Cambridge 1946), esp. pp. lxxv–lxxxvi.

24 Singer-Rabin, *Prelude to Modern Science*, lxxvii.

25 Singer-Rabin, ibid.

translations of Ibn Sīnā's *K. al-Qānūn fī al-ṭibb*. Take for example, their discussion on p. 24, n. 131, regarding the term זרוע:

> "ZĔROA' is biblical, being mostly applied to the forearm. It is thus employed by Meathi and Lorci. The printed Hebrew edition of the Canon of Avicenna (1491), however, following Graciano (= Zeraḥyah Ḥen), used it for the upper arm. Doubtless on account of this confusion, Vesalius or Lazarus in the Fabrica give the phrase of the printed Hebrew Avicenna QĔNEH HA-ZEROA' = shaft of the upper arm."

One more study was devoted to the Hebrew elements in Vesalius' *Fabrica* by Juan Jose Barcia Goyanes and published under the title 'Los terminos osteologicos de la Fabrica y la evolucion del lenguaje anatomico Hebreo en la edad media' in 1982.[26] As the title indicates the author, contrary to Etzioni, dealt with the origin of medieval Hebrew terminology featuring in the *Fabrica*, book one. Thus he consulted the Hebrew translations of Ibn Sīnā's *K. al-Qānūn fī al-ṭibb*, by Nathan ha-Me'ati, Zeraḥyah Ben Isaac Ben She'altiel Ḥen, and Joshua Lorki. The following comparative table clearly shows the differences in approach by both scholars:

Goyanes	Etzioni
Ibid.:	Fabrica, ed. 1543, p. 166, l. 20:
Suturae...שלבים scelauim: The proper transliteration is shlabim meaning mortised boards, steps of a ladder, plural of שלב shalv or shalav, of the root שלב, joint.[27] N (= Nathan): שלב y שלבים šalab̲, šĕlab̲îm. L (= Joshua Lorki): idem, Az.[28] : idem; Z: חוליה ḥulyâ, member, joint, vertebra. Av (= Avicenna) uses the terms درز and دروز, which are transliterated by Alpago[29] as adorem and feature in Vesalius as direzan, adorem. AH[30] has: šĕleb̲, pl. šĕlab̲îm, pl. c. šilb̲ê. The term darz used by Avicenna is a translation of the Greek ῥαφή as used by Galen...	Suturae...שלבים scelauim: The proper transliteration is shlabim meaning mortised boards, steps of a ladder, plural of שלב shalv or shalav, the derivative of the root שלב join, fit in with mortise and tenon. Compare the synonym with מחוברים mechubarim, Tabula VI, 1. For שלב see Jastrow, Taanith Yerushalmi, IV 68.

26 J.J. Barcia Goyanes, 'Los terminos osteologicos de la Fabrica y la evolucion del lenguaje anatomico Hebreo en la edad media'. *Sefarad* 42 (1982), 299–326.

27 For this term see the extensive discussion in H. Rabin, 'Toledot Targum Sefer ha-Qanun le-Ivrit', *Melilah* III–IV (Manchester 1950), 132–46, p. 146.

In a second article entitled 'Medieval Hebrew Anatomical Names: A contribution to their history', published in 1985,[31] Goyanes studied nineteen, (mainly anatomical) terms in the previously mentioned translations of Ibn Sīnā's *K. al-Qānūn fī al-ṭibb*, and in Shem Tov Ben Isaac's Hebrew translation of al-Rāzī's *K. al-Mansūrī*.[32]

The usefulness of the published studies is unfortunately very limited because they discuss so few terms. Thus, they do not contribute significantly to our knowledge of the medieval medical terminology in general and do not make it easier to read the pertinent texts. Moreover, none of them is devoted to the technical vocabulary or translation technique of one translator in particular. These eclectic studies do not help the reader of medieval Hebrew medical literature solve the most common problem, namely, that many of the extant medical texts do not name their translator.

The articles collected in this volume deal with four prominent translators, all of them active in the thirteenth century: Hillel Ben Samuel of Verona, Moses Ben Samuel Ibn Tibbon, Shem Tov Ben Isaac of Tortosa, and Zeraḥyah Ben Isaac Ben She'altiel Ḥen.[33] In the case of Hillel of Verona the source for the novel terminology was the *Sefer Keritut* (Surgery), i.e. his translation (dating from the year 1254) of the *Cyrurgia magna* composed by Bruno Longobucco (Longoburgensis), a practitioner from Padua. For the novel

---

28 Az. is the abbreviation used by Goyanes to refer to Azriel Ben Joseph of Gunzenhausen, who with his father Joseph Ben Jacob printed the Hebrew edition of the *K. al-Qānūn* (Naples 1491–2). However, this edition is, according to Richler (*Manuscripts of Avicenna's Kanon*, 148), based on the translation of Nathan for Books II–V, while the edition of Book I is based mainly on Lorki's translation, which is a revision of that by Nathan. Thus, Az. is nothing else but N. In an earlier comparative study Rabin (*Toledot Targum Sefer ha-Qanun le-Ivrit*, 137) came to the conclusion that this edition is mainly based on Nathan's translation, but that the editor sometimes prefers the version of Joshua Lorki or Zeraḥyah.

29 I.e. Andrea Alpago (sixteenth century), who revised the Latin translation by Gerard of Cremona.

30 AH, i.e. The Academy of the Hebrew Language.

31 J.J. Barcia Goyanes, 'Medieval Hebrew Anatomical Names: A contribution to their history', *Koroth*, vol. 8, no. 11–12 (1985), 192–202.

32 For Shem Tov Ben Isaac, see below. For this translation, see M. Steinschneider, *Die hebräischen Übersetzungen des Mittelalters* (Berlin 1893, repr. Graz, Akademische Druck- u. Verlagsanstalt 1956), 725–6.

33 The terminology of one more prominent thirteenth century translator, namely Nathan ha-Me'ati will be analysed separately in the forthcoming edition of his translation of Maimonides' *Medical Aphorisms*.

terminology used by Moses Ibn Tibbon I consulted his translation of Ibn al-Jazzār, *Zād al-musāfir*, which Moses Ibn Tibbon called *Sefer Ẓedat ha-Derakhim* and completed in the year 1259. The novel terminology used by Shem Tov Ben Isaac is gleaned from his translation of book 30 of the *Kitāb al-taṣrīf li-man 'ajiza 'an al-ta'līf* (The Arrangement of Medical Knowledge for One Who is Not Abel to Compile a Book for Himself), which was composed in the tenth century by the Andalusian physician Abū l-Qāsim Khalaf ibn ʿAbbās al-Zahrāwī. Shem Tov started his translation of the *Kitāb al-taṣrīf*, which he called *Sefer ha-Shimmush*, in 1254 and completed it at an unknown date.[34] And finally for the novel terminology used by Zeraḥyah Ḥen I consulted his translation (dating from the year 1279) of Maimonides' *Medical Aphorisms* (Fuṣūl Mūsā fī l-Ṭibb).

34 The current section on Shem Tov is a corrected and updated version of the article published previously as: 'Medical terminology in the Hebrew tradition: Shem Tov Ben Isaac, *Sefer ha-Shimmush*, book 30, *JSS* LV/1 (2010), 53–101.

1. Hillel Ben Samuel of Verona, *Sefer Keritut*

Introduction

Hillel Ben Samuel (*c.* 1220–95) was a talmudic scholar, philosopher, physician and translator of medical works.[35] He is also called Hillel Ben Samuel of Verona on the basis of the assumption that he lived in that city. But actually only his grandfather Eliezer Ben Samuel lived there. We do not have much personal information about Hillel, nor about his place of birth or life. Most of the relevant information comes from the correspondence between him and his friends. However, according to Sermoneta this correspondence cannot always be regarded as a reliable historical source for the reconstruction of his biography. Thus, his testimony that he studied medicine in Montpellier finds no corroboration in other sources. What we do know for certain, however, is that he lived in Rome, where he was in contact with the translator and philosopher Zeraḥyah Ben Isaac Ben She'altiel Ḥen mentioned above, and befriended the physician Isaac Ben Mordecai Gaio. In a letter to Isaac, Hillel shows his great regard for Maimonides' *Medical Aphorisms* and *Commentary on Hippocrates' Aphorisms*. Of the latter work he remarks that although he already possesses the Latin translation by Constantine the African (which he regarded to be inferior)[36] and the commentary by Burgundius of Pisa, he still wanted the commentary by Maimonides in order to solve the 'hundred' queries he had and entreats Gaio: 'Do not care about the cost, and make a scribe copy them, and I shall immediately send you the scribe's salary and [the price] of the paper and the corrections, as much as demanded. Even if it turns out to be a substantial expenditure it will become smaller [in my mind] when considering how much I love them [the books]'.[37] Subsequently, he lived in Naples and

---

35 The main data regarding Hillel's biography are taken from the account by J. Sermoneta in *Encyclopaedia Judaica*^{2}, vol. 9 (Detroit 2007), 113–15. As my article concentrates on Hillel's activity as a translator of medical works, I only provide those bio-bibliographical data that are relevant for that activity.

36 Cf. Hebrew text in B. Richler, 'Another Letter from Hillel Ben Samuel to Isaac the Physician?', *Kiryat Sefer* 62: 1–2 (1988–9): 450–2, p. 451: אבל אותם של קושטנטינו אין בהם מתום (but that [i.e. the translation] by Constantine is imperfect).

37 Translation J. Shatzmiller, *Jews, Medicine, and Medieval Society* (Berkeley-Los Angeles-London 1994), 46.

Capua, where he practised medicine and studied philosophy with Abraham Abulafia. While Hillel is foremost known as a philosopher and author of the *Tagmulei ha-Nefesh* (composed between 1288–91),[38] a work which deals with the nature of the soul, the intellect and the question of the soul's retribution, he was also active as a translator. Thus he translated the pseudo Aristotelean *Liber de Causis* under the title *Ma'amar Lamed Bet Haqdamot*, which survives in extracts in *Tagmulei ha-Nefesh* and in the manuscript Bodleian Library, Mich. 82.[39]

However, he was especially active as a translator in the field of medicine, as he translated some important medieval medical works from Latin into Hebrew. Apart from the *Chirurgia* by Bruno Longobucco, to be discussed below, Hillel translated the following medical works into Hebrew: 1. Hippocrates' *Aphorisms* with Galen's commentary in the Latin translation by Constantinus Africanus[40]. Under the title 'Aphorismi' this work is extant in manuscripts in Paris, BN heb. 1111, 1112; Berlin, Staatsbibliothek (Preussischer Kulturbesitz) Or. Qu. 511, 517; Jerusalem, Mossad Harav Kook 202; Firenze, Biblioteca Medicea Laurenziana Plut. 88. 54; and Rome, Biblioteca Casanatense 2834.[41] 2. Galen's *Ars Medica*, also called 'Ars parva' or 'Microtegni', according to the Latin translation by Gerard of Cremona.[42] The text survives in two manuscripts, namely Rome, Biblioteca Casanatense 2834[43] and Paris BN heb. 1111; 3. Ibn Sīnā's *K. al-Qānūn fī al-ṭibb*. Of this (partial?) translation only Book 4, until Fann 2 (the end of the section on crises) has been preserved in one manuscript in Boston, F.A. Countway Library of Medicine heb. 2.[44]

---

38 A critical edition with introduction and commentary was published by J. Sermoneta, (Jerusalem 1981).

39 Cf. Steinschneider, *Die hebräischen Übersetzungen*, p. 262f; see as well J.P. Rothschild, 'Les traductions du Livre des causes et leurs copies', *Revue d'Histoire des Textes*, 24 (1994). I thank David Wirmer for this reference.

40 Cf. Steinschneider, *Die hebräischen Übersetzungen*, 660.

41 Steinschneider, ibid. For information about MSS not mentioned by Steinschneider see the online Catalogue of the Institute of Microfilmed Hebrew Manuscripts.

42 Cf. J. Sermoneta, entry 'Hillel Ben Samuel', *Encyclopaedia Judaica*[2], vol. 9 (Detroit 2007), 115. For this work and its translations cf. Fichtner, *Corpus Galenicum. Verzeichnis der galenischen und pseudogalenischen Schriften* (Tübingen 1989), no. 7. Hillel's translation is missing from the list by Fichtner.

43 Cf. Steinschneider, *Die hebräischen Übersetzungen*, 734.

44 According to the online Catalogue of the Institute of Microfilmed Hebrew Manuscripts.

Bruno Longobucco (Longoburgensis) Cyrurgia magna and the Hebrew Translation by Hillel

Bruno Longobucco (Longoburgensis), a practitioner from Padua, is the author of two works, the *Cyrurgia magna*[45] and *Cyrurgia parva* (or minor). The *Cyrurgia magna* was composed at the proposal of a friend, Andreas da Vicenza, to produce a book bringing together the teachings of 'Galen, Avicenna, Almansor, Albucasis, Haly, and other skilled ancients' and he finished the task in January 1252.[46] Major sources consulted by the author were Galen's *De Methodo medendi* (in the abbreviated paraphrase prepared from the Arabic by Constantinus Africanus), the fourth book of Avicenna's *Canon*, and Albucasis' *Surgery*. Bruno divided his work into two parts of exactly twenty chapters each. The first part deals with those problems which Galen and Avicenna refer to as 'solutio continuitatis': wounds, ulcers, fistulas, fractures and dislocations; the second part with mostly nontraumatic complaints: illnesses of the eye and ear, growths and swellings, dropsy and hernia, haemorrhoids, bladder stone and the like. McVaugh characterizes the work as 'an explicit manifesto for the kind of rational surgery—rational in its search for causes, rational in its structure, rational in its insistence that it can be read and taught from texts—towards which Teodorico[47] seems to have been hesitantly groping'.[48] The *Cyrurgia magna* was prescribed for study in the university of Bologna (possibly also in the university of Ferrara),[49] and was also recommended for study in Paris.[50] Almost the whole of the work was taken over by Teodorico in his surgical work without acknowledgment.[51]

45 For a critical edition of the work cf. S.P. Hall, *The Cyrurgia Magna of Brunus Longoburgensis*. Ph.D. (Oxford 1957).

46 Cf. M. McVaugh, *The Rational Surgery of the Middle Ages* (Firenze 2006), 25.

47 I.e. Teodorico Borgognoni, author of a surgical work that survives in three versions: *Vulnera*, possibly composed in the mid-1240s; *Tractaturi*, composed in the early 1250s and *Venerabili*, composed in the early 1260s; cf. McVaugh, *Rational Surgery*, 16-24, esp. p. 21. For an English translation cf. E. Campbell and J. Colton, *The Surgery of Theodoric*. 4 books in 2 volumes (New York 1955–60).

48 McVaugh, *Rational Surgery*, 27.

49 Hall, *Cyrurgia Magna*, VI.

50 McVaugh, *Rational Surgery*, 231.

51 Following the fundamental and innovative study by Monica Green, *Moving from Philology to Social History: The Circulation and Uses of Albucasis's Latin Surgery in the Middle Ages* (forthcoming); Hall, *Cyrurgia Magna*, p. VI, only lists the three translations into French, Italian and German.

Except for the Hebrew translation by Hillel Bruno's work was translated into eight other languages, amongst which are French, Italian and German.[52]

Hillel Ben Samuel's Hebrew translation entitled *Sefer Keritut* (Surgery) was written in the year 1254.[53] The translation was widely distributed amongst the Jews as it survives in 15 manuscripts. The demand for it seems to have been especially high amongst the Jews in Italy in the fourteenth-fifteeth century as ten manuscripts were copied in Italian script in that period.

These 15 manuscripts are the following:[54]

1. Strasbourg, Bibliothèque Nationale et Universitaire 4106; copied in the sixteenth century.
2. Oxford - Bodleian Library MS Opp. 688 (cat. Neubauer 2123); fols 1–106a; copied in 1469 in a Byzantine script.[55] The manuscript is a medical miscellany bound with an anonymous Hebrew translation of Roger Frugardi of Palermo's *Chirurgia* (fols 117b–142b).
3. Moscow - Russian State Library, Ms. Guenzburg 165; fols 261a–359b; Italian script, dated 1442.
4. Rome - Biblioteca Casanatense 2756; Italian script; fifteenth–sixteenth century.[56]
5. Moscow - Russian State Library, Ms. Guenzburg 164; fols 1a–43b; Italian script, fifteenth century.
6. Vatican - Biblioteca Apostolica ebr. 376; fols 1r–101r; Italian semi-cursive script, fifteenth century. The manuscript is a medical miscellany bound with an anonymous Hebrew translation of Roger Frugardi of Palermo's *Chirurgia* (fols 108r–150r).[57]
7. Munich - Bayerische Staatsbibliothek, Cod. hebr. 463; 13 fols (fragmentary, beginning of the preface and middle of Bk. 1, ch. 10 until end is missing); Sephardic cursive script.[58]

---

52 Cf. Hall, *Cyrurgia Magna*, p. VI; see as well Green, *Moving from Philology to Social History*.

53 The date is that given by Sermoneta, *Hillel Ben Samuel*, 115. Note that according to Steinschneider, *Die hebräischen Übersetzungen*, 788, it was translated in the 1252.

54 For the data of these manuscripts see the online Catalogue of the Institute of Microfilmed Hebrew Manuscripts, in addition to the catalogues mentioned below.

55 See A. Neubauer, *Catalogue of the Hebrew Manuscripts in the Bodleian Library* (Oxford 1886, repr. 1994). And *Supplement of Addenda and Corrigenda* compiled under the direction of Malachi Beit-Arié and edited by R.A. May (Oxford 1994).

56 See G. Sacerdote, *Catalogo dei codici ebraici della Biblioteca Casanatense*, in *Cataloghi dei codici Orientali di alcune Biblioteche d'Italia* (Firenze 1878), 475–665, no. 192.

57 Cf. B. Richler, *Hebrew Manuscripts in the Vatican Library. Catalogue*. Palaeographical and Codicological Descriptions: Malachi Beit-Arié in collaboration with Nurit Pasternak. (Città del Vaticano 2008).

58 E. Roth, *Verzeichnis der Orientalischen Handschriften in Deutschland. Teil 2: Hebräische Handschriften*, Wiesbaden 1965, No. 257.

8. Paris - Bibliothèque Nationale heb. 973; fols 22b–199b; copied in 1378; Italian script.[59]
9. Parma - Biblioteca Palatina Cod. Parm. 2115 (= cat. Richler 1529); fols 138r–215v; fourteenth century; Italian script. Medical miscellany.[60]
10. Firenze - Biblioteca Riccardiana, Ricc. 26; fourteenth century; Italian script.
11. Vatican - Biblioteca Apostolica ebr. 368 (cat. Richler); fols 1r–18v (Bk 1, middle of chapter 3 to Bk 2, middle of ch. 1); fifteenth century; Italian semi-cursive script. Medical miscellany.
12. Vatican - Biblioteca Apostolica ebr. 462 (cat. Richler); fols 7r–129v; fourteenth century; Italian semi-cursive script. The manuscript is a medical miscellany bound with an anonymous Hebrew translation of Roger Frugardi of Palermo's *Chirurgia* (fols 131r–169r).
13. Vatican - Biblioteca Apostolica ebr. 550 (cat. Richler); fols 1v–112r; early fourteenth century; Sephardic semi-cursive script.
14. Parma - Biblioteca Palatina Cod. Parm. 2475 (cat. Richler 1530); early fourteenth century; Italian semi-cursive script. The manuscript is a medical miscellany bound with an anonymous Hebrew translation of Roger Frugardi of Palermo's *Chirurgia* (fols 54v–74r).
15. Parma - Biblioteca Palatina 2468 (cat. Richler 1522); fols 4a–72a; fourteenth century; Italian semi-cursive script.

Next to these translations Bruno's Cyrurgia magna was also available in a summary entitled כלל קצר מקצת מאמרי ברונו that is extant in Oxford - Bodleian Library MS Mich. 343 (cat. Neubauer 2285/4), fols 50b–62a which dates from the sixteenth century and was copied in Italy in a Sephardic script.

59 Cf. H. Zotenberg, *Catalogues des Manuscrits hébreux et samaritains de la Bibliothèque Impériale* (Paris 1866).

60 B. Richler, *Hebrew Manuscripts in the Biblioteca Palatina in Parma.* Catalogue. Palaegraphical und codicological descriptions: Malachi Beit-Arié (Jerusalem 2001).

Hillel's Poem on a Doctor's Fees

Hillel translation of Bruno's Chirurgia is preceded by the following poem:[61]

לכל אדם היה נודר לשרת	בחכמתך ואל לרפא תדור
הליכתך[62] שאל ושכר עבודה	אם ימות ואם רפא ירפא
ותשאל פי שנים לו בקומו	והשען במשכון לא בעל פה
עבוד שרים למזל או למרפא	ונדבתם כמו מלקוש תצפה
ואם תתעל(?) לרפא הגבירות	אזי תעדה עדי זהב וישפה

Translation:

Promise any man to serve him with your skill, but do not promise to heal

Ask for travel expenses and payment for work, regardless whether [the patient] dies or is healed (cf. Ex. 21: 19)[63]

Ask for a double compensation if he recovers fully. Rely on a collateral, not on a verbal promise

Serve princes [whether] for fate or for actually healing, and their generosity expect like rain

And if you rise up(?) to cure noble women, you will adorn yourself with ornaments of gold and jasper

61 The poem was published by B. Peyron, *Codices Hebraici manu exarati regiae bibliothecae quae in Tarinensi Athenaeo asservatur recensuit* (Romae, Taurini, Florentiae 1880), codex CCXLIII. A. VII. 31, and by Moritz Steinschneider in *Leopold Zunz. Jubelschrift zum 80. Geburtstag* (Berlin 1884), 96; My edition is based on MS Parma 2475 where the poem features at the end, on fol. 54a. For the subject of a doctor's fees see, for instance, J. Shatzmiller, 'Doctor's Fees and Their Medical Responsibility. Evidence from Notarial and Court Records', *Sources of Social History* (1984), 201–8; Y. Tzvi Langermann, 'Fixing a cost for medical care: Medical ethics and socio-economic reality in Christian Spain as reflected in Jewsh sources', in S. Kottek and L. García-Ballester (eds), *Medicine and medical ethics in medieval and early modern Spain. An intercultural approach* (Jerusalem 1996), 154–62; F. Rosner and J. Widroff, 'Physician's Fees in Jewish Law', *The Jewish Law Annual* vol. XII (1997), 115–26.

62 הליכתך: ארוחתך (maintenance), MS Paris 973; Peyron, *Codices,* codex CCXLIII. A. VII. 31 fol. 22b

63 The verse in Ex. 21: 19 is the basis for the law of medical compensation when someone injures someone else. I thank my friend Eric Pellow for his help in the interpretation of this poem.

In other words Hillel gives the physician the following advice:

1. Do not promise a cure when you cannot be sure of it.
2. Make sure your payment includes both travel expenses and work whether you are successful or not.
3. Ask for a double payment in case of success.
4. Rely only on collateral and not on mere words.
5. If you work for princes, whether successful or not, the reward will be like rain.
6. And if you heal noble women, your reward will be extraordinary.

Hillel's advice is, except for a partial similarity, quite different from that found in other Jewish sources. For instance, a contemporary of Hillel, Moses Ben Nahman (Nahmanides; 1194–1268) remarks that the physician may charge for his time and exertion, but not for the cost of his education. Thus it is only similar to Hillel's advice which features in the first part of no. 2, but misses the second part 'whether successful or not'. The third and fourth piece of advice is similar to that found in documents on doctor-patient agreements hailing from the fifteenth century. In these agreements, two sums of money are quoted: one in the event of a successful cure and another, evidently lower sum, in the event of failure.[64] In one case, a Jewish lady, Dona Lelal of Sevilla, maestra de sanar ojos, received 600 of the 1200 maradivi promised if her treatment would eventually be successful.[65] Hillel's advice is thus an early example of a mode of agreement which according to Shatzmiller, might have been referred to as early as the fourteenth century by Kalonymos Ben Kalonymos of Arles in his Hebrew critique on the doctors of his day when he quoted a doctor stipulating: 'Make a downpayment now and pay the rest when he recovers'.[66]

The first piece of advice though is, as Michael McVaugh informed me, very widespread all through Latin medicine of the same period, and the third has parallels in some writers, like Henry of Mondeville.

---

64 Cf. Shatzmiller, *Doctor's Fees and Their Medical Responsibility*, 204.

65 Cf. K. Wagner, *Regesto de documentos del archivo de Protocolos de Sevilla referentes a judios y moros* (Seville 1978), 37 (no. 120), following Shatzmiller, *Doctor's Fees*, 204.

66 Kalonymos Ben Kalonymos, *Even Boḥan* (Hebrew), A.M. Habermann (ed.) (Tel Aviv 1956), 45; following Shatzmiller. ibid.

Study of the technical terminology employed by Hillel in his translation of Bruno's Cyrurgia

The following study of the technical terminology employed by Hillel is based on MS Oxford Bodleian Library MS Opp. 688 (= O). In cases of omissions or corruptions I consulted Paris BN heb. 973 (= P) and Biblioteca Palatina Cod. Parm. 2115 (= R). The folio numbers refer to the Oxford manuscript, unless otherwise indicated. Every Hebrew entry is followed by the Latin equivalent derived from the critical edition of Bruno's *Cyrurgia* prepared by Hall mentioned above (= H). Next to the analysis of the terminology employed by Hillel, I shall refer to parallel terms gleaned from the following texts: 1) the Hebrew translations of Maimonides' *Medical Aphorisms* by Nathan ha-Me'ati, active in Rome between 1279–83, and Zeraḥyah Ben Isaac Ben She'altiel Ḥen; 2) Shem Tov Ben Isaac, *Sefer ha-Shimmush*; 3) Moses Ben Samuel Ibn Tibbon, *Sefer Ẓedat ha-derakhim*; 4) Moses Ben Samuel Ibn Tibbon's translations of Maimonides' treatises *On Poisons*,[67] and *On Hemorrhoids*[68] completed at an unknown date. The following list of terms consists of three parts: 1) Hebrew terms that for the major part do not feature in the current dictionaries, or that can be found in them but are registered as either Biblical and/or Rabbinic and/or Modern; 2) Hebrew[69] transcriptions of Latin terms; 3) Mixed terms; i.e. terms that are partly Hebrew, partly Latin, and mostly belong to the field of medicine.

List of Terms

I. Hebrew terms

אבנט = Latin braccale 'truss'; cf. fol. 93b (H 278, l. 20): ומונעין אותו שלא ירחב בתקון האבנט[70] (And prevent it [i.e. the hernia] from getting larger by applying a truss). Hebrew אבנט only features in the sense of 'girdle' (BM 32–3) or

67 See Maimonides, *On Poisons and the Protection against Lethal Drugs*. A New Parallel Arabic-English Translation by Gerrit Bos with Critical Editions of medieval Hebrew translations and Medieval Latin translations by by Gerrit Bos and Michael R. McVaugh. (Provo 2009).

68 See Maimonides, *On Hemorrhoids*. A New Parallel Arabic-English Translation by Gerrit Bos with Critical Editions of medieval Hebrew translations by Gerrit Bos and Latin translations by Michael R. McVaugh. Provo (forthcoming).

69 Only a small selection has been made of the many transcriptions featuring in the text.

70 האבנט: האמבטי O.

'belt' (JD 7) in the current dictionaries. Masie (MD 738) mentions the following terms for 'truss': חגורת שבר and סמך.

אֵבָר: האיברים המיוחסים = Latin membra principalia vel nobilia 'the principal or noble organs'; cf. fol. 40b (H 113, ll. 10–12): ובאמת הנגע הבא אל המעים או אל השלפוחית או אל האיברים המיוחסים לא יבריא לגמרי (Indeed a fistula that affects the intestines or the urinary bladder or the noble organs cannot be cured completely. The Hebrew term האיברים המיוחסים does not feature in the current dictionaries. The Arabic parallel to the Latin term, i.e. الأعضاء الشريفة is translated by N as האברים הנכבדים or האברים המעולים and by Z as האברים המעולים (MA 3: 79; 10: 2).

אִמּוּן = Latin administratio 'administration; application'; cf. fol. 38b (H 108. ll. 11–12): אימון הרפואות המצמיחות בשר שכתבנו בשער שעבר (The administration of the flesh-growing remedies that we mentioned in the previous chapter). Hebrew אִמּוּן does not feature in this sense in the current dictionaries.

אימן (אמן) = Latin administrare 'to administer, apply'; cf. fol. 22b (H 61, ll. 10–12): אם כן הוא כמו שאמרנו שאם מזג האבר יהיה יבש צריך שתאמן בו הרפואה המיבשת (Therefore, if, as I said, the temperament of the organ is dry, one should administer a drying medication). Hebrew אימן does not feature in this sense in the current dictionaries. Cf. entries נהג and הרגיל.

אריגה: אריגת העכביש = Latin aranee tela 'a spider's web'; cf. fol. 27b (H 76, l. 14). The Hebrew term is attested in medieval literature in the *Tales of Ben Sira.*[71] It does not feature in the current dictionaries. The regular Hebrew term for 'a spider's web' is the Biblical קורי עכביש (KB 1091).

בגד, Plur. **בגדים** = (a) Latin velamina, panniculi 'membranes'; cf. fol. 46a (H 128, ll. 14–16): המוח יש לה ב' בגדים אחת נקרא דורא מטרי ואחרת נקרא פיאה מטרי (The brain has two membranes, one called 'dura mater' and one called 'pia mater'. Hebrew בגד does not feature in the sense of 'membrane' in the current dictionaries. The Arabic equivalent to 'velamina' i.e. أغشية, is translated by both N and Z as קרומים or קרומות (MA 1: 11, 14, 18, 49, 56, 68 et passim). Jacob Ẓahalon, *Oẓar ha-Ḥayyim* calls one of the membranes of the brain with the term עור; cf. העור הדבק על המוח נקרא פיאה מאדרי (The

71 Eli Yassif (ed.), *Sippurei Ben Sira bi-Yemei ha-Benayyim. The Tales of Ben Sira in the Middle Ages* (Jerusalem 1984), 238, ll. 4–5.

membrane that adheres to the brain is called 'pia madre' (following HA 88–9, n. 16). See as well entry כתנת below; (b) (singular בגד) = Latin pannus 'pannus'; cf. fol 66b (H 195, ll. 10–11): הבגד המתילד בעינים מחמת המכות או מחמת פישטולי הוא מכת נמנעי הרפואה (Pannus that affects the eye because of a blow or a fistula is one of those afflictions that cannot be cured). Hebrew בגד does not feature in the sense of 'pannus' in the current dictionaries; For the synonym קרום מכסה see below; (c) (singular בגד) = Latin pellicula '(small) skin'; cf. fol. 95a (H 283, ll. 18–19): אחר כן יחתוך הבגד שעל הביצה לאורכו (Then cut the skin lengthwise above the testicle).

בחינה = Latin experimentum 'experience'; cf. fol. 24a (H 65, ll. 17–18): הרפואות המחברות שסמכתי מטובם ומרוב הבחינה ומעדות הקדמונים הם אלו (Incarnative medicines, concerning the goodness of which I have relied [on] the lengthy experience and testimony of the ancients are the following). Hebrew בחינה is attested in medieval philosophical literature as meaning: 1. examination, test; 2. viewpoint, criterion (cf. EP 13). In the sense of experience it is a non-attested semantic borrowing from the Latin experimentum which can mean both 'test' and 'experience'; cf SSH 242.

גיד = (a) Latin nervus 'nerve'; cf. fol. 5a (H 5, l. 8): כגון בבשר ובגידים ובורדים (...like in the flesh, the nerves, and the veins); (b) Latin virga 'penis'; cf. fol. 97a (H 291, ll. 5–6): שער ארבע עשר. מן הוורוג'י והפורי הבאים בגיד (Chapter fourteen. On warts and tubercles occurring on the penis). For the different meanings of the term גיד cf. BM 751; S s.v. גיד and especially Lieber, *Asaf's Book of Medicines*[72]: 'As in the Bible it may indicate any elongated, but not necessarily hollow, structure in the body, including vessels of all kinds, nerves, sinews, tendons and, when qualified, even the penis'. Both N and Z have Hebrew עצב for Arabic عصب (nerve) (MA 1: 1, 2, 6–11, 13, 21–3 et passim); likewise S (s.v. התלבדות). גיד in the sense of 'penis' also features in N, next to אמה, while Z only has the latter term (MA 3: 62; 16: 10; 23: 18).

גֻּמְמוּת = Latin concavitas 'concavity'; cf. fol. 11a (H 24, ll. 7–9): ואם בחבלה יתחדש שום גוממות ועומק אז לא תהיה כוונתך על הדרך שזכרנו (But if the wound is deep and concave you should not [treat] it in the way we mentioned before).

---

72 E. Lieber, 'Asaf's Book of Medicines: A Hebrew Encyclopaedia of Greek and Jewish Medicine, Possibly Compiled in Byzantium on an Indian Model', in J. Scarborough (ed.), *Symposium on Byzantine Medicine* (Dumbarton Oaks Papers. Number 38, 1984. Washington 1985), 233–49.

Hebrew גוממות for ‘concavity’ is not attested in secondary literature. The common medieval term for ‘concavity’ was קערירות (cf. BM 6051), while Z uses the term חללות; thus he translates مقعّر الكبد (the concave side of the liver) as חללות הכבד, while N translates it as מקוער הכבד or קערירות הכבד or קערורית הכבד (MA 6: 57; 9: 70, 75; 10: 48; 11: 14; 25: 12). The term חללות for ‘concavity’ also features in S. See as well MD 177: קעירות.

גֻּמְמִי: החבלות הגממיות = Latin vulnera concava ‘concave wounds’; cf. fol. 23b (H 64, ll. 14–18): וענין אימון הרפואה בדברים הנזכרים היא שבחבלות הגוממיות שבהן חסרון בשר וכן בחבלות העמוקות שנאבד משם עצם הבשר תניח תחילה מן המולידות בשר (The method of applying the aforementioned medications should be [as follows]: in concave wounds, in which flesh is lacking and likewise in deep wounds in which there is a loss of essential flesh one should first apply a medicine that produces flesh). Hebrew גממי does not feature in this sense in the current dictionaries.

גפרית חי = Latin sulphur vivum ‘natural sulphur’; cf. fol. 41b (H 117, l. 9). The Hebrew term is not attested in the current dictionaries, but features as well in CN 171 and BL 277, l. 7 (heb.), 213 (french trans.). The same Hebrew term can be found in Shem Tov’s glossary as a translation of Arabic كبريت غير مطفأ (SG Gimel 11). Maimonides’ *On Poisons* (BMP 53) calls this kind of sulphur: الكبريت الذي لم يدنو من النار (sulphur that has not been in the fire). Moses Ibn Tibbon translates this term as: השולפרי אשר לא קרב לאש.

גרידה = Latin scarificatio ‘scarification’; cf. fol. 5a (H 5, ll. 13–14): אבל אותה הנעשית באיברים הרכים היא נחלקת לשלשה פנים: א’ הנעשית בבשר לבד ונקרא’ גרידה (But the [surgery] applied to the soft parts is divided into three parts: 1) that which is done in the flesh only and is called ‘scarification’. Hebrew גרידה in the sense of ‘scarification’ features in BM 841 in a quotation from Nathan ha-Me’ati’s Hebrew translation of Ibn Sīnā’s *K. al-Qānūn fī al-ṭibb*. In addition to גרידה in the sense of ‘scarification’, we find שריטה; cf. BM 7619.

גירש (גרש) = Latin impellere ‘to push (upon)’; cf. fol. 63a–63b (H 185, l. 19–186, l. 2): עם כל זה יהיה הרופא משגיח שיגרש הפרק בידיו ורגליו עד שיושב למקומו הטבעי (But let the physician be careful to push upon the joint with his feet or hands until it [i.e. the hip] is reduced to its natural postion). See as well fol. 62a (H 182, ll. 17–18): ויגרש האמיננציאה לצד פנים עד שישוב למקומו (and he should push the protruding part inward until it returns to its place). Hebrew

גירש only features in the sense of 'to drive away; to expel; to divorce' in the standard dictionaries (cf. BM 851–2).

דֶּבֶק, Plur. דבקים Latin iuncturae 'joints'; cf. fol. 40b (H 113, ll. 13–16): וכאשר יגיע לאחד מן האשפונדלי חוליות בלשון הקודש או אל הצלעות או אל אחד מן הדבקים ביד או ברגל או בגיד או בווריד גדול או בווייתן בכל אלה לפי הרוב הם מכות נמנעות מרפואה (When [a fistula] affects one of the vertebrae or ribs or one of the joints in the hand or foot, or [affects] a nerve, large vein or artery, it is an affliction that cannot be cured in most cases). Hebrew דֶּבֶק features in Rabbinic literature in the sense of: 1) glue, paste; 2. junction (TB Ḥullin 50a: מקום הדבק [the place where the entrails adhere to the hip]); 3) nexus, cause (JD 1: 278). The Arabic aequivalent to 'iuncturae', i.e. مفاصل is translated by both N and Z as פרקים (MA 3: 21; 8: 19; 9: 35, 99 et passim). Next to דבקים for 'joints' Hillel uses מודבקים for 'joints' (see below).

-: דבק היד = Latin iunctura manus, lit. 'joint of the hand', i.e. 'wrist'; cf. fol. 61b (H 180, ll. 2–3): וכאשר תבוא ההשמטה בדבק היד השבתו קלה (When the dislocation affects the wrist, it is easily reduced). Hebrew דבק היד is a literal translation of Latin iunctura manus. The Arabic equivalent to 'iunctura manus', i.e. معصم is translated by Shem Tov (S) as פרק קנה הזרוע הסמוך ליד or as פרק היד. This last term is also used by Hillel (see below). Masie (MD 781) mentions שורש היד or רסג היד for 'wrist', featuring in Nathan ha-Me'ati's Hebrew translation of Ibn Sīnā's *K. al-Qānūn fī al-ṭibb.*

דְּבֵקוּת: See **התרה**.

דבש: דבש מְקֻצָּף = Latin mel dispumatum 'skimmed honey'; cf. fol. 41b (H 117, l. 2). The Hebrew term דבש מְקֻצָּף does not feature in the current dictionaries. The Arabic equivalent العسل المنزوع الرغوة is translated by N and Z as (ה)דבש (ה)מוסר קצפו (MA 21: 61).

דחיקה = Latin strictura 'bandage'; cf. fol. 57b (H 166, ll. 7–9): וכבר ידעת אופן דחיקת הקשר בכלל כלומר כשתהיה הדחיקה על מקום השבר יותר חזקה (You already know about the way of bandaging in general; that is that the bandage should be tighter over the point of the fracture). Hebrew דחיקה does not feature in this sense in the current dictionaries. Another term for 'bandage' employed by Hillel is קֶשֶׁר (see below).

דחק = Latin stringere 'to bind, to bind tightly'; cf. fol. 56a (H 161, ll. 1–2): אחר כן יוחבש כראוי וידחוק השבר עם לוח אם יצטרך (Then cover the fracture with a suitable medication, and bind it tightly with a splint if that is necessary). Hebrew דחק does not feature in this sense in the current dictionaries (cf. BM 918–19: 'to press'; JD 293: 'to press, to squeeze; to crowd; to stamp'). It is possible that דחק in the sense of 'to bind' is a semantic borrowing from Latin 'stringere' which has the basic meaning of 'to squeeze' (cf. root 'strig', Greek στράγξ; LSD 1766). Zeraḥyah uses the same term דחק as an equivalent to Arabic ضغط (to compress, to press on) (MA 7: 28; 15: 45; 16: 16). A second term used by Hillel to translate Latin 'stringere' is עצר (see below).

בדֹחַק: דֹחַק = Latin fortiter 'strongly; forcefully'; cf. fol. 62b (H 182, ll. 18–19): ויניח פסותיו על האשפונדלי[73] ויעצור בדוחק עד שובם (And he [i.e. the physician] should put the palms of his hands on the vertebrae and press upon them forcefully until they return [to their proper place]). Hebrew בדֹחַק only features in EM 297 in the sense of 'with difficulty'.

הדבקה = Latin agglutinatio 'agglutination'; cf. fol. 92b (H 275, ll. 18–20): ואימון רפואתו שיחבוש השבר במה שמגרש הרוחות ושיהיה בהן קבצות חזקה עם הדבקה קונגולוטינציאוני (It [i.e. the hernia] should be treated by applying [medicines] to it which expel the ventosity, have a strong astringency and [some] agglutination). The Hebrew term does not feature in this sense in the current dictionaries. BM 4711 refers to the term as featuring in a supplement to the edition of Hillel's *Sefer Tagmulei ha-Nefesh*, Lyck 1874, fol. 46b, where Hillel speaks about the הדבקה (cleaving) of the soul to matter (חומר).

הזרה = (a) Latin refrenatio 'restraining'; cf. fol. 78a (H 228, l. 20–229, l. 1): אלא שאין צריך בתחלה הזרה גדולה (but in the beginning it does not need intense restraining [treatment]). The Hebrew term does not feature in this sense in the current dictionaries. It does feature, however, in Zeraḥyah's translation of Arabic رَدْع (restraining, repelling) in addition to הזיר and כח הזרה, while Nathan has ארתעה/הרתעה/הרתיע (MA 3: 85, 110; 9: 121; 15: 2); (b) repercussio 'rebounding, repelling'; cf. fol. 96b (H 288, ll. 5–7): ורפואת המורסא הקרה היא ההתכה לבד בלא הזרה[74] (But the treatment of a cold abscess is merely to dissolve it, not to 'repel it'. Cf. entry זור.

73 האשפונדלי: Lat. Spondali.

74 הזרה: הסרה O.

העדפה: העדפות = Latin superfluitates 'superfluities'; cf. fol. 85a (H 249, ll. 14–15): שער השביעי מן האישקורופולו ומשאר ההעדפות הדומות להם (Chapter seven: On scrofula and other superfluities that are similar to them). העדפה features in Rabbinic literature in the sense of 'surplus, addition, increase' (JD 360). In a medical sense it is attested for Nathan's Hebrew translation of Ibn Sīnā's *K. al-Qānūn* in BM 1143. העדפות is also used by Shem Tov as a translation of the Arabic equivalent to 'superfluitates', i.e. فضول (cf. S). N translates the Arabic term as מותרים/מותרות, Z as ליחות (MA passim), and M (BIZ 17: 4) has מותרות.

התהפך (הפך) = Latin diversificari 'to vary, to be different'; cf. fol. 37b (H 104, ll. 15–16): אמנם הנגעים יתהפכו לפי התהפך הזמן כי מהן יש שהן חדשים ומהן ישנים (Ulcers differ according to the difference in time, for some are recent and others are old). Hebrew התהפך does not feature in this sense in the current dictionaries.

הפשטה = Latin ulceratio 'ulceration'; cf. fol. 42b (H 120, ll. 13–15): וממנו שיתילד משחורה שהיא משרפה מאדומה טבעית וכאבו חזק מרוב הפשטה ([Another kind of cancer] is that which originates from black bile which results from burnt natural yellow bile; it is very painful because of its severe ulceration). Hebrew הפשטה does not feature in this sense in the current dictionaries. The Arabic equivalent to 'ulceratio', namely تقريح is translated by N as השחנה and by Z as חבלה (MA 6: 7).

השבה = Latin restauratio 'restoration'; cf. fol. 51a (H 145, ll. 19–20): באמת הרפואות שאנו רגילים בם אחר ההשבה מכל השברים ומן ההשמטות ומן העקומים הם אותם שמיבשות ומדביקות עם מעט חום (Indeed the medicines which we employ in the restoration of all fractures and dislocations and sprains are those that have drying and gluing [qualities] with some heat). Hebrew השבה is not attested in the current dictionaries. Shem Tov uses the term in the combination השבת השברים for Arabic جَبْر: 'setting of bones' (cf. S).

השבון = Latin restauratio 'restoration'; cf. fol. 32b (H 90, ll. 3–5): אמר הגופים שמקבלים בחבלותיהן ההשבון במהרה הם ממזג יותר טוב עם דם מובחר מבלתי לחות עודפת ולא יובש (He says that bodies that quickly achieve restoration from ulcers have a better temperament and good blood that is not excessively moist or dry). The Hebrew term only features in the sense of 'making amends for robbery, fraud; restitution' in the current dictionaries (JD1: 369; BM 1202; EM 412).

השמטה, Plur. **השמטות** = Latin dislocationes 'dislocations'; cf. fol. 51a (H 145, ll. 19–20): באמת הרפואות שאנו רגילים בם אחר ההשבה מכל השברים ומן ההשמטות ומן העקומים הם אותם שמיבשות ומדביקות עם מעט חום (Indeed the medicines which we employ in the restoration of all fractures and dislocations and sprains are those that have drying and gluing [qualities] with some heat). In a medical sense Hebrew השמטה features in EM 415 in a quotation from Rashi on TB Hulin 28: השמטה בגרגרת (when the gullet has slipped from its place). It is used by Zeraḥyah to translate the Arabic equivalent of Latin 'dislocatio', namely خَلْع 'dislocation', whereas N has שמט (MA 15:46), S has a variant שמיטה (S, s.v. חִבּוּשׁ) and M has הקעה (BIZ 15:1).

הַשְּׁמָעוּת = Latin obedientia 'susceptibility'; cf. fol. 52b (H 150, ll. 14–15): ועוד מתהפך השבר לפי ההשמעות ובלתי ההשמעות מן המיתוח ומן ההשבה (Fractures vary also according to their susceptibility to traction and reduction). Hebrew הַשְּׁמָעוּת only features as modern in EM 415.

התהפך = Latin diversitas 'diversity, difference'; cf. fol. 7a (H 11, ll. 15–16): השער השני מן התכונה הכללית מהתרת הדבקות לפי התהפך האברים (Chapter two: On a general [discussion] [disputatio] of the dissolution of continuity according to the different parts of the body). Hebrew התהפך does not feature in this sense in the current dictionaries. The Arabic aequivalent to 'diversitas', i.e. اختلاف, is translated by N as התחלפות and by Z as השתנות or שנוי (MA 4: 7, 8, 15–17, 19, 31, 40; 23: 21, 38; 25: 44, 57, 58, 59, 64). From the same root as Hebrew התחלפות we find התחלף and חלוף for Latin 'diversitas' in, for instance Kalonymus Ben Kalonymus' Hebrew translation of Aristotle's *De generatione et corruptione*.[75]

התחכחות = Latin crepitatio 'crepitus'; cf. fol. 55b–6a (H 160, ll. 13–16): כשיבוא לצלעות השבר הזה אינו נעלם במישוש הידים בעבור שיש[76] שעירות שם וחוש לא ימצא שם בשוה ולפעמים ישמע התחככות שברי העצם זה בזה (When the ribs are affected by this fracture it is not hidden when it is palpated with the hands, because

75 Cf. the glossary on p. 178 in F.A. Fobes and S. Kurland (eds), *Averrois Cordubensis Commentarium Medium in Aristotelius De Generatione et Corruptione Libros*. (Cambridge, Mass. 1956).

76 שיש: editor emendation שאין O.

roughness and unevenness are felt at the point and sometimes one can hear crepitus of the bone fragments). Hebrew התחכחות does not feature in this sense in the current dictionaries; cf. BM 1225; EM 427.

התרה: התרת הדבקות = Latin solutio continuitatis 'dissolution of continuity';[77] cf. fol. 15a (H 37, l. 20–38, l. 3): אמר גלינו ושאר החכמים התרת הדבקות בגידים מרוב הרגשתם והדבקתם במוח ממהרות להביא הקיוץ (Galen and the other learned [physicians] say that a dissolution of continuity in the nerves will quickly lead to spasms, because of their extreme sensitivity and their connection with the brain). Hebrew התרת הדבקות is not attested in secondary literature. N translates the Arabic aequivalent تفرّق الاتّصال as פרוק חבור and Z as הפרדת הדבקות (MA 7: 6; 25: 21).

ויתן, Plur. **ויתנים** = Latin. arteriae 'arteries'; cf. fol. 7b (H 12, ll. 12–14): וזה מנוסח דברי גליני' באמרו רבים חשב<ו> שיהיה מן הנמנע שעצם הויתנים יתחבר אם יותר (This is according the statement of Galen who says that many [physicians] held the opinion that the substance of the arteries cannot be healed once it has become apart). Hebrew ויתן features as וָתִין in BM 1273 in the sense of 'aorta', Cf. KA 3: 259, s.v. וְוּתָן: 'Herzader' and Nathan's quotation from the *Sefer ha-Refu'ot* by Asaph ha-Rofe (ibid.): וותן הוא גיד בספר הרפואות (WWTN is vein according to the *Book of Medicines* [composed by Asaph]). See as well the Aramaic counterpart וַתְנָא (DA 122), or וְותָנָא (LC 209) 'vein'.

(זור) הזיר: המזירים = (a) Latin refrenatio 'restraint'; i.e. restraining ingredients; cf. fol. 78a (H 228, ll. 6–8): וזה יעשה בדברים מרככים ומתירים וקלים ועם כל זה תמיד תקדים המזירים (And this should be done with softening, dissolving and light ingredients, but always give precedence to restraining ingredients); (b) Latin repercussiva, i.e. repercussive remedies; cf. fol. 79b (H 233, ll. 10–11): ועם כל זה שים המזירים עליו בהתחלה (Nevertheless, put repercussive remedies on it in the beginning. The Hebrew term does not feature in these meanings in the current dictionaries. A similar Hebrew term features in Zeraḥyah's translation of the Arabic الأدوية التي تمنع وتردع (the detaining and restraining drugs) as הרפואה אשר תזיר ותמנע, while Nathan has: הרפואות המונעות והמרתיעות (MA 9: 121).

77 For this Galenic notion known as 'συνεχείας λυσίς' see Phillip de Lacy, 'Galen's concept of continuity', *Greek, Roman and Byzantine Studies*, vol. 20 (Spring 1979, no. 1; Duke University, Durham, North Carolina), 355–69.

זינה = Latin nutrimentum 'nutriment, nourishment'; cf. fol. 32a (H 89, ll. 5–8): אמר ואין צריך שתניח שם רפואה מצמחת עד שתטהר תחילה החבלה או שימשך שם הזינה אם יהיה שם חסרון באיזה מקום שיהיה ([Avicenna] says: One should not apply remedies that make the flesh grow unless the ulcer be first cleansed, or nourishment may be drawn to it if it should have diminished wherever it may be). Hebrew זינה only features as modern in EM 468.

זמן = Latin etas 'age'; cf. fol. 92b (H 275, ll. 7–9): ואז תשגיח בגודל השבר וישנו וזמן החולה (Then consider the size of the rupture, how long it has been there, and the patient's age). The Hebrew term does not feature in this sense in the current dictionaries. The Arabic equivalent to Latin 'etas', namely سِنّ is translated by both N and Z as שנים (MA 12: 22, 26).

חבלה, Plur. **חבלות** = Latin ulcera 'ulcers'; cf. fol. 31a (H 85, ll. 15–16): אחר כן אומר לפי דברי ב''צ שהחבלות אותן נראות או הן נעלמות (Then I say according to Avicenna that ulcers are either visible or hidden). Hebrew חבלה is not attested in the sense of 'ulcer' in the current dictionaries. Even Shoshan (EM 497) lists the term as Rabbinic in the sense of 'wound' or 'fine', and as modern in the sense of 'trauma'. The parallel Arabic term, i.e. قرحة which can mean both 'ulcer' and 'wound' is translated by N, Z (MA 3: 13, 93; 6: 41, 51, 71 et passim), and M (BIZ, ch. 22) as נגע. Additionally Z has חבלה. Another term used by Hillel for Latin 'ulcus' is מכה (see below).

רפואה מחברת: חִבֵּר (חבר) = Latin medicamen incarnativum 'incarnative medicine'; cf. fol. 21a–b (H 58, ll. 6–8): הרפואה המחברת כמו שאמר ב''צ היא מה שמקבץ בין שני חלקים רחוקים (An incarnative medication, according to Avicenna, is that which builds flesh between two widely separated parts. Hebrew חִבֵּר does not feature in this sense in the current dictionaries.

חלאת הים: חלאה = Latin spuma maris, lit. 'froth of the sea' ; cf. fol. 86b (H 254, l. 18). The Latin term corresponds to Greek ἁλκυόνιον 'bastard-sponge' (LS 67) and designates according to Dioscurides (5:118) 'a mixture of sponges, algae and polypiers rejected by the sea'.[78] Hebrew חלאת הים, literally meaning 'filth of the sea' is not attested in secondary literature, but is used by Shem Tov as a translation of Arabic زبد البحر (sea foam); cf. SG Ḥet 33.

78 Cf. *Pedanii Dioscuridis Anazarbei De Materia Medica Libri Quinque*, ed. M. Wellmann, 5 books in 3 vols. (Repr. in 1 vol., Berlin 1958).

החליק (חלק): דברים מחליקים = Latin lenificantia 'mollifacients'; cf. fol. 96a (H 283, ll. 4–6): וחובש המקום בדברים מתיכים מחליקים כמו כממילא[79] קמח פולים ודומיהם (Then one should poultice the spot with solvents and mollifacients such as camomile, bean meal and the like). Hebrew החליק features in the current dictionaries in the sense of 'to glide, to smooth' (BM 1600–1; JD 473). The term מחליק features in Zeraḥyah as a translation of Arabic الدواء الملّين, i.e. a softening remedy (MA 21: 64).

-: רפואה מחליקה = medicina abstersiva "detergent remedy"; cf. fol. 26b (H 74, ll. 2–4): ויש לך לדעת שהמכות הנמסות הטריות צריכות רפואה מחליקה יותר מאותה שמניחין בשאר המכות (You should know that sordid wounds need remedies that are more detergent than those needed for the other wounds).

חלקות = Latin abstersio 'detergence'; cf. fol. 22a (H 60, ll. 10–14): כמו שנאמר בחלקות גם כן שלא תהיה חזקה אבל מעוטה בכמות מספקת לטהר העפוש בלי נשיכה (As it is also said, there should not be a strong detergent power in it (i.e. in a medication that makes the flesh grow), but very little, so that it cleanses the filth without biting). The Hebrew term does not feature in this sense in the current dictionaries.

טֹרַח: בטֹרַח = Latin raro 'rarely'; cf. fol. 82a (H 240, ll. 7–8): ודע כי המורסות בעלות הליחה הפשוטות בטורח יבואו לידי עפוש (know that simple flegmatic ulcers rarely putrefy). The Hebrew term does not feature in this sense in the current dictionaries.

יציקה = Latin embroca 'embrocation'; cf. fol. 84b (H 248, ll. 7–8): ראוי שתניח היציקות מקמח חיטים עם דבש ומיץ כרפס[80] אפיאו (It is proper for you to administer embrocations of wheat flour with honey and parsley juice). יציקה is only attested for Rabbinic literature in the sense of 'casting, pouring' (JD 589). It is used by Nathan as a translation of the Arabic equivalent of Latin 'embroca', namely تنطيل, whereas Zeraḥyah has נטילות (MA 13:38). Shem Tov translates plural تنطيلات as הטפות (S). For 'embrocation' in Rabbinic literature we find the term משיפה (bShabbat 77b; JD 853).

כורת, Plur. כורתים = Latin cyrurgici 'surgeons'; cf. fol. 4b (H 5, l. 1): כונת הכורתים צריך שיהיה על ג' מינים: האחד הדבקת החלקים שנפרדו (The intention of the

79 כממילא: emendation editor כרמילא MSS

80 כרפס אפיאו: כרפס אופיאו L O apium.

surgeons should be threefold: 1) Joining the parts that were separated). The term is not attested in this sense in secondary literature. A more common term for 'surgeon' is מְנַתֵּחַ; cf. EM 975 with an attestation from the *Sefer ha-Kuzari* by Judah ha-Levi.

כלי: כלי הממשש = Latin tenta 'probe'; cf. fol. 37a (H 104, ll. 4–7): ואף על פי כן הנגע הבא אל הבשר אינו מכאיב כל כך כמו הבא אל הגיד ובסגולה כאשר יגע בעומקה בכלי הממשש הוא טנטא בלעז (nevertheless a fistula affecting the flesh is not as painful as a fistula that affects the nerves, especially not when it can be touched deep within with a probe). Hebrew כלי הממשש does not feature in the current dictionaries. To translate the Arabic parallel to Latin 'tenta', i.e. مدس or مسبار Shem Tov uses Hebrew מחפש (cf. S). Masie (MD 598) mentions as synonyms בוחן and מחדר. Cf. entries ממשש and טנטא.

כמהים or **כמהין** (JD 646) (from Sing. כמה [BM 2416] or כמהה [EM 746]) = Latin fungus 'fungus'; cf. fol. 89b (H 265, ll. 16–18): והיא מורסא בשרית גדולה ורכה ודומה לכמיהים פונגו בלעז (And it is a large, fleshy, soft abscess resembling a fungus). Hebrew כמהים only features in the current dictionaries in the sense of 'truffle'; cf. JD 646; BM 2416. The current term for fungus is פטרייה (cf. EM 1420).

כף = Latin rotula 'patella; kneecap'; cf. fol. 63b (H 187, ll. 12–14): ומצד פנים לא תעשה השמטה בעבור הכף שמונעה (it [i.e. the knee] cannot be dislocated anteriorly because of the protection of the patella). As an anatomical term כף features in the current dictionaries as: 1. the hollow, the flat of the hand; 2. the whole hand; 3. the sole of the foot (כף הרגל); 4. socket of the hip (כף הירך); cf. KB 491–2; BM 2477–81; Low LVI. Aramaic כפא features in the sense of 'shoulder' in Rabbinic literature (SDA 594). In the Hebrew translation of Ibn Sīnā's *K. al-Qānūn* by Nathan ha-Me'ati we find כף הארכובה for 'patella' (cf. MD 551).

כריתות = Latin cyrurgia 'surgery'; cf. fol. 3a (H 1, l. 1): זה ספר כריתות אשר חברו מאשטרו ברונו בלשון נוצרי (This is the book on surgery compiled by Master Bruno in Latin). The term is attested in this sense in BM 2516 who quotes our text. Both N and Z translate Arabic عمل اليد (surgery) as מלאכת היד (MA 0; 9: 102, 124; 15: 0).

כֻּתֹּנֶת, Plur. **כתנות** = Latin tunicae 'membranes, tunics'; cf. fol. 7b (H 12, l. 16): שני הכתנות של וותנים (the two membranes of the arteries) and fol. 67a: (H 196, ll. 17–20): ועם כל זה פעולת הכריתות בעין מסוכנת מאד מפחד פן יגע בכתונת הנקרא קורניאה (Nevertheless, surgery of the eye is very dangerous because it is to be feared that one touches the cornea). Hebrew כתנת only features in BM 2558 in a medical context as כתנות העיניים; i.e. the tunics of the eyes. In the sense of 'membranes' כתנות also features in *Sefer ha-Refu'ot* by Asaph (following Kaufmann, *Die Sinne*, p. 86, n. 4).[81] N uses the same term as a translation of Arabic صفاقات (membranes). In addition to this term N uses: עורות and קרומות, while Z uses קליפות or קרומות (MA 2: 19; 3: 53; 23: 25). See as well entry בגד.

לוח, Plur. **לוחות** = Latin astellae 'splints'; cf. fol. 50 (H 142, ll. 13–14): אמנם על הקשירות הנזכרות ישים לאלתר הלוחות הנקרא' שקלולי (on the mentioned pads one should immediately put splints called ŠQLWLY[?]). Hebrew לוח does not feature in this sense in the current dictionaries. The Arabic equivalent to Latin 'astellae', namely جبائر is translated by N as חבישות, by Z as דבקות (MA 15: 69) and by S as קשישים (S). The last term already features in the sense of 'splints' in Rabbinic literature (JD 1431). See as well entry דחק.

מְדָבָּק, Plur. **מְדֻבָּקִים** = Latin iuncturae 'joints'; cf. fol. 59a (H 171, ll. 6–7): ההשמטה היא ההפרדה או יציאת[82] המודבקים ממקומם (A dislocation is a separation or departure of the joints from their [normal] position). Hebrew מְדֻבָּק does not feature in this sense in the current dictionaries. See entry דבק above.

מוצא = Latin anus 'anus'; cf. fols 98a–b (H 294, ll. 1–3): והם על שני פנים או שיהיו בתוך המוצא ואז יוצא הדם מהם תמיד או שהם מחוץ לו (There are two types [of haemorrhoids]): either they are inside the anus, and the blood issue from them constantly; or they are outside it). Hebrew מוצא does not feature in this sense in the current dictionaries. In Rabbinic literature we find the Plural נקבים for the 'orifices' (anus, urethra) (Low LXV), and בית נקובה next to נקב בית הרעי for the 'anus' (MD 51). The Arabic equivalent for Latin 'anus', i.e. مقعدة is translated by N as טבעת and by Z as פי הטבעת (MA 1: 28; 6:81; 9:97; 13: 39; 22: 54, 60, 63; 24: 2, 16) (cf. MD ibid.). Synonyms for 'anus' used by Hillel are המעי התחתון and הנקב התחתון (see a.l.).

---

81 D. Kaufmann, *Die Sinne. Beiträge zur Geschichte der Physiologie und Psychologie im Mittelalter aus hebräischen und arabischen Quellen* (Jahresbericht der Landes-Rabbinerschule in Budapest für das Schuljahr 1883–4. Budapest 1884).

82 יציאת: emendation editor יוציא L OP egressio.

מזלג = Latin uncinus 'hook'; cf. fol. 28a (H 77, l. 16–18): וכשהדם יוצא מן הוותנים או מן הורידים הגדולים והדברים הנזכרים לא יועילו צריך שתאחוז במזלג אחד דק אותו הקצה מן הווייתן או אותו הוריד (When blood flows from the arteries or the large veins and the mentioned [remedies] are not beneficial [to stop the bloodflow] one should grasp the end of that artery or vein with a fine hook). Hebrew מזלג is attested as '(meat) fork (for taking meat out of the cauldron)' (KB 565; JD 755), and as an instrument for taking the child out of the womb (forceps?) (BM 2885). Shem Tov uses the term מזלג to translate Arabic نشل 'lancet' (cf. S and SG, Mem 34).

מחבר: See **חבר**.

מְחִלָּה = Latin caverna 'cavity'; cf. fol. 32a (H 88, ll. 17–19): ובאמת החבלות העמוקות שיש בהן סתרים ומחילות לא ינקו ברפואות מצמיחות בשר (Indeed, deep ulcers in which there is a recess or cavity are not cleansed by remedies that make the flesh grow). The Hebrew term is only attested in the sense of 'cavity' for the Bible and Rabbinic literature (cf. KB2: 569; JD2: 761: 'hole, cave'; BM 2914–15: 'underground hollow').

מחליק: See **חלק**.

מיוחס: See **אֵבָר**.

מכה, Plur. **מכות** = Latin ulcera 'ulcers'; cf. fol. 32a (H 88, ll. 10–11): וזאת היא חזקה אמנם המכות שהן מעופשות מעט לא יסבלוה (This is a strong [cleanser] which is not tolerated by ulcers which are but slightly dirty). Hebrew מכה features in the sense of wound, plague, stroke, and blow in the Bible and Rabbinic literature (KB 579; JD 781). Another term used by Hillel for Latin 'ulcus' is חבלה (see above).

מכסה: **הַמְּכַסֶּה הַמַּבְדִּיל** = Latin diafragma 'diaphragm'; cf. fol. 5a (H 5, l. 19): או שבמכסה המבדיל ונקרא שבר (or that which is in the diaphragm and which is called fracture). The Hebrew term is not attested in secondary literature, but note that in the Bible we find the hapax legomenon מְכַסֶּה in Lev. 11:19 in the sense of 'the fatty tissue covering the internal organs' (KB 581). Next to הַמְּכַסֶּה הַמַּבְדִּיל, Hillel has דיאפרגמא for Latin 'diafragma'; cf. fol. 14b (H 36, l. 5): וגלינו אמר במכות הריאה או בדיאפרגמא (Galen said regarding wounds in the lungs or the diaphragm). N translates the parallel Arabic term حجاب 'diaphragm' a.o. as מסך or טרפשה, and Z a.o. as המסך המבדיל הנקרא דיאפרמה

(MA 1: 2, 28–30; 3: 40 et passim). M translates it as המסך המבדיל (MZ fol. 86a); cf. S, s.v. טרפשה.

מלקחים = Latin forceps 'forceps'; cf. fol. 47a (H 133, ll. 2–4): אם העצם נשבר ונפרד כלו במהרה תוכל להוציאו עם פיציקרולי או במלקחים והשמר מאד שלא תיגע הכתונת (If there is a complete fracture in the bone [of the head, the fractured part] can be taken out with a [piczicarolum?] or forceps, but be very careful not to touch the membrane). Hebrew מלקחים in the sense of forceps is attested as 'modern' in EM 956. The term also features in Shem Tov's translation of al-Zahrāwī's *Kitāb al-taṣrīf* as an equivalent of the Arabic كلاليب (S).

ממשש = Latin tenta 'probe'; cf. fol. 39a (H 108, ll. 18–19): ואז צריך הממשש מן העופרת כשהוא יותר רך ונכפף (Then you should use a leaden probe because it is softer and more pliable). Cf. entries טנטא and כלי הממשש.

מעי: המעי התחתון = Latin anus 'anus'; cf. fol. 83a (H 243, ll. 10–11): אמנם מאלה כלומר המורסות הנולדות במעי התחתון לא תאחר בהן הבקוע עד עת הבשול (but one should not delay perforating abscesses that appear in the anus until the time of [complete] digestion). The Hebrew term does not feature in this sense in the current dictionaries. Other terms used by Hillel for 'anus' are מוצא and הנקב התחתון (see a.l.).

מְעֻנָּג: מעונג = Latin delicatus 'soft'; cf. fol. 11a (H 23, ll. 5–8): וזכור כי כאשר יהיה האבר יותר נכבד ויותר מעונג כפי זה צריך שיתחברו חלקיו בעונג (And note that the more a part of the body is more prominent and more soft, the more it is necessary that the parts [of a wound in it] should be sewn up delicately). Hebrew מעונג does not feature in this sense in the current dictionaries, cf. BM 4576. Of the Arabic parallels to 'delicatus', namely لَيِّن and رخص, the former term is translated by N as רך /רזה and by Z as דשן/ לח (MA 16: 7); the latter term is translated by both N and Z as רך (MA 22: 23).

מעצור = Latin abstinentia 'abstinence'; cf. fols 89a–b (H 265, ll. 6–7): והמעצור משתיית המים ומכל מזונות הקרים ומן הקשים להתעכל (and abstinence from water and all cooling and indigestible foods). Hebrew מעצור is not mentioned in this sense in the current dictionaries, but cf. SSH 246. It features in the Bible (KB 615) and apocryphal literature (EM 1004) in the sense of 'impediment, limitation' and in modern literature (EM ibid.) in the sense of 'stoppage, inhibition'. See as well entry עצר. For Hebrew מעצור in the sense of 'diet' cf. Moses Ibn Tibbon.

מֻפְשָׁט = Latin ulceratus 'ulcerated'; cf. fol. 81a (H 237, ll. 5–6): ואם כל זה אם המקום מופשט לא תקררנו אלא מסביב (nevertheless, if the place is ulcerated, apply cooling only to the surrounding area). Hebrew מֻפְשָׁט does not feature in this sense in the current dictionaries. Cf. entry פשט.

מְקֻצָּף: See **דבש**.

מְשִׁיחוּת = Latin unctuositas 'greasy quality'; cf. fol. 30b (H 84, ll. 18–20): משיחות שמרככות ומחליקות האבר בלחותם ומשיחותם (ointments which soften and relax the part by reason of their wet and greasy quality). The Hebrew term does not feature in this sense in the current dictionaries. Cf. entry חלק.

משלחת = Latin effusio 'pouring, flowing'; cf. fol. 96a (H 287, ll. 3–6): הבשרית האות עליה הכובד והקושי והעובי עם[83] כאב גדול וסבתה משלחת החומר מן המעים אל הבצים או הכאה (fleshy [hernia]: its symptom is heaviness, hardness and puffiness with severe pain; and its cause is the flowing of matter from the intestines to the testicles or a blow). Hebrew משלחת does not feature in this sense in the current dictionaries.

מתאים: See **תאם**.

מתלעת (= **מלתעת**/ **מלתעה**) = Latin mandibula 'jaw' or 'jaw bone'; cf. fol. 59b (H 172, ll. 15–16): ההשמטה מעצם המתלעת תבוא לעתים רחוקות וההוראה על זה היא בהיות שורת השנים התחתונים בלתי שוה בעליונה (A dislocation of the jaw bone occurs rarely; its symptoms are: the lower row of teeth do not line up evenly with the upper ones…). Hebrew מלתעה, Plur. מלתעות and מתלעת, Plur. מתלעות feature in the Bible in the sense of 'jaw bone' (cf. KB 595 and 654). According to Ben-Yehuda (BM 3062) מלתעה is identical with Hebrew ניב, i.e. canine tooth (BM 3645). Ben-Yehuda (BM 3062) adds that according to some מלתעה can also mean 'jaw bone', as, for instance, in the encyclopaedic work *Shilṭei Gibborim* composed by Abraham Portaleone (1542–1612). The Arabic equivalent to Latin 'mandibula', i.e. لحي is translated by N as לחי and by Z as לחי or לחיים (MA 1: 21; 9: 42; 15: 62), which has the standard meaning of 'cheek' (cf. BM 2051–2).

נֶגַע = (a) Latin fistula 'fistula'; cf. fol. 36b (H 101, ll. 16–18): הנגע היא חבלה עמוקה וצרה מעוקלת כלומר במקום אחד רחבה ובמקום אחר צרה עם קושי הבשר שסביבה והיא כמו קנה נוצת אווז בענין הכנסה (A fistula is a deep, narrow and curved ulcer,

83 עם כאב גדול: L cum parvitate doloris (with slight pain).

i.e. wide in one place and narrow in another, with hard flesh around it. It is similar to the feather of a goose in the way it penetrates [into the part]). Hebrew נגע is only attested in the sense of 1. 'onset of illness': i.e. affliction, plague, infestation, and 2. 'blow' (KB 669; see as well BM 3520–1: 'plague, leprosy'). S translates the Arabic equivalent ناصور as Hebrew גרגתני, N transcribes the same Arabic term as נאצור and Z translates it as Romance פישטולא (MA 15: 29, 44); cf. S, s.v. גרגתני; (b) Latin pustula 'pustule'; cf. fol. 30b (H 84, ll. 9–10): אמר ב''צ החבלות הישנות המעופשות מתילדות מן המכות ומן המורסא הנפסדת ומן הנגעים (Avicenna says that putrid chronic sores [ulcers] arise from wounds and corrupt abscesses and pustules). The Arabic parallel term to Latin 'pustula', i.e. بثر is translated by S as השחין הדק (cf. S), by M as שחין (BIZ 8: 4) and as אבעבעות (BIZ 22: 1), by N as צמח, while Z transcribes it as בתר (MA 6: 24).

נהג = Latin administrare 'to administer' (a remedy); cf. fol. 16b (H 42, ll. 2–3): ואפילו בגופים הקשים והיבשים מאד הסרפינו עם טירבינטינה תנהוג (Even in extremely hard and dry bodies you should administer sagapenum with turpentine). Hebrew נהג does not occur in this sense in the current dictionaries. Cf. entries אימן and הרגיל.

נמלה = Latin formica 'shingles'; cf. fol 81a (H 236, ll. 14–15): הנמלה היא מורסא קטנה המתילדת מחומר מרירי (shingles consists of small pimples that originate from bilious matter). As a disease the Hebrew term features in *Sefer ha-Refu'ot* by Asaph ha-Rofe as quoted by Ben Yehuda (BM 3678): שיחוש האדם בחלי כמו נמלים הלכים על בשרו ([in this disease] it feels as if ants creep over one's flesh). The same Hebrew term is used by both N and Z as a translation of the Arabic aequivalent نملة (MA 9: 105, 106; 22: 25; 23: 35).

נסירה = Latin incisio 'incision'; cf. fol. 70a (H 206, ll. 5–6): ואז אם תהיה הנסירה גדולה תתקבץ מחוץ בתפירה (And then, if the incision is large, gather it up [i.e. the eyelid] from the outside with a suture). Hebrew נסירה does not occur in this sense in the current dictionaries. The Arabic aequivalents for 'incisio', namely بطّ and شقّ are translated by N as חתך and שסוע and by Z as פתיחה and הקזה (MA 15: 49; 23: 32; 24: 47). See as well S s.v. פֶּלָה.

נסורת: נסורת ברזל = Latin limatura ferri 'filings of iron'; cf. fol. 41a (H 115, ll. 9–10). Hebrew נסרת only features in the current dictionaries in the sense of sawdust (EM 1165; BM 3699; JD 915). Instead of נסורת in the sense of 'filings' Shem Tov has קלפה; cf. SG Quf 43: קליפי הנחשת (copper filings), while Hillel uses the term קלפה in the sense of 'dross'; cf. entry קלפה below.

נקב: הנגעים הנוקבים = Latin fistule penetrantes 'penetrating fistulas'; cf. fol. 100a (H 299, ll. 11–13): ואל תחשוב שיש דרך אחרת בנגעים הנוקבים (Do not think that there is another way to heal penetrating fistulas). Hebrew נקב does not feature in this sense in the current dictionaries.

נֶקֶב: הנקב התחתון = Latin anus 'anus'; cf. fol. 65a (H 191, l. 7): שער הי"ו מן הנגעים הבאים בנקב התחתון (Chapter sixteen: On anal fistulae). Hebrew הנקב התחתון does not feature in the current dictionaries. Synonyms for 'anus' used by Hillel are המעי התחתון and מוצא (see a.l.).

-: נקב אותו מקום של אשה = Latin vulva mulieris 'vulva of a woman'; cf. fol. 97a (H 290, 9–12): הראשון שבאנשים שנראה בעור הבצים באותו שהוא באמצע שניהן תבנית נקב אותו מקום של אשה ויש שם שערות (The first [kind] of a male [hermaphrodyte] is that there is the appearance of the shape of a vulva in the middle of the scrotum [between the testes] and that there are hairs over there). The Hebrew term does not feature in the current dictionaries. Shem Tov (*Sefer ha-Shimmush*, ch. 70 [MS Paris 1163, fol. 220b]) translates the Arabic equivalent فضاء as נקבת אשה. The general Hebrew term for the female (and male) genitals is ערוה; cf. KB 882: 'nakedness, genital area of a man or a woman'; MD 778. The specific term for vulva featuring in Rabbinic literature is פרוזדור; cf. Low LXXII.

נֻקָּה (נקה) = Latin curatus esse 'to heal'; cf. fol. 36b (H 101, l. 20–102, l. 3): וסבותיה שתים אחת פנימית ואחת חיצונית הפנימית היא מלחות נפסדות והחיצונית היא ממכות או מחבלות מבלתי נוקו כהוגן (Its causes [i.e. of a fistula] are twofold, one internal and one external. The internal [cause] is corrupt moisture and the external cause is a wound or an ulcer that have not sufficiently healed). Hebrew נֻקָּה is not attested in this sense in the current dictionaries. For נִקָּה in the common sense of to 'cleanse' or to 'purge', cf. entry חובל.

לְהִנָּקוֹת: נִקָּה = Latin ad curandum 'to heal'; cf. fol. 5b (H 7, l. 18): שער שמני יבקש למה המכות מתאחרות להנקות ומתחבולות הנקיות מאותן המכות (Chapter eight: About the reason why wounds are slow to heal and about means to cure those wounds). Hebrew להנקות is not attested in this sense in the current dictionaries. See entry נקיות.

נקיון = Latin curatio 'cure, therapy'; cf. fol. 5b (H 7, l. 12): שער חמישי מן סוג הכולל הנקיון מן החבלות שבגידין (Chapter five: On the general therapy of wounds of the nerves). Hebrew נקיון is not attested in this sense in the current dictionaries. In the context of diseases it can have the specific meaning of 'crisis' in medieval medical literature; cf. BM 3796: נקיון המחלה 'crisis of a disease'. Cf. entry פרח for נקיון in the sense of 'cleansing remedy'.

נקיות = Latin curatio 'cure, therapy'; cf. fol. 5b (H 7, l. 18): שער שמני יבקש למה המכות מתאחרות להנקות ומתחבולות הנקיות מאותן המכות (Chapter eight: About the reason why wounds are slow to heal and about means to cure those wounds). Hebrew נקיות is not attested in this sense in the current dictionaries. See entry נִקָּה.

סור = Latin cavere 'to be on one's guard, to take care, to guard against'; cf. fol. 84b (H 247, ll. 10–12): וסור מאד שלא יבוא שמן או מים או שום דבר שמן אחרי שנפתחה (Be very careful that no oil, water or any fatty substance comes into contact with it once the [abscess] has been cut open). The Hebrew term is not attested in this sense in the current dictionaries. The Arabic equivalent to 'cavere', i.e. تحفّظ is translated by both N and Z with the standard term נשמר (MA 7: 15).

סיד: הסיד החי = Latin calx viva 'quicklime'; cf. fol. 16a (H 41, l. 15). Hebrew סיד means 'lime, plaster' and features in the Bible (e.g. Num. 27:2) and Rabbinic literature, e.g. in mShab 8.4 (KB 750; JD 976). Hebrew סיד חי which is attested in EM (1788) as modern is possibly coined as a loan translation of Latin 'calx viva'. It also features in the glossary compiled by Shem Tov Ben Isaac (SG, Samekh 21).

סינן (סנן) = Latin instillare 'to pour in by drops, to drip'; cf. fol. 48b (H 138, ll. 3–4): וגם יסונן שמן רוסטו באזנים (and rose oil should be dripped into the ears). Hebrew סינן does not feature in this sense in the current dictionaries; cf. JD 1008: 'to smelt, to refine'; BM 4125: 'to filter'. The Arabic counterpart to Latin 'instillare', i.e. قطّر is translated both by N and Z as הטיף (MA 9: 27, 126; 15: 28; 22: 12, 47).

עלילה = Latin vitium 'fault, defect, blemish'; cf. fol. 104a (H 314, ll. 12–13): על כאב ועלילת הכבד תכוה על הכבד (Against pain and a blemish [disease] of the liver, apply cautery over the liver). Hebrew עלילה does not feature in this sense in the current dictionaries.

עצירה: אופן העצירה = Latin modus stringendi ‘the mode of binding (tightly)’; cf. fol. 57a (H 164, ll. 6–8): אחר כן כשתקל המורסא עצור השבר כמו שאמרנו ואופן העצירה הוא כמו שאמרנו (Then, when the abscess has been alleviated, bind up the fracture as we have said. The mode of binding it has been outlined [in a previous chapter]). Hebrew עצירה does not feature in this sense in the current dictionaries; cf. JD 1102: 1) closing up, obstruction of orifices; 2) locking up, detention.

עצר = Latin stringere ‘to bind, to bind tightly’; cf. fol. 56b (H 163, ll. 9–10): ואם יהיה השבר קרוב לכתף תעצרהו עמו (If the fracture [in the humerus] is close to the shoulder, bind up [the shoulder] tightly with it). Hebrew עצר only features in the current dictionaries in the sense of: 1. to restrain, to keep back; 2. to press, to squeeze (BM 4659–62). Another term used by Hillel for ‘to bind’ is דחק (see above). The Arabic parallel to ‘stringere’, i.e. ربط is translated by both N and Z as קשר (MA 1: 56, 60, 64; 15: 40, 47, 69; 25: 23).

עצר: לעצור עצמו מן = Latin abstinentia ‘to abstain from, abstention from’; cf. fol. 82b (H 241, ll. 8–10): וצוה לחולה שיעצור עצמו מן המאכלים הרעים והמולידים אותה (and tell the patient to abstain from bad foodstuff and from that which produces [black bile]). The Hebrew term does not feature in this sense in the current dictionaries. However, Nathan translates the Arabic equivalent to ‘abstinentia’, namely إمساك عن as לעצור מן or המנע מן while Z has המנע מן or לעמוד מן (MA 19: 20, 23). See as well entry מעצור.

עִשּׁוּן = Latin balneum ‘bath’; cf. fol. 61b (H 179, ll. 16–19): ואם תרצה תניח עליו חלב מן האנטרי[84] עם חמאה חם במזג וישאהו לפני העשון ואחר העשון (And if you wish, apply melted goose[85] fat with butter, moderately warm, using it both before the bath and after). Hebrew עשון could not be identified in this sense. See entry עשן.

עשן: עישן במים = (a) Latin humectare in balneo ‘to soak in the bath’; cf. fol. 61b (H 179, ll. 13.15): ואם אחרי הבריאות ישאר כובד בתנועתו אז יעושן במים חמים (If, after healing, [the joint] still moves with difficulty, then soak the part in the bath); (b) Latin fomentare ‘to foment’; cf. fol. 61b (H 180, ll. 14–17): ואם תכבד תנועתו אז יעושן במים חמים (And if it is difficult to move it [i.e. the hand],

84 חלב מן האנטרי: חלב מן האנדרי L R sepum arietinum.

85 goose: ‘ram’ L.

then it should be fomented with hot water). Hebrew עישן could not be identified in this sense. Cf. entry עשון.

פרח: פרח הנחשת = Latin flos eris 'verdigris'; cf. fol. 14b (36, ll. 17–19): ושמור שלא תרגיל בו נקיון חזק כמו פרח הנחשת (Be careful not to apply a strong cleansing remedy to it, such as verdigris). The term is not attested in the current dictionaries but features in Shem Tov Ben Isaac's glossary (SG, Pe 11) and subsequently in Judah ben Solomon Natan's *Kelal Qaẓar mi ha-Sammim ha-Nifradim* (JNK 210:50).

פרק: פרק היד = Latin iunctura manus, lit. 'joint of the hand', i.e. 'wrist'; cf. fol. 61b (H 180, ll. 7–9): וישתוה עוד שיונח פרק היד על שום לוח ויפשטנו[86] בפשוט ראוי (There is another method of realigning it (i.e. a dislocated wrist), and that is to place the wrist upon a flat surface and to apply the proper traction). See entry דבק היד above.

(פשט) פִּשֵּׁט המעים: פִּשֵּׁט Latin excoriare intestina 'to excoriate the intestines'; cf. fol. 86a (H 252, ll. 17–18): וזה כמו שאמר ב''ס שזאת הרפואה אינה מחממת ולא מפשטת המעים (And [one should use] this remedy because, as Ibn Sīnā says, it neither heats nor excoriates the intestines). The Hebrew פשט is attested in the Hiphʿil in the sense of 'to strip, to flay, to skin' for the Bible (KB 980–1) and Rabbinic literature (JD 1246; BM 5272).

(פשט) נפשט = Latin ulcerari 'to ulcerate'; cf. fol 43b (H 123, ll. 5–7): אבל אם הסרטן נפשט לא יתרפא בדברים הקרים אבל צריך שיחתוך ויאומנו בו רפואות חמות מאד כמו הכויה באש (If the cancer has ulcerated it cannot be cured with cold things, but should be cut and treated with very hot means, such as cauterization). Hebrew נפשט does not feature in this sense in the current dictionaries. The Arabic equivalent to 'ulcerari', i.e. تقرّح is translated by N as התחבל or השחין, by Z as התחבל, חבל or התנגע (MA 6: 72; 23. 46) and by S as נתבעבע (S). M (BIZ 13:3) translates the Arabic أقرح (to ulcerate) as לנגע. See as well entry מֻפְשָׁט.

צמח = Latin apostema (from Greek ἀπόστημα 'abscess' (LS 119)) 'the separation of corrupt matter into an ulcer, an abscess, imposthume' (LSD 139); cf. fol. 45a (H 38, ll. 9–11): עוד בעבור שכל כאב מקבץ הריאומה ששם נעשה

86 ויפשטנו: ויפשוט O.

הנפח והצמח שבעבורים יבוא הקווץ אל נקלה (Moreover, every pain concentrates[87] the rheum from which tumours or [other] morbid growths originate which easily lead to cramps). Hebrew צמח means 1) 'growth, sprout, plant', and 2) 'morbid growth, swelling, ulcer, eruption' (JD 1287; BM 5521f., Low LXXIV s.v. צמחים). In the latter sense the term features in medieval medical literature (cf. BM 5522). Plural צמחים features in Shem Tov Ben Isaac's glossary as a translation of Arabic أنبات, Sing. نبت, meaning 'abcess, ulcer, boil' (D 2: 633), and of Arabic دماميل, Sing. دمّل meaning 'a kind of purulent pustule, or imposthume' (L 915, SN 96); cf. SG Ẓade 28.

קִוּוּץ = Latin spasmus 'spasm'; cf. fol. 15a (H 37, l. 20–38, l. 3): אמר גלינו ושאר החכמים התרת הדבקות בגידים מרוב הרגשתם והדבקתם במוח ממהרות להביא הקווץ (Galen and the other learned [physicians] say that a dissolution of continuity in the nerves will quickly lead to spasms, because of their extreme sensitivity and their connection with the brain). Hebrew קווץ, derived from the root קוץ, to shrink (cf. BM 5862) does not feature in the current dictionaries. The Arabic aequivalent تشنّج is translated by N as כויצה, Z as כווץ or התכווץ (MA passim), while M (BMR 4: 18, 27) has the same term as Hillel, namely קיווץ; cf. KZ 65; SG Kaf 21; BS, s.v. כווץ.

קליבוסתא = Latin ancha 'coccyx, femur'; cf. fol. 62b (H 183, l. 19–184, l. 2): השמטת הקליבוסתא היא מד' פנים א' שיושמט מצד פְּנים ב' מצד חוץ ג' מצד פָּנים ד' מצד אחור (A dislocation of the femur occurs in four ways. It is dislocated internally, externally, forward or backward). Aramaic קליבוסתא is only attested for Rabbinic literature (cf. SD 1018: 'os innominatum'). The Arabic counterpart عصعص is translated by Shem Tov as עָצֶה or סוף הפרשות (S); see as well SG Quf 43.

קלפת עופרת: קלפה = Latin scoria plumbi 'dross of lead' (cf. GS 137); cf. fol. 25b (H 69, l. 13). The Hebrew term קלפה does not feature in this sense in the current dictionaries. Shem Tov uses the same Hebrew term in the sense of 'filings'; cf. SG Quf 43: קליפי הנחשת (copper filings). Cf. entry נסרת above.

87 'concentrates': exacuit L, i.e. makes sharp.

קנה: קנה משמרת = Latin canellum emboti 'tube, funnel'; cf. Hunt, *Medieval Surgery*,[88] no. 36: 'chalmel qui est appele embottun' (Anglo-Norman). The Hebrew term does not feature in the standard dictionaries.

קרום: קרום מכסה = Latin pannus 'pannus'; cf. fol. 64b (H 192, 3–4): חליי העינים מתהפכים כי מהן חוליי הדמעות ומהן אודם ומהן קרום מכסה (There are different eye diseases such as tears [epiphora], redness and pannus). The Hebrew term does not feature in the current dictionaries. Masie (MD 541) gives as the Hebrew equivalent for 'pannus' תבלול which features in the Bible (cf. KB 1684–5) and Rabbinic literature (cf. Low LXXXIV: 'cataract of the eye'). Another term for 'pannus' used by Hillel is בגד (see entry above).

קשירה, Plur. **קשירות** = (a) Latin ligamenta 'ligaments'; cf. fol. 61a (H 177, ll. 12–14): ההשמטה מן הגומברו היא יותר חזקה מן השאר ודומה[89] גם כן השבתו ויהיה מחוזק הקשירות וקטנם[90] ומהתנגדות גוממותו (the dislocation of the elbow is harder than all others and similarly its reduction. This is the case because of the strength and shortness of the ligaments and because of the diversity of its concavities). Hebrew קשירה does not feature in this sense in the current dictionaries. Ben Yehuda (BM 6265) refers to the term קֶשֶׁר for the meaning of ligament. Shem Tov (S) mentions קשירה, next to אסר as a translation of the Arabic رباط (ligament). N and Z translate the Arabic term, amongst others, as קשירה, קשורים, קשור (MA 1:8, 9–11; 3: 21, 52; 7: 33; 15: 29 et passim) and M as קשרים (BIZ 15: 5); (b) Latin ligatura 'bandage'; cf. fol. 61b (H 179, ll. 12–13): ואם לאו תוסיף לעשות התחבושת והקשירות עד שיתחזק (And if not, repeat the poultice and bandaging until it grows strong). Ben Yehuda (BM 6251) refers to קשירה in the sense of 'bandage, dressing', quoting from the Hebrew translation of Ibn Sīnā's *K. al-Qānūn* by Nathan ha-Me'ati.

קֶשֶׁר = Latin ligatura 'bandage'; cf. fol. 61b (H 179, ll. 9–12): ויתלה זרועו אל צוארו ויונח כן כמה ימים אחר כן תתיר ואם תראה שנתחזק הדבק במקומו אז תתיר הקשר (suspend the forearm from the neck and leave it for some days. Then remove [the sling] and if you see that the joint has grown stiff in that position, then remove the bandage). Hebrew קשר does not feature in this sense in the

88 Tony Hunt, *Medieval Surgery* (Woodbridge 1992).

89 ודומה גם כן השבתו: om. O.

90 וקטנם: om. O.

current dictionaries. Another term for 'bandage' employed by Hillel is דחיקה (see above).

רִבּוּעַ: רבוע הראש = Latin cornu capitis 'the prominence of the head'; cf. fol. 103b (H 313, ll. 4–6): על חולי הישן מכאב הראש תכוה על כל ריבועי הראש (Against chronic pain in the head, apply the cautery over each prominence of the head). Hebrew רבוע does not feature in this sense in the current dictionaries. The Arabic equivalent قرن الرأس is translated by Shem Tov as קרן הראש (cf. S).

רגיל: היה רגיל = Latin uti 'to use, to apply'; cf. fol. 51b (H 146, ll. 13–16): ונחבוש תחבושות משיבות השבר וההשמטה בלי גמורה והוא אותו שהיו בו רגילין הקדמונים מאבק הרחים (And we apply plasters that heal a fracture and an incomplete dislocation, such as [the plaster] which the ancients used that is [made] of milldust). Hebrew רגיל is only attested in the current dictionaries in the sense of 'accustomed to, common, regular'; cf. BM 6409–11. Shem Tov uses the term as a translation of the Arabic حاذق: 'having skill', i.e. skilled (S).

הרגיל (רגל) = Latin administrare 'to administer'; cf. fol. 12b (H 28, ll. 6–9): ואם התולה יהיה מעט בשום פנים לא תחתכנו והרפואה המצמיחה תרגיל שם (If [the piece of flesh] that hangs [from the wound] is small, you should not cut it in any way, but administer a remedy that makes the flesh grow. Hebrew הרגיל does not feature in this sense in the current dictionaries. But it does occur in the same sense in Shem Tov's translation of al-Zahrāwī's *Kitāb al-taṣrīf*, Bk. 30; cf. S. M translates the Arabic equivalent استعمل as עשה or לקח (BMR 3:5,7,8), while N translates the Arabic استعمال as עשיה, and Z as עשיה or עשות (MA 16:18, 30; 17: 8). Cf entry נהג above.

-: הרגיל במרחץ = Latin uti balneo 'to bathe in the bathhouse; to take a bath'; cf. fol. 82b (H 241, ll. 16–17): וישמור[91] החולה שלא ירגיל מאד במרחץ בעבור שהוא מתיך החומר הדק ומקשה העב (The patient should take care not to frequent the bathhouse because it dissolves the soft matter and hardens the thick matter). The Hebrew term does not feature in this sense in the current dictionaries. The Arabic equivalent to 'uti balneo', namely استحمّ is translated by both N and Z as רחץ or התרחץ (MA 10: 4; 17: 12; 19: 13).

רפואה: See **חבר**, **תאם**.

---

91 וישמור...העב: om. O.

שכיבה = sedari 'to be alleviated'; cf. fol. 79a (H 231, ll. 4–6): ואותות המורסא הקשה הוראה עליה שכיבת הכאב וקושי מתרבה (The symptoms of a hard tumour are that the pain is alleviated and that it becomes [even] harder). The Hebrew term does not feature in this sense in the current dictionaries. The Arabic equivalent to 'sedari', i.e. سكن is translated by N as נח and שקט, by Z as עמד, סר, נח, שכך (MA 9: 92; 10: 46; 13: 47 et passim), and by M as שכך (BIZ 15: 4).

שמירה or **הנהגת השמירה** = Latin dieta 'diet' (H 2, ll. 16–20–3, l. 1); cf. fol. 4a: כי חלקי הרפואה הם שלשה שבאמצעותם יוכל הרופא מסיבות החולי לעזור: הראשון הנהגת השמירה הב' הנהגת המשקיות הג' הכריתות. השמירה הוא הראשון והמובחר כמאמר גלינו בספר הנהגת החדות (For medicine has three [instruments] by means of which a physician can combat the causes of a disease: 1. diet [regimen in food]; 2. regimen in drinks; 3. surgery. A diet is the first and best [instrument] as Galen has said in the book 'Regimen in Acute Diseases'). Both terms are not attested in the sense of 'diet' in the current dictionaries. Hebrew שמירה is used by both N and Z for Arabic حمية 'abstinence' (MA 8: 8).

שעיר = Latin asper 'rough'; cf. fol. 100b (H 302, ll. 4–6); ומיני האבן רבים ממנה קטנה וממנה גדולה וממנה חלקה ממנה שעירה וממנה קצרה וממנה ארוכה (There are different types of stones [in the bladder]: some are small, some large, some smooth, some rough, some short, and some long). Hebrew שעיר only features in the current dictionaries in the sense of 'hairy'; cf. BM 7593. Next to Hebrew גס Zeraḥyah uses שעיר to translate the Arabic equivalent of Latin 'asper', i.e. خَشِن, while Nathan has נחור (MA 7: 67).

שעירות = Latin asperitas 'roughness'; cf. fol. 20a (H 52, ll. 1–19: אם מיובש אותותיו הקושי והשעירות ומעט הטרי (If [a dyscrasy] of the flesh in which there is a wound] hails from dryness, its symptoms are hardness, roughness and a small quantity of pus). שעירות only features in the current dictionaries in the sense of 'hairiness'; cf. BM 7594–5. Next to Hebrew גסות Zeraḥyah has שעירות as a translation of the parallel Arabic term خشونة, while N has נחירות (MA 6: 37, 41; 7: 67; 25: 8).

שעיעות = Latin lenificatio 'softening'; cf. fol. 86b (H 254, ll. 4–5): אמנם צריך שעיעות לניפיקציאון בלע' למען ישועע העב (However, a softening [remedy] [emollient] is necessary in order to soften [thin] the thick [matter]). Hebrew

שעיעות is only attested in the sense of 'smoothness' for Rabbinic, medieval and modern literature (cf. EM 1869, BM 7353).

שִׁעֲשַׁע (שעע) = Latin lenire 'to soften'; cf. fol. 82b (H 241, ll. 10–12): אחר כן תשוב אל הרפואה המקומית[92] במה שיתיך וישעשע ביחד (Then you should return to the local treatment with that which both dissolves and softens). Hebrew שעשע only features in the current dictionaries in the sense of 1) to smooth, paste over; 2) to appease, console (JD 1611). The Arabic equivalent to Latin 'lenire', namely لَيَّن is translated by N as ריכך and by Z as החליק (MA 9. 72).

שִׁפּוּל = שפולי הבטן = Latin inguen 'groin'; cf. fol. 62b (H 184, ll. 6–8): ואין החולה יכול לכוף ברכו לצד שפולי בטנו ומקום השפול נפוח בנפיחה נגלית (and the patient cannot bend his knee [and bring up his foot] towards his groin, and the area of the groin is obviously bulged). Hebrew שפול, meaning 'the lower part, extremity' features in an anatomical context, for instance in mNid 9.8 as שפולי מעיים (the lower part of the abdomen) (cf. JD 1566; Low LXXXIV: 'groin, lower intestines, sexual organs'). Instead of שפולי הבטן we find שפולי האצטומכא in Shem Tov's glossary (SG Shin 65) as a translation of the Arabic خمل المعدة 'the lining of the stomach' (cf. D 1: 406). The proper Arabic term for 'groin', namely أربية is translated by N as אורבים and by Z as אנגוינליא (MA 15: 48).

רפואה מתאימה: התאים (תאם) = Latin medicamen consolidativum 'a consolidative remedy'; cf fol. 21b (H 59, ll. 2–5): והרפואה המתאימה היא אותה שמיבשת שטח המכה עד שיעשה שם קליפה שישמרנה מן הדברים המזיקים (a consolidative remedy is that which dries the surface of a wound until a scab is formed which protects it from harmful things). Hebrew מתאים does not feature in this sense in the current dictionaries.

תוצאה, Plur. **תוצאות** = Latin egestio 'emptying, voiding; excretion'; cf. fol. 100a (H 300, ll. 2–4): ולי נראה שיבוא זה מהטרדת התוצאות ומן הליחות המשוקעות בשולי[93] הנגע (it seems to me that it occurs because of the hindrance to excretion and because of the fluids contained in the margins of the fistula). Hebrew תוצאה, Plur. תוצאות does not feature in this sense in the current dictionaries. The Arabic equivalent to 'egestio', i.e. خروج is translated by both N and Z as צאת or יציאה (MA 7: 40, 45, 62, 63 et passim).

---

92 המקומית: om. O.

93 בשולי: in profunditate (in the depth) L.

תחת: תחת השחי = Latin subascellas 'armpits'; cf. fol. 15b (H 39, ll. 14–17): ולכן צריך שנקיז בחולה מבלתי שנשגיח על כוחו והעורף והחוט השדרה ותחת השחי תמשה תמיד בשמן חם (Therefore one should bleed the patient without allowing for his strength, and one should constantly rub his neck, spinal column and armpits with hot oil). Hebrew תחת השחי, a literal translation of Latin subascella does not feature in secondary literature. N translates the Arabic parallel إبطان (armpits) as אצילים or ארבות הידיים והרגליים, and Z as שחי or תחת לזרועות (MA 7: 71; 15: 48; 23: 56).

תחבושת = Latin emplastrum 'plaster, poultice'; cf. fol. 61b (H 179, ll. 12–13): ואם לאו תוסיף לעשות התחבושת והקשירות עד שיתחזק (And if not, repeat the poultice and bandaging until it grows strong). For תחבושת in this sense cf. MD 593. Both Ben Yehuda (BM 7715–16) and Even-Shoshan (EM 1927) only mention this term in the sense of 'bandage, bandaging'. תחבושת also features in both N and Z as a translation of Arabic ضماد (poultice/ cataplasm) (MA 9: 33, 77, 91, 115; 10: 5; 15: 2, 52; 19: 17).

תער = Latin novacula 'a sharp knife'; cf. fol. 40a (H 112, ll. 4–7): ואם החולה לא יסבול חתוך הבשר המעופש בתער אז תעשה זולתי החתוך של הפתוח עד העומק (if the patient cannot tolerate cutting away the putrid flesh with a knife, one should only open [the ulcer] by making a deep incision). Hebrew תער is not attested in a medical context in the current dictionaries; cf. KB 1771; BM 7840; S.

תפירה = Latin ligatura 'suture'; cf. fol. 10b (H 21, ll. 13.15): אבל אם המכה תהיה כל כך גדולה שלא תוכל לאסוף החלקים הנפרדים אז צריך לך התפירה (but if the wound is that large that one cannot join the separated parts, then suture is necessary). The Hebrew term תפירה is only attested in this sense as modern in AD 158. See as well S.

II. Hebrew transcriptions of Latin terms

אדרופיקי = Latin ydropici 'dropsy patients'; cf. fol. 32b (H 90, ll. 12–14): לכן כבדה רפואת האדרופיקי אשר לחותם עודפת והיא לחות זרה (And therefore the cure of dropsy patients is difficult because of their superfluous, external moisture). The Arabic parallel to Latin ydropici , i.e. مستسقين is translated by N as בעלי השקוי and by Z as בעלי ההדרוקן (MA 22: 24).

ווירוס = Latin virus 'poisonous liquid'; cf. fol. 30b (H 84, l. 20–85, ll. 1–2): עוד אמר שאותן שהן מעפוש דק נקראות וורוס ומעפוש עב נקראות שורדיציאיש (He further said that the putrid substance that is thin is called 'virus' and the putrid substance that is thick is called 'sordities').

וינטוסי = Latin ventose 'cupping glasses'; cf. fol. 19a (H 50, ll. 12–15): ואם הרצוץ יהיה עמוק והדם קפוי או אין ההקזה מספקת ואז צריך הוינטוסי עם שריטה והעלוקות (If the contusion is deep and the blood has congealed and if bleeding is not sufficient, one should [apply] cupping glasses with incision and also leeches); cf. ונטוזא in CN 157. The Arabic parallel to Latin 'ventose', namely محاجم is translated by N as קרני המציצה and by Z as כוסות (MA 3: 85, 106; 12: 37, 46; 16: 11, 12).

זיפק = Latin syphac/siphac (= Arab. صفاق) 'peritoneum' (FA no. 3031, HA 221–4); cf. fol. 13b (H 32, l. 4–6): וכשתשיב המעים מבפנים תאחוז החבלה באצבעותיך והזיפק יתפור ככתוב (Once you have returned the intestines [to their position] take hold of the wound with your fingers and suture the peritoneum as I have written before). N and Z transcribe the Arabic صفاق as ציפאק, but also translate it, a.o., as קרום (cf. MA 1: 44; 7: 65; 9: 90; 15: 36; 23: 24, 25, 75; 24: 34; 25: 2).

זירבו = Latin zirbus 'omentum' (HA 247–50); cf. fol. 12b (H 30, l. 1): שער הרביעי להשיב המעים והזירבו (Chapter 4: On returning the intestines and the omentum [to their place]). The parallel Arabic term ثرب is translated by both N and Z as חלב (MA 1: 54, 55, 60; 9: 102), while Shem Tov Ben Isaac has החלב המכסה את הקרב (cf. S); cf. MD 522: פדר (= AD 113).

טיסיס = Latin ptisis 'phthisis'; cf. fol. 18a (H 10, ll. 10–15): ואני אומר שחבלת הריאה תילקח על שני פנים או מעילה[94] חיצונית או מעילה פנימית. הפנימית נקראה טיסיס ואינה מקבלת רפואה (I say that a wound in the lungs can [happen] in two ways,

94 מעילה: editor emendation מעילת O מעילות P.

either through an external cause or through an internal one. The internal [cause] is called phtisis and this one cannot be cured). A similar transcription, namely טיציש or טישיש features in Z's translation of the Arabic term for phtisis, i.e. سلّ, while N has Hebrew שדפון or a combined transcription of both the Arabic and Latin term: הסל הוא טישי (MA 6: 51; 8: 58; 22: 44, 70; 23: 17).

טנטא = Latin 'tenta' probe; cf. fol. 29a (H 80, ll. 8–10): וצריך שתשים עוד הטנטא בחבלה למען תכיר בעבור הדרך שלקח לו החץ (You should also put the probe into the wound in order to explore the path of the arrow [into the body]). See entry כלי הממשש above.

טשטי (= Ital. tessuti) = Latin licinia 'lints' (for dressing wounds); cf. fol. 14b (H 36, l. 11); 27b (H 77, ll. 5–7): ויזרה מזה במספיק על המכה ויבלול הטשטי באבק זה בעבור שזה האבק מופלא (Strew a sufficient amount of this [medicine] on the wound and cover the lints with this powder because it is a wonderful powder).

לצרטי = Latin lacerti, plural of lacertus 'upper arm, arm'; cf. fol. 18b (H 48, ll. 13–14): והחבלות הבאות בקצווי הלצרטי (The wounds occurring to the extremities of the arms). Both N and Z translate the Arabic parallel to Latin lacertus, i.e. عضد as זרוע (MA 15: 62).

מוסקולו = Latin musculi 'muscles'; cf. fol. 18b (H 48, ll. 18–19): ודע כי אמרו גלינו ואלמנסור כי המוסקולו הם מורכבים מבשר וגידים ומקשרים (Know that Galen and Almansor (= al-Rāzī, author of the *K. al-Mansūrī*) said that the muscles are composed of flesh, nerves and ligaments). The Arabic parallel to Latin musculi, namely عضلات is translated by N as עצלים and by Z as מושקולי (MA 16: 15).

מירק = Latin mirac, mirach (= Arab. مراقّ) (FA no. 2077; HA 177–81) 'abdominal wall, abdomen'; cf. fol. 13b (H 32, ll. 6–10): והטוב בתפירתו הוא כמו שלמדנו גלינו בספר תחבולות הבריאות שאמ' היה כונתך בשברון הבטן שהזיפק תתפור בתפירה מדבקת עם המירק (The best way to suture [the wound] is that which Galen taught us in the book *De methodo medendi* where he said: In the case of an abdominal rupture take care to suture the peritoneum with the abdominal wall).

פישטולא = Latin fistula 'fistula'; cf. fol. 15a (H 37, ll. 12–16): ואם תתאחר רפואת החבלה בעניינים האלה אז תדע כמו שאמר אלבוקשין שכבר נעשה שם פישטולא והיא מכת הכבידות להרפא (But if this wound takes a long time to heal with these ingredients, know that, as Abulcasis said, a fistula will develop in that spot, and this is an affliction that is hard to cure). פישטולא also features in Z as a translation of Arabic ناصور 'fistula', while N transcribes the Arabic term as נאצור (MA 15: 29, 44).

ריאומה = Latin reuma 'catarrh, rheum' (BP 70); cf. fol. 45a (H 38, ll. 9–11): עוד בעבור שכל כאב מקבץ הריאומה ששם נעשה הנפח והצמח שבעבורם יבוא הקווץ אל נקלה (Moreover, every pain concentrates[95] the rheum from which tumours or [other] morbid growths originate which easily lead to cramps). The Arabic parallel term to Latin 'reuma', i.e. نظلة is translated by N as נזילה/ נזל/ נזלים and Z as נזילה/ נזל/ קטרא (MA 3: 66; 6: 41; 8: 38; 9: 7; 13: 13; 16: 30). Plural نظلات is translated as הזלות הראש by S (cf. S). See as well צמח above.

III. Mixed terms

זפת גריקא = Latin colophonia, id est pix Greca 'colophonia, i.e. Greek pitch (= resin)', so called because it was allegedly imported from Ionic Colophon; cf. DT 1: 31, n. 4; GA 175; cf. fol. 24b (H 67, ll. 2–3).

טירה חתומה = Latin terra sigillata 'sigillate earth'; cf. fol. 15a (H 37, l. 4). The term is a combination of the Hebrew transcription of Latin terra (earth) with Hebrew חתום (sealed). Moses Ibn Tibbon's equivalent for the parallel Arabic term الطين المختوم is הטין החתום, i.e. a combination of the Hebrew transcription of Arabic *ṭīn* with Hebrew חתום (BMP 19). In Shem Tov Ben Isaac's glossary we find the Arabic term translated as טיט חתום (SG, Ṭet 1). Terra sigillata, i.e. 'sealed earth or clay', was so called because the pastilles prepared from these kinds of earth or clay were marked with a seal.

קמח אורובי = Latin farina orobi 'meal of bitter vetch'; cf. fol. 24b (H 67, l. 6). The term consists of the Hebrew קמח, i.e. meal and the Latin orobi, Sing. Gen. of orobus, from Greek ὄροβος i.e. bitter vetch (Vicia ervilia Willd.); cf. AL 182.

---

95 'concentrates': exacuit L, i.e. makes sharp.

קמח לופיני = Latin farina lupinorum 'meal of lupines'; cf. fol. 24b (H 67, l. 6). The term consists of the Hebrew קמח, i.e. meal and the Latin lupini, Sing. Gen. of lupinus, i.e. lupine; for its different varieties see AL 148; R 379.

2. Moses Ibn Tibbon, *Sefer Ẓedat ha-Derakhim*

Introduction

Moses Ben Samuel Ben Judah Ibn Tibbon (fl. 1244–83) was the grandson of Judah Ben Saul Ibn Tibbon (*c.* 1120–90), called the 'father of translators', who was born in Granada, but — because of the Almohad persecutions — fled to southern France. There he settled in Lunel and was active as a physician, merchant and translator. His son Samuel Ben Judah Ibn Tibbon (*c.* 1165–1232), the father of Moses Ben Samuel Ibn Tibbon, was born in Lunel but subsequently lived in Marseilles where he was, just like his father, active as a physician, merchant and translator. As a translator he is foremost known for his translation of Maimonides' *The Guide of the Perplexed.*

Moses Ben Samuel Ibn Tibbon lived in Marseilles approximately until the year 1252 and moved to Montpellier some time between 1252 and 1254, but also spent some years in Naples with his brother-in-law Jacob Anatoli.[96] Moses was a prolific translator; however, to what extent he was able to earn a living from his translation activities is uncertain. Steinschneider remarks that it is very probable that the art of translation involved a certain remuneration.[97] However, he admits at the same time that no references to concrete payments have been found. Freudenthal remarks that we do not know much of the economic aspects of the translation activity, but that it seems that the translators were not paid for their labours.[98] According to Halkin, translators who were requested by a patron to translate a certain work presumably received some payment from their patrons.[99] In addition to being a translator, it seems reasonable to assume that Moses Ibn Tibbon was trained as a physician in the light of the large number of medical treatises translated by him and in

96 Cf. J.T. Robinson and U. Melammed, entry 'Ibn Tibbon (Tibbonids)', *Encyclopaedia Judaica*[2] vol. 19 (Detroit 2007), 712–14, p. 712.

97 Steinschneider *Die hebräischen Übersetzungen*, p. XVII: 'Es ist sehr wahrscheinlich dass auch jene Kunst "nach Brot ging"'.

98 G. Freudenthal, *Science in the Medieval Hebrew and Arabic Traditions* (Ashgate 2005), 31.

99 A.S. Halkin, entry 'Translation and Translators', *Encyclopaedia Judaica*, 16 vols. (Jerusalem 1971), vol. 15, p. 1319; cf. O. Fraisse, *Moses Ibn Tibbons Kommentar zum Hohelied und sein poetologisch-philosophisches Programm*. Synoptische Edition, Übersetzung und Analyse (Studia Judaica. Forschungen zur Wissenschaft des Judentums Band XXV. Berlin-New York 2004), 35.

the light of the references to the medical profession in his own writings. For instance, in the *Sefer ha-Pe'ah* (a commentary on selected Rabbinic Aggadot) he remarks:

> כדרך הרופא הטוב כשיראה חולי רע ביד האדם או ברגלו או בזרועו או בשוקו ויפחד ממנו שיתפשט יחתכהו פן יפסיד הגוף וימיתהו לא שישנא האבר החולה אבל אוהב אותו תכלית האהבה
>
> (Just as a good doctor when he sees someone suffering from an evil disease in one of his hands, feet, arms or legs and fears that it might spread, and therefore amputates that limb so that it does not corrupt his body and kills him, does not hate the diseased bodily part but loves it dearly).[100]

Moses Ibn Tibbon was possibly one of several Jewish physicians active in Marseilles and subsequently in Montpellier in spite of the secular and ecclesiastical legislation in both France and Spain in the thirteenth century directed against Jewish medical practice.[101] According to Shatzmiller, Jewish doctors played an impressive role in the city of Marseilles. During the hundred years preceeding the Black Death, we find fifteen Jews in the profession.[102] As for Montpellier, the legislation concerning the Jews in general promulgated in 1267 by James I, king of Aragon and Majorca, who also ruled over the Duchy of Montpellier, was, according to Blumenkranz-Weinberg, fairly favorable. Especially noteworthy was the clause prohibiting their prosecution on the basis of an anonymous denunciation. Those who accused or denounced Jews were to provide two guarantors and were threatened with being condemned themselves if they could not prove their accusation. Bail was to be granted to the accused Jew if he could provide a satisfactory guarantee.[103] The city of Montpellier was also a centre for the teaching of medicine. William VII of Montpellier established a faculty of medicine in 1180, recognised by Pope Nicholas IV; the city's university was established in 1220.[104] However, we do not have any

---

100 Cf. Fraisse, *Moses Ibn Tibbons Kommentar zum Hohelied*, p. 34.

101 Cf. M. McVaugh, *Medicine before the plague. Practitioners and their patients in the Crown of Aragon, 1285–1345* (Cambridge 1993), 59.

102 J. Shatzmiller, *Jews, Medicine and Medieval Society* (Berkeley-Los Angeles-London 1994), 107.

103 Cf. B. Blumenkranz and D. Weinberg, entry 'Montpellier', *Encyclopaedia Judaica*^{2}, (Detroit 2007), vol. 14, 462–3.

104 Cf. V. Nutton, 'Medicine in Medieval Western Europe', in *The Western Medical Tradition. 800 BC to AD 1800* (Cambridge 1995), 153.

documentary evidence that Jews participated in the intellectual life of the medical faculty during the twelfth and thirteenth centuries.[105]

Moses Ibn Tibbon was a prolific translator producing translations both in the field of philosophy and natural sciences.[106] As for medicine, he translated the following works from the Arabic into Hebrew:

A. Dated Translations

1. Maimonides, *Fī tadbīr al-ṣihḥa* (On the Regimen of Health), translated in the year 1244 under the title מאמר בהנהגת הבריאות.[107]
2. Al-Rāzī, *al-Aqrābādin al-kabīr* (Antidotarium), translated in the year 1257 as אקראבדין.
3. Ibn al-Jazzār, *Zād al-musāfir wa-qūt al-ḥāḍir* (Provisions for the Traveller and the Nourishment for the Sedentary), translated in the year 1259 as צידת הדרכים.[108]
4. Ibn Sīnā, *al-Urjūza fī l-ṭibb* (Poem on Medicine with the commentary by Ibn Rushd), translated in the year 1260 as באור ארגוזה.[109]
5. Maimonides, *Šarḥ fuṣūl Abuqrāṭ* (Commentary on Hippocrates' Aphorisms), translated under the title פרקי אבוקראט in the year 1260.[110]
6. Ibn Sīnā, *K. al-Qānūn al-ṣaghīr* (Small Compendium of the Canon). This pseudepigraphical work that has been lost in the original Arabic and has no relationship to Ibn Sīnā's *Qānūn* whatsoever was translated in the year 1272 under the title הסדר הקטן.[111]

---

105 Cf. J. Shatzmiller, 'Etudiants juifs à la faculté de médecine de Montpellier, dernier quart du XIVe siècle', *Jewish History*, vol. 6, nos. 1–2, 243–55, p. 243.

106 For a survey of all his translations see Fraisse, *Moses Ibn Tibbons Kommentar zum Hohelied*, 40–3.

107 Cf. Maimonides, *On the Regimen of Health.* A New Parallel Arabic-English Translation by Gerrit Bos with Critical Editions of medieval Hebrew translations by Gerrit Bos and Latin translations by Michael R. McVaugh (forthcoming).

108 Cf. *Ibn al-Jazzār on Skin Diseases and Other Afflictions of the Outer Part of the Body.* A New Parallel Arabic-English translation of Bk. 7 chs. 7–30 with a Critical Edition of Moses Ibn Tibbon's Medieval Hebrew Translation by Gerrit Bos and a study of the Romance terminology by Guido Mensching and Julia Zwink (forthcoming). On Ibn al-Jazzār and his works see Gerrit Bos, *Ibn al-Jazzār on Sexual Diseases: A critical edition, English translation and introduction of* Zād al-musāfir wa-qūt al-ḥādir. Provisions for the Traveller and the Nourishment of the Settled. Book 6. The original Arabic text with an English translation, introduction and commentary. (London 1997), 8–11.

109 Cf. M. Kozodoy, 'To Sing the Body: Medieval Hebrew Medical Poetry in Context' (forthcoming: *Aleph*).

110 Cf. Maimonides, *Commentary on Hippocrates' Aphorisms.* A New Parallel Arabic-English Translation by Gerrit Bos with Critical Editions of medieval Hebrew translations (forthcoming).

111 Cf. Steinschneider, *Die hebräischen Übersetzungen*, 695–6.

7. Al-Rāzī, *K. al-taqsīm wa l-tašgīr* (Liber divisionum), translated in the year 1274 under the title ספר החילוק והחילוף.

B. Undated translations:

1. Maimonides, *K. al-sumūm wa l-taḥarruz min al-adwiya al-qattāla* (On Poisons and the Protection against Lethal Drugs), translated at an unknown date.[112]
2. Maimonides, *Fī l-bawāsīr* (On Hemorrhoids). The identification of Moses Ibn Tibbon as one of the translators of this treatise not featuring in Fraisse's list is based on the colophon in MS Moscow Guenzburg 462:

   נשלם המאמר הזה העתקת החכם הכולל ר' משה בן החכם הכולל ר' שמואל אבן תבון ברוך נותן לעיף כח ולאין אונים עצה ירבה ב"ה וב' שמו יתברך

   (This is the end of this treatise, translated by the erudite scholar Moses, the son of the erudite scholar Samuel ibn Tibbon, may He be blessed who gives strength to the tired and rich counsel to the weary).[113]

As I stated above, one of the goals of the Jewish translators' project is to give a description of the medical terminology characteristic for each of them to facilitate the identification of anonymous translations. In addition to the technical terminology peculiar to Moses Ibn Tibbon, his translations are characterised by a striking feature, namely that in several cases he gives the equivalent of the Arabic names of certain remedies or plants in Latin or Romance, often Occitan. In other cases he adds an explanatory note to these terms possibly out of fear for a confusion.

Some examples of Romance equivalents gleaned from his translation of Maimonides' *K. al-sumūm* are[114]:

1. إيرسا وهو أصل السوسن الأسمانجوني : אירסא והוא שורש אל סוסן אל אסמנגוני ונק' גלביול

   גלביול is the is the O.Occ. glaujol (< Lat. GLADIOLUS) for 'gladiolus'.[115]

---

112 Cf. Maimonides, *On Poisons* (ed. Bos-McVaugh).

113 The ascription of this translation to Moses Ibn Tibbon confirms Zotenberg's conjecture that the anonymous translator of Maimonides' *On Hemorrhoids* as featuring in MS Paris héb BN 1173, 3 is identical with Moses Ibn Tibbon, the translator of the next treatise in the same MS, namely Maimonides' *On Poisons* (cf. Zotenberg, H. (ed.), *Catalogues des Manuscrits hébreux et samaritains*. At the same time this explicit ascription refutes Steinschneider's rejection of Zotenberg's conjecture. (cf. Steinschneider, *Die hebräischen Übersetzungen*, 763). Cf. Maimonides, *On Hemorrhoids* (ed. Bos-McVaugh).

114 Cf. Maimonides, *On Poisons* (ed. Bos-McVaugh), 27–8. For the interpretation of the meaning of the Romance terms I thank my colleagues Guido Mensching and Julia Zwink at the Freie Universität, Berlin.

2. הורג אביו שנקרא בלעז מטרונה: قاتـــل أبيـــه

   מטרונה is possibly a transcription of Romance *maṭronyo* (= *madroño*).[116]

3. הבנג' הוא הקניליידה.

   הקנילייאדה is the O.Occ. *canelhada* or *canilhada* for Hyoscyamus.[117]

4. הטחלב הוא לינטילייש דבלאט.

   The compound vernacular term לינטילייש דבלאט could not be found in our sources, but should be read as O.Occ. *lentilhes de blat*, literally 'lentils of wheat'. The first element is the O.Occ. plural *lentilhes* for 'lentils', documented for example in Corradini Bozzi's *Ricettari medicao-farmaceutici medievali*.[118] The second element is the O.Occ. *blat* for 'wheat'.[119]

5. חוקן הוא קלישתירי.

   The vernacular term קלישתירי is the O.Occ. *clisteri* for 'clysters'.[120]

The following examples hail from his translation of Ibn al-Jazzār, *Zād al-musāfir wa-qūt al-ḥāḍir*:

1. אויל ('WYL") (29.1): 'WYL might represent the O. Occ. form *uelh* (variant of *olh*, *ulh*, 'eye'),[121] but here it takes the meaning of 'corn, clavus'. In Mod. Occ., this kind of callus at the toes or fingers is called *oelh pegui*.[122]
2. איפורבי ('YPRBY) (18.7): 'YPRBY is O. Occ. *eforbi*, a variant of the more common *euforbi*, 'spurge (Euphorbia amygdaloides)' (< Lat. EUPHORBIA).[123]
3. לאורייר (L'WRYYR) (11.7): L'WRYYR matches the O. Occ. *laurier*, 'laurel, laurel tree (Laurus nobilis L.)'[124] (FEW 5:208b) or *laureir* (DAO l.c.). Ibn Tibbon's term is obviously

---

115 Cf. W. von Wartburg, *Französisches Etymologisches Wörterbuch* (Bonn, Leipzig, Tübingen, Basilea), 1922 ff., 4:143a–b.

116 Cf. Miguel Asín Palacios, *Glosario de Voces Romances registradas por un botánico anónimo Hispano-Musulmán* (siglos XI–XII). Edición facsímile. Introducción de V. Martínez Tejero (Zaragoza 1994), nos 340 and 430.

117 Cf. K. Baldinger (ed.), *Dictionnaire onomasiologique de l'ancien occitan*, 10- fasc. (Tübingen 1975–), 7:522.

118 Cf. M.S. Corradini Bozzi, *Ricettari medico-farmaceutici medievali nella Francia meridionale* (Florence 1997), 300, line 9.

119 Baldinger (ed.), *Dictionnaire onomasiologique*, 5:376.

120 Cf. F.J. Reynouard, *Lexique: Ou dictionnaire de la langue des troubadours comparée avec les autres langues de l'Europe latine* (1836–45. Repr. Heidelberg 1960), 1:417b.

121 Cf. von Wartburg, *Französisches Etymologisches Wörterbuch*, 7:310a.

122 Cf. von Wartburg, *Französisches Etymologisches Wörterbuch*, 7:319b.

123 Cf. von Wartburg, *Französisches Etymologisches Wörterbuch*, 3:249b; Corradini Bozzi, *Ricettari medico-farmaceutici medievali*, 305.

124 Cf. von Wartburg, *Französisches Etymologisches Wörterbuch*, 5:208b.

the diphthongised variant, which existed in O. Occ. besides *laurer/ laurel* and simple *laur.*[125]

4. פניגריג (PNYGRYG) (15.7; 27.5) or פנגריג (PNGRYG) (30.2): The Romance term for 'fenugreek' (Trigonella foenum graecum L.) appears in two variants in Ibn Tibbon's translation: PNGRYG, i.e. O. Occ. *fengrec*,[126] and a variant with an epenthetic vowel, PNYGRYG, which corresponds to O. Occ./ O. Cat. *fenigrec*[127] or O. Occ. *finigrec*.[128] The final -c of the Occ. and Cat. word is the result of a final devoicing rule in these languages (GRAECUM > *grego > greg > grec). In the Hebrew spelling of O.Occ. words this devoicing is often not reflected and the voiced consonants are used instead.[129]

The following explanatory notes feature in his translation of Ibn al-Jazzār, *Zād al-musāfir wa-qūt al-ḥādir*:

1. مغاث (*moghat*)[130] (ch. 25:5), i.e. the root of Clossostemon Bruguieri D.C.: ומעאד הוא שרשי אילן הרמונים ויש אומרים שהוא שורש הפלפל ועושין ממנו דבק (M''D, i.e. the root of the pomegranate tree, and according to some it is the root of the pepper [bush], from which glue is prepared).
2. حصف (heat-spots) (24.0): חצף הוא הצפניתא הוא חמרמרות העור וברידלוש (*ḥaṣaf*), i.e. heat-spots: it is *ḥazpanita*,[131] that is redness of the skin WBRYDLWŠ.
3. كشمش (seedless raisins [currants]) (18.6): כשמאש שהוא צמוקים קטנים שאין להם גרעינים *kišmiš*, i.e small raisins that have no seeds).

125 Ibid.

126 Cf. von Wartburg, *Französisches Etymologisches Wörterbuch*, 3:461b.

127 Cf. A.M. Alcover and F. de B. Moll, *Diccionari català-valencià-balear*[2], 10 vols (Palma de Mallorca 1980–5), 5:795a.

128 Cf. C. Brunel, 'Recettes médicales d'Avignon en ancien provençal', in *Romania* LXXX (1959), 145–90, p. 164.

129 Cf. C. Aslanov, *Le Provençal des Juifs et l'Hébreu en Provence: Le dictionnaire Šaršot ha-Kesef de Joseph Caspi* (Paris-Louvain 2001), and Introduction to *Sefer ha-Šimmuš, bk. 29, Shem Tov Ben Isaac medical synonyms (list 1)*, ed. by G. Bos and G. Mensching in collaboration with F. Savelsberg and M. Hussein (forthcoming).

130 The identification of *mughādh* as *moghat* is the result of modern research, undertaken by Schweinfurth. In medieval Arabic medical literature the term is erroneously used for the bark of the root of the wild pomegranate tree; cf. A. Dietrich, *Dioscurides Triumphans. Ein anonymer arabischer Kommentar (Ende 12. Jahr. n. Chr.) zur Materia medica.* Arabischer Text nebst kommentierter deutscher Übersetzung hrsg. (Abh. der Akad. der Wiss. in Göttingen, Phil. Hist. Klasse, Dritte Folge, Nr. 172). I–II (Göttingen 1988), 1:82, n. 2. For the term *moghat* cf. EL S. Amin, Olfat Awad, M. Abd El Samad and M.N. Iskander, 'Isolation of estrone from moghat roots and from pollen grains of Egyptian date palm', *Phytochemistry* 8, (1969), 295–7.

131 Cf. M. Sokoloff, *A Dictionary of Jewish Babylonian Aramaic of the Talmudic and Geonic Periods* (Ramat Gan 2002), 441, s.v. חוספניתא: 'a skin disease'.

4. ورس (*wars*)[132] (24.2): ורס והוא זרע כמו זרע שומשמין (*wars*, it is a seed similar to the sesame seed).

Study of the technical terminology employed by Moses Ibn Tibbon in his translation of Ibn al-Jazzār, Zād al-musāfir, Bk. 7, Chs 7–30

The following study of the technical terminology employed by Moses Ibn Tibbon is based on my forthcoming critical edition mentioned above. Every Hebrew entry is followed by: a) the Arabic equivalent as it features in Ibn al-Jazzār's text, b) an attestation from Moses Ibn Tibbon's translation; c) the English translation. In addition to the analysis of the terminology employed by Moses Ibn Tibbon, I shall refer to parallel terms gleaned from the following texts: 1) the Hebrew translations of Maimonides' *Medical Aphorisms* by Zeraḥyah Ben Isaac Ben She'altiel Ḥen and Nathan ha-Me'ati;[133] 2) Shem Tov Ben Isaac, *Sefer ha-Shimmush*, bks. 29 and 30; 3) Hillel Ben Samuel of Verona, *Sefer Keritut*. The list has been arranged alphabetically and consists of a major section of technical terms followed by a minor section of materia medica.

List of Terms

בלל = Arab. بَلّ 'to moisten'; cf. 26.5: תאר אבק לסוקרא או למי שהוכה בסיף או סכין או במקל: יקח אלובי ומירא ואמוניאק וסרקא קולא מ"א אוקיא וירדיט וסוכר קשה מ"א שני שקלים יודק היטב וימלא בו הנגע או הסוקרא ואחר כן יבלול חתיכת בגד דק ברוק ויושם עליו (A powder beneficial for a head wound or for someone struck by a sword, stabbed by a knife or beaten by a stick: Take one ounce each of aloe, myrrh, gum ammoniac and sarcocol, two *mithqāl*s[134] each of verdigris and *ṭabarzad*[135] sugar. Pound [these ingredients] well, then fill up the wound or

---

132 'wars'; Traditionally it is thought to be a red colouring material derived from Memecylon tinctorium WILLD.; it was recently discovered to be the product of Flemmingia rhodocarpa BAK. The term is also used for the biliary calculus of cattle in Marocco; cf. F. Rosner, *Moses Maimonides' Glossary of Drug Names*. Translated and annotated from M. Meyerhof's French edition (Maimonides' Medical Writings 7, Haifa 1995), no. 123.

133 Critical editions of both translations are forthcoming in the series: 'The Medical Works of Maimonides', published by Brigham Young University Press.

134 One *mithqāl* is 4.46 grams; cf. O. Kahl, Sābūr ibn Sahl, *Dispensatorium Parvum* (al-Aqrābādhīn al-saghīr), analysed, edited and annotated. (Leiden-New York-Köln 1994), 228.

135 '*ṭabarzad* sugar'; according to Maimonides, *Sharḥ asmā' al-'uqqār,* trans. F. Rosner: *Moses Maimonides' Glossary of Drug Names* (Haifa 1995), no. 289, it is solid hard sugar which is

the head wound with it, then moisten a piece of fine cloth with saliva and put it on [the wound]). Hebrew בלל does not feature in this sense in the current dictionaries. N translates the Arab. بلّ as בלל and טבל and Z as טבל (MA 4.41; 8.35; 9.99; 21.93).

ברזל = I. Arab. مبضع 'scalpel'; cf. 13.3: ואם היה צר הנה ראוי שנפתח שפתיו בברזל ונרחיב ראשו ונשרוט סביב הנגע שריטות גדולות כדי שיצא הדם יציאה רבה או יכוה המקום באש כי היא תעצור ותעכב הארס ממרוצת הגרתו וימנענו מהכנס תוך הגוף (When [the wound] is narrow, we should [cut] open its edges with a scalpel, widen its upper part, make a deep incision around the wound so that much blood will stream forth and cauterize the spot because this will prevent the poison from streaming and penetrating into the interior of the body). Hebrew ברזל does not feature in this sense in the current dictionaries. The common term for 'scalpel' is אזמל (cf. MD 642, Low XXXVI). Shem Tov translates the Arab. مبضع as מסמר הגרע (cf. S); II. Arab. حديدة 'scalpel'; cf. 16.3: ואם סרו במה שזכרנו טוב ואם לא יעקרם בברזל או בכויה ויכוה בקני הדס כמו שאמר אפלטון (If they disappear through the mentioned [remedies] fine, but if not, remove them with a scalpel or with the fingers[136] and cauterize [the spot] with myrtle branches, as Plato stated).

גיד: הגיד האמצעי = Arab. الأكحل 'the median cubital vein'; cf. 17.3: ואם ראינו שהדם הוא הגובר נצוה להקיז הגיד האמצעי אם לא ימנע ממנו מונע ויצא הדם כל זמן שהתמיד לצאת נפסד והכח סובל אותו (If we see that the blood is the dominant [humour], we order to bleed from the median cubital vein, if there is no hindrance from [doing so]. We let the blood flow as long as it is corrupt and as long as the strength [of the patient] endures it). Hebrew הגיד האמצעי does not feature in the current dictionaries. N transcribes Arab. أكحل as אכחל while Z has הגיד הנקרא אכחל והוא האמצעי/ גיד האלאכחל והוא הגיד האמצעי שיבוא מהגוף כולו/ הגיד הנקרא אכחל/ האמצעי הנק' אכחל/ גיד האכחל (MA 10.64; 12.23,33,40); For the different meanings of גיד cf. Shem Tov.

---

the same as that which is called by the Egyptians 'sukkar al-nabāt' (sugar candy). See as well *The Encyclopaedia of Islam*, New ed. (Leiden and London 1960ff.), vol. 9, 804b–805a, s.v. 'sukkar' (D. Waines) who remarks that *sukkar ṭabarzad* is probably that which is set hard in moulds, while *nabāt* is set on palm sticks placed in the recipient where it was being prepared.

136 'with the fingers': translated after the Arabic بالإصبع.

הקעה = Arab. خَلْع 'dislocation'; cf. 15.1: הנה כל מורסא תתחדש מהגרת ליחה אל אבר מהאברים וסבות ההגרה מהם מתחילות באות מחוץ ומהם קודמות פנימיות והמתחילות כמו הכאה או נגע או ריצוץ או הקעה או שבר או סדק (Every tumour arises from the streaming of matter to some part of the body. The causes of the streaming [of matter] are partly evident,[137] [namely] external, and partly hidden,[138] [namely] internal. Examples of evident[139] [causes] are a blow, wound, contusion, dislocation, fracture or bruise[140]). Hebrew הקעה in the sense of 'dislocation' features in BM 1173 in an attestation from Nathan ha-Me'ati's translation of Ibn Sīnā's *K. al-Qānūn* prepared in Rome in 1279. N translates Arabic خَلْع as שמט, Z as השמטה (MA 15.46), and S as שמיטה. This last term also features in Moses Ibn Tibbon's חרוזי אבן סינא (BM 7238), i.e. the Hebrew translation of Ibn Sīnā's *'Urǧuza fī al-ṭibb* which Moses Ibn Tibbon prepared in the year 1260.[141] Hillel translates the Latin parallel 'dislocatio' as השמטה.

התלהבות = Arab. التهاب 'inflammation'; cf. 12.1: אולם הצרעה והדבורים הנה ארסם חם חד ובעבור זה יקרה ממנו כאב חזק והתלהבות ונקודות קטנות שחורות (The poison of wasps and bees is hot and sharp. For this reason it causes a severe pain, inflammation and small black dots). Hebrew התלהבות in the sense of 'inflammation' is a non-attested semantic borrowing from Arab. التهاب. Shem Tov translates Arab. التهاب, just like Moses Ibn Tibbon, as התלהבות (cf. S).

התרה = Arab. استطلاق 'diarrhoea'; cf. 8.5: וכאשר עברו על החולה שבעה ימים ראוי לו להזהר ממה שירכך הטבע כלל כי ההתרה מדרכה לבוא בקדחת הזאת מעצמה ויטה ההנהגה אל מה שיעצור הטבע (When the patient has been ill for seven days, he should be cautious not to take any laxative under any circumstance, because diarrhoea has the property to occur spontaneously during the fever [accompanying this disease]. He should tend in his regimen to astringent [foodstuff]). Hebrew התרה does not feature in this sense in the current dictionaries. Arab. استطلاق is translated by N as שלשול and by Z as התרת הבטן (MA 7.42).

חי: יין חי = Arab. شراب صرف 'unmixed wine'; cf. 11.1: או יקח שרש זעפראן גנים הוא אלקרטם או פריו או עלהו ויכתשהו עם מעט פלפל וישתהו ביין חי (Or take the root, fruit

---

137 'evident': translated after the Arabic بادية.

138 'hidden': translated after the Arabic باطنة.

139 'evident': translated after the Arabic بادية.

140 'bruise' = Arab. وثء. Cf. entry רסוק below.

141 Cf. M. Steinschneider, *Die hebräischen übersetzungen des Mittelalters und die Juden als Dolmetscher* (Berlin 1893, repr. Graz 1956), 699.

or leaves of wild safflower (*Carthamus lanatus*), pound it with some pepper and let him drink it with unmixed wine). Hebrew יין חי is only attested for Rabbinic literature in the sense of 'unmixed wine'; cf. JD 450. N translates Arab. الشراب الصرف as היין החי and Z as היין החי and היין בלתי מזוג (MA 19.24).

חולי האריה :חלי = Arab. داء الأسد 'leontiasis'; cf. 17.1: והוא מתחלק לארבעה חלקים אחד מהם המתילד מן הדם ויקרא חולי השועל הנקרא אלופיציא והשני המתילד מליחת מרה כרכומית ויקרא חולי האריה הנקרא לאוניאה והשלישי המתילד מליחה מרה שחורה ויקרא חולי הפיל והרביעי מתילד מליחת הליחה הלבנה ויקרא חולי הנחש. [Leprosy] consists of four varieties; the first [variety] originates from blood and is called 'alopecia'; the second originates from the humour of yellow bile and is called 'leontiasis'; the third originates from the humour of black bile and is called 'elephantiasis'; the fourth originates from the humour of phlegm and is called 'ophiasis'. The Hebrew term is a non-attested loan-translation of the Arabic داء الأسد.

חולי הנחש:- = Arab. داء الحية 'ophiasis'; cf. previous entry. Hebrew חולי הנחש, a loan-translation of Arabic داء الحية is quoted in BM 1868, a.o. in an attestation from Nathan's Hebrew translation of Maimonides' *Medical Aphorisms*, where Z has סרפין בעברי חלי הנחש (MA 23.53).

חולי הפיל:- = Arab. داء الفيل 'elephantiasis'; cf. entry חלי: חולי האריה. Hebrew חולי הפיל, a loan-translation of Arabic داء الفيل is quoted in BM 1868, a.o. in an attestation from pseudo Abraham Ibn Ezra, *Sefer ha-Nisyonot* (cf. ed. J.O. Leibowitz and S.Marcus [Jerusalem 1984], 276).

חולי השועל:- = Arab. داء الثعلب 'alopecia'; cf. entry חלי: חולי האריה. Hebrew חולי השועל, a loan-translation of Arabic داء الثعلب features in BM 1573 in an attestation from Maimonides' commentary on *Mishnah Nega'im* 12.5. The term also features in N and Z (MA 22.2; 23.53).

חמרמרות = Arab. سحج 'abrasion'; cf. 29.1: ואם יהיה החמרמרות מבלתי נפח ומורסא יקח מן התחתון מן המנעל וישרפהו וישחקהו ויזרהו על החמרמרות (If [the pressure of the shoe] causes an abrasion that is not accompanied by an inflammation, one should take the old, worn-out part (Arab. الخلقة) from the bottom of the shoe, burn and pulverize it and sprinkle it on the abrasion). Hebrew חמרמרות features in BM 1639 in an attestation from Meir Aldabi's *Shevilei Emunah* which he completed in 1360. The verb سحج 'to abrade' is translated by N as הפשיט and by Z as הוליד פונט (MA 6.90).

חספניתא = Arab. حصف 'heat-spots'; cf. 24.3: והחספניתא אמנם תצא בקיץ כשיתחזק החום עם רוב הזיעה והיותו מחומר ידמה המותר אשר מדרכו שיתך בכל יום מן הגופות וכאשר יתעבה יום אחר יום על נשומי הגוף ונקבי העור יסתמם ויהיה עליו כגלד והקלפה ולכלוך ויביא זה לחספניתא ואל כנים וחכוך ואם יארך זה ישוב גרב גמור (Heat-spots break out in the summer when it gets very hot and one sweats severely. It originates from matter that is similar to the superfluity that has the property to be dissolved from the body every day, and if it becomes thicker day after day on the skin and pores of the body, it closes it off and turns into something similar to dirt, scab and filth from which heat-spots, lice, and pruritus develop. If it becomes chronic, it turns into inveterate mange). Aram. חספניתא is only attested for Rabbinic literature in the sense of 1) scaly skin, 2) scab, eruption (JD 489) or of 'a skin disease' (SDA 441, s.v. חוספניתא/חולפניתא/חספנותא). See as well Low LII: 'a drying of the skin'.

חפיפה = Arab. غمز 'massage'; cf. 14.1: ותהיה החפיפה לאלו האברים באלו השמנים בנחת ומצוע ויכנסו במרחץ ממוצע החום (The application of massage with these oils to [the affected] parts of the body should be soft and moderate and [the patient] should take a bath of moderate heat). Hebrew חפיפה features in Rabbinical literature in the sense of 'cleansing the head' (JD 491). As 'massage' it features in BM 1686 in an attestation from Nathan ha-Me'ati's translation of Ibn Sīnā's *K. al-Qānūn*.

חִתּוּם = Arab. إلحام 'growing together' (of fractured parts); cf. 25.2: ואחר כך נכון בסוף להולדת החתום (And in the end one should seek [a regimen] that makes [the fractured parts] grow together [again]). Hebrew חִתּוּם does not feature in this sense in the current dictionaries.

חתם: החתים = I. Arab. ألحم 'to close up'; cf. 25.1: וכאשר הותרו החתולים והקשרים ביום השביעי או קרוב ממנו תעיין בו ואם ראית האבר בריא מן הנפח או ראית אותו קטן ממה שהיה לפנים בעת בריאותו שים כונתך להחתים העצם ושים עליו המחתימים כדי שיצמח הבשר אשר יתחתם בו ויקשרהו (If you loosen the bandage on the seventh day or the like, you should check: if you see the limb free from swelling or that it is thinner than normal, then seek to close up the bone and put splints on it so that the flesh will grow by which it will be closed up and put a bandage on it). Hebrew החתים does not feature in this sense in the current dictionaries. In the Bible (Lev. 15:13) we find: החתים בשרו מזובו (to have an obstruction in the penis [KB 364]). N translates the Arab. ألحم as הדביק and Z as עשה מה שיעלה בשר

(MA15.17); II. Arab. جبر 'to mend, set'; cf. 25.5: ומזה תאר טיחה מחתימה העצמות והפרקים (Composition of a salve that mends [broken] bones and joints). Hebrew החתים does not feature in this sense in the current dictionaries. N translates Arab. جبر as חבש and Z as דיבק (MA 15.67). See as well entry מחתים.

-: **התחתם**= I. Arab. التحم 'to be closed up'; cf. entry חתם: החתים. Hebrew התחתם does not feature in this sense in the current dictionaries. N translates Arab. التحم as דבק or התדבק and Z as עלה בשר/ העלה בשר or התרקם (בשר) (MA 15.46,56,62; 25.17). II. Arab. جُبِّرَ 'to be mended'; cf. 25.2: וזה כי מזון מימי אי אפשר שיתילד ממנו בשר אשר יתחתם בו העצם אבל במזון עב אשר אין בו דבקות (For watery food cannot produce such a growing[142] together by which the [broken] bone is mended, but fat food that is not viscous [can do so]). Hebrew התחתם does not feature in this sense in the current dictionaries. N translates Arab. جبر I 'to set' as חבש and Z as דיבק (MA 15.67). Shem Tov translates Arab. انجبر as התחבש (cf. S).

טיחה = I. Arab. لطوخ 'salve'; cf. 16.3: והנה יעשו מן המירא וקשיא ליניאה ודבש טיחות ליבלות (One may also apply myrrh, cinnamon and honey as a salve on the warts); II. = Arab, طلاء 'liniment'; cf. 18.3: וכאשר עשינו בנקוי הגוף והוצאת החומר הנפסד ממנו נשוב אל הטיחות מחוץ (Once we have effected the cleansing of the body and expelled the corrupt matter from it, we turn to [the application of] liniments on the outside). Hebrew טיחה is quoted by BM 1868 in an attestation from the *Qibbuẓei Galenus*, the Hebrew translation of a summary of Galenic works by Shimshon Ben Shlomo in 1322. Just like Moses Ibn Tibbon Shem Tov Ben Isaac uses טיחה both for Arab. لطوخ and Arab. طلاء 'liniment' (cf. SG Tet 6).

יציאה: יציאות = Arab. خراجات 'abscesses'; cf. 23.2: פתילות ליציאות ולחזירים ואלרישה ([A compress[143] beneficial] for an abscess, scrofula and lacrymal fistula). Hebrew יציאה in the sense of 'abscess' features in BM 2120, a.o. in an attestation from Nathan ha-Me'ati's translation of Ibn Sīnā's *K. al-Qānūn*. The term recurs in Nathan's translation of Maimonides' *Medical Aphorisms*, in addition to מורסא and נגע, while Z has יציאה and צמח (MA passim).

---

142 'growing together': translated after the Arabic الحام.

143 '[compress]': The corresponding Arabic term فتائل has the general meaning of 'suppositories'.

כלב: כלב שוטה = Arab. الكَلْب الكَلِب 'a mad dog'; cf. 13.1: והטובה שבראיות והאותות עליו גם כן לקחת פת לחם ולמשוח אותה מן הדם היוצא מן המקום הנשוך ואחר כן ישליכנה לכלבים ואם לא יאכלוה ידע כי הנשיכה נשיכת כלב שוטה ואם יאכלוה ידע כי הכלב אשר נשכו משאר הכלבים (One of the most genuine symptoms [to recognize a mad dog] is also that if you take a piece of bread and smear some of the blood that dripped out of the spot that was bitten on it and then throw it to a [healthy] dog, if it does not eat it, we know that the bite is that of a mad dog, but if [the healthy dog] eats it, we know that the bite is that of another dog [that is not mad]). Hebrew כלב שוטה is only attested for Rabbinic literature; cf. EM 1790; BM 2370.

מדביק = Arab. لصوق 'a sticking plaster'; cf. 26.6: אבק יולש ברוק יאכל הבשר המת ויצמיח הבשר החי וכשהיה הנגע מכה טריה בדמו ימלאהו בו בראש או בפנים או בגוף פעם אחת יבריאהו: יקח דם שני האחים וסרקא קולא מ"א אוקיא כאנפר דרהם יודק וינופה ויולש ברוק וימלא ממנו הנגע וישים עליו מדביק ויזרה זריה. ([Composition of] a remedy that should be kneaded with saliva [and that] eats the dead flesh away and makes the healthy flesh grow. If the wound is fresh and bleeding and one fills it up once [with this remedy] whether [the wound] is in the head, the face or the [rest of] the body, it (i.e. this remedy) will cure it. Take one ounce each of dragon's blood and sarcocol, and one *dirham*[144] of camphor. Pound, sieve and knead these ingredients with saliva and fill up the wound with it. Put a sticking plaster on it, once you have sprinkled some of this remedy on it). Hebrew מדביק does not feature in the current dictionaries.

מחוכם = Arab. محكم 'firm, solid, precise'; cf. 10.2: וראוי להתחיל ברפואתו בקשור למעלה ממקום הנשיכה קשירה מחוכמת כדי שלא יעבור הארס בעורקים אל האברים הראשים וימית (One should start his treatment by tightly tying the spot above the bite so that the poison does not progress through the vessels to the major organs and becomes fatal). Hebrew מחוכם as 'firm, solid, precise' is a non-attested semantic borrowing from Arab. محكم.

מחתים: מחתימים = Arab. جبائر 'splints'; cf. entry חתם: החתים. Hebrew מחתים does not feature in the current dictionaries. Shem Tov translates Arab. جبائر as the Rabbinic term קשישים (cf. SG Qof 28). N translates the same term as חבישות

144 The standard *dirham* is 3, 125 grams; see W. Hinz, *Islamische Masse und Gewichte umgerechnet ins metrische System* (Handbuch der Orientalistik I, Ergänzungsband I, 1. Photomechanischer Nachdruck mit Zusätzen und Berichtigungen Leiden/Köln 1970), 3.

and Z as דבקות (MA 15.69). Hillel translates the Latin parallel 'astellae' as לוחות. See entry חתם.

מיתר: אבר שיש לו מתרים רבים = Arab. عضو عضلي 'a limb with many muscles'; cf. 25.10: ואם היה הרצוץ באבר שיש לו מתרים רבים או עצבים שים עם מה שספרתי מעט שמן איריאוש או שמן נרקיט ומעט יין ריחני (If the bruise occurred to a limb with many muscles or nerves, one should add to the remedy I described some oil of lily or oil of narcissus and some fragrant wine). As a medical-anatomical term Hebrew מיתר features in the current dictionaries only in the sense of 'sinew' (cf. EM 930–1). Arab. عضل is translated by N as עצל or עצלים and by Z as מוסקולו or מוסקולי (MA passim). The latter Hebrew term is used by Hillel for Latin musculi.

מנגע: סמים מנגעים = Arab. الأدوية التي تُقْرِح 'ulcerating drugs'; cf. 13.3: וראוי שנתחיל ברפואתו קודם שיראו בו האותות הרעות שנשתדל לשרוף המקום הנשוך בכויה עמוקה מרחבת הנשיכה או בסמים מנגעים ומרחיבים אותה ולא יושם עליה רפואה שתנגבה ויסתמה ויעשה הארס לפנים (We should begin his treatment before the bad symptoms appear by burning the bitten spot through cauterization that penetrates deeply [into the wound] and makes it wider, or by [applying] drugs that make [the wound] ulcerate and make it wider. But one should not apply a drug to it that dries it up and closes it, so that the poison can be active from within). Hebrew מנגע does not feature in this sense in the current dictionaries. Arab. قرح I 'to develop an ulcer' is translated by N as התחבל or השחין and by Z as חבל and התחבל and התנגע (MA 6.72; 23.46). See as well entry מתנגע.

מעצור = Arab. حمية 'diet'; cf. 17.5: ויתמיד השמירה ויעזוב התערובות במאכלים וכבר שאלו לגאליה מה היא הרפואה היותר גדולה? אמר המעצור (They should adhere to a diet and avoid eating different kinds of food at the same time. Galen was asked: what the best [kind of] treatment? He answered: a diet). Hebrew מעצור is not attested in the sense of 'diet' in the current dictionaries. The term features in Hillel as a translation of Latin abstinentia, i.e. 'abstinence'. Cf. entry שמירה below.

מצנפות = I. Arab. رباط 'bandage'; cf. 26.2: וראוי שתושם הרפואה הזאת על העורק עצמו אשר יגר ממנו הדם ואחר כן יושם ממנו הרבה על הנגע כלו ואחר כך יקשרהו במצנפות מבגד פשתן על הרפואה (This remedy should be applied to the very vessel from which the blood streams, then a large quantity of it should be put on the whole of the wound. Then one should put a bandage of linen rags on the remedy); II. Arab. خِرَق 'rags'; cf. 25.3: ואולם הקעת הפרקים הנה ראוי לשפוך עליו מים חמים ואחרי כן יושבו בדקות עד שישוב אל ענין השווי ויחותל במצנפות חתול שוה וישים עליו אחת מאלו הרפואות המורכבות המועילות (In the case of a dislocated joint one should pour hot water on it and then move it back gently until it returns to its normal position and tie it with rags, not too tight and not too loose. One should put one of those compound, beneficial remedies on it); III. Arab. رفائد 'rags'; cf. 26.3: כבר זכר בן מאסויה בספר התועלת רפואה תפסיק הדם מן הנגעים וזה תארה: יקח אלובי אוקיא קלפת לבונה שתי אוקיות דם שני האחים וסרקא קולא מ"א שמונה שקלים וירדיט חמשה שקלים יודק וינופה ויושם על המקום בלובן ביצה ושער ארנבת ולחם שחוק ויחותל במצנפות (In his work [*al-Nujḥ*] *(Favourable outcome)* Ibn Māsawayh mentions a remedy which stops the bleeding of wounds. This is its composition: Take one ounce of aloe, two ounces of bark of the frankincense tree, eight *mithqāl*s each of dragon's blood (red resin of *Dracaena draco*) and sarcocol, five *mithqāl*s of verdigris. Pound and sieve [these ingredients], put them on the [affected] spot with egg white, the hair of a hare and pulverized quicklime,[145] and apply it with a piece of rag). The Hebrew term does not feature in these meanings in the current dictionaries.

מַרְאֶה = Arab. لون 'colour'; cf. 7.1: והשתנותה באיכותה יהיה לפי המותר המורק ותהיה משתנה אם במראה כמו שיקרה כשתהיה אדומה או כרכומית או ירוקה או לבנה (Its [i.e. sweat] change in quality occurs according to the nature of the superfluity that is evacuated; its colour changes according to what [is evacuated], whether it is red, yellow, green or white). Hebrew מראה is attested in the sense of colour in Rabbinic literature only; cf. JD 834. Both N and Z translates the Arabic لون as מראה, while Z also has זיו and צבע (MA passim).

מְשַׁכֵּךְ: הרפואות אשר יודעו במשככות = Arab. الأدوية التي تعرف بالردّاعة 'remedies which are known as restraining'; cf. 15.3: וכאשר הריקונו כל הגוף נשוב אל הרפואות אשר יודעו במשככות והדוחות בהתחלה (Once we have evacuated [all the superfluities] from the body, we turn in the beginning [of the tumour] to those remedies which are known as restraining and repelling). Hebrew מְשַׁכֵּךְ does not feature in this sense in the current dictionaries; cf. EM 1824, s.v. שָׁכֵךְ. Z uses the term מְשַׁכֵּךְ in the combination הרפואה המשככת as a translation of Arab الأدوية المسكنة, i.e. alleviating remedies, whereas N has הרפואות המשקיטות (MA 8.38).

145 'quicklime': translated after the Arabic جير.

Arabic الأدوية التي تمنع وتردع (the drugs that detain and restrain) is translated by N as הרפואות המונעות והמרתיעות and by Z as הרפואה אשר תזיר ותמנע (MA 9.121).

מתנגע = Arab. متقرّح 'ulcerous'; cf. 20.3: וזכר שהוא כשיעורב גפרית עם גומא טרבנטינה יסיר הגרב המתנגע והקובא והרשמים הלבנים אשר יקרו בצפרנים (He remarks that if one mixes sulphur with resin from the turpentine tree, it exterminates ulcerous scabies, eczema, and the white spots happening to the nails). Hebrew התנגע does not feature in this sense in the current dictionaries. Arab قرح I 'to ulcerate' is translated by N as התחבל or השחין and by Z as חבל/ התחבל/ התנגע (MA 6.72; 23.46); see entry מנגע.

נֶגַע = I. Arab. قرحة 'ulcer'; cf. 14.2: ואם הרתיחה ולא תתעפש תחדש המין אשר יתחדש עמו דומה בכאב הנגע בכל שטח הגוף ותהיה עמו עקיצה דומה לעקיצת המחטים (If [the humours] become boiling hot but do not putrefy, it results in the kind [of fatigue which comes with] something similar to the pain caused by ulcers on the whole outside of the body. It also comes with [a sensation of] pricking similar to the pricking of a needle). II. Arab. جراحة 'wound'; cf. 15.1: הנה כל מורסא תתחדש מהגרת ליחה אל אבר מהאברים וסבות ההגרה מהם מתחילות באות מחוץ ומהם קודמות פנימיות והמתחילות כמו הכאה או נגע או ריצוץ או הקעה או שבר או סדק (Every tumour arises from the streaming of matter to some part of the body. The causes of the streaming [of matter] are partly evident,[146] [namely] external, and partly hidden,[147] [namely] internal. Examples of evident[148] [causes] are a blow, wound, contusion, dislocation, fracture or bruise).[149] Hebrew נֶגַע features in BM 3520–1 in the sense of 'plague' or 'leprosy' (cf. JD 875) and in Low LXIII as 'Morbus contagiosus (eg. a skin disease = leprosy); communicable disease'. נֶגַע features in N and Z as a translation of Arabic قرحة 'wound, ulcer', whereas N also uses שחין and Z חבלה (MA passim). See as well entry עשה הנגע.

נקיון = Arab. بحران 'crisis'; cf. 7.1: והזיעה הטבעית היא כמו הזיעה אשר תהיה מן הנקיון הטוב (Natural sweat is equivalent to the sweat that occurs in a wholesome crisis). Hebrew נקיון is attested in this sense in BM 3796 in a quotation from *Perush Ibn Rushd 'al Ḥaruzei Ibn Sina* (Ibn Rushd's commentary on Ibn Sīnā's *'Urǧūza* in the Hebrew translation prepared by Solomon Ibn Ayyub in

146 'evident': translated after the Arabic بادية.

147 'hidden': translated after the Arabic باطنة.

148 'evident': translated after the Arabic بادية.

149 'bruise' = Arab. وثء.

the year 1261. N translates Arabic بحران as גבול, plur. גבולים and also transcribes it as בחראן, while Z has בחראן, קרישיש and טירמיני or טירימיניאו (MA passim). For נקיון in the sense of 'cure, therapy' cf. Hillel.

סְבוּב = Arab. سدر 'dizziness'; cf. 10.1: ויקרה לו עלוף רב וסבוב וזיעה קרה ועוצר השתן ועצור ויקיא מרה כרכומית (Extreme feebleness, dizziness, cold sweat, dysuria, cramps,[150] and vomiting of yellow bile befall him). In the sense of 'dizziness' Hebrew סבוב features as סבוב הראש in BM 3913 in an attestation from Nathan ha-Me'ati's translation of Ibn Sīnā's *K. al-Qānūn* (cf. EM 1209). Nathan translates the same Arabic term as ערבוב in MA 25.11, while Arabic السدر والدوار (the vertigo and dizziness) is translated by him as סְבוּב (בראש) ובלבול בראש (MA 6.34), while Z has השקוטומיאה.

סְנַפִּיר: סנפירות = Arab. خشكريشة 'eschars'; cf. 22.1: הנגעים אמנם יתילדו ממשיכת הדם וכל שכן הנגעים האדומים והם נגעים רעים שיש עמהם קדחת ועליהם סנפירות ומראיהם אדום ואדמימותם נוטה למראה אפר (Ulcers, especially red ulcers originate from the attraction of blood [to a certain spot]. These are malignant ulcers which are accompanied by fever and eschars, and their redness [tends] somewhat towards ash-grey). Hebrew סְנַפִּיר, Plur. סנפירות features in BM 4128 in the sense of 'ichtyosis'. Arab. خشكريشة is transcribed by N as כשכרישה and translated by Z as המקום בעצמו אשר שם כעין סובין (MA 15.9).

עִגּוּל = Arab. شياف 'collyrium'; cf. 15.3: וכאשר הריקונו כל הגוף נשוב אל הרפואות אשר יודעו במשככות והדוחות בהתחלה כמו שנדל ובול ארמיני ועגול ממיטא ואופי ומה שדומה לזה (Once we have evacuated [all the superfluities] from the body, we turn in the beginning [of the tumour] to those remedies which are known as restraining and repelling, such as red sandalwood [*Santalum rubrum*], Armenian earth, horned poppy [*Glaucium corniculatum*],[151] opium, and the like). Hebrew עִגּוּל only features in the current dictionaries in the sense of 'circle, equator' (BM 4301–3). In Rabbinical literature we find the term קילור in the sense of 'collyrium' or 'eye-salve' (cf. JD 1360; Low LXXVI, Shem Tov and SG Qof 22).

עוגה = Arab. قرص 'pastille'; cf. 18.4: והנה יודק שורש אשקריולא מדברית ויולש בדבש ויעשה עוגות ויצניעם ויקח עוגה אחר עוגה ויתיכה במים ושלניטרי ויטוח אותה על הבהק וינקה אותו (One may also pound wild endive root, knead it with honey, make

150 'cramps': translated after the Arabic مغص.

151 Lit. horned poppy (*Glaucium corniculatum*) collyrium.

pastilles of it, store them, and take one pastille at a time, dissolve it in water and natron and rub it on the [spot affected by] *bahaq* and it will make it clean). Hebrew עוגה in the sense of 'pastille' features in BM 4300, a.o. in an attestation from Nathan ha-Me'ati's translation of Ibn Sīnā's *K. al-Qānūn*. In Moses Ibn Tibbon's translation of Maimonides' *On Hemorrhoids* 3.1 עוגה features in the sense of 'omelette' for Arabic عجّة.

עִצּוּר = I. Arab. عصر 'pressure'; cf. 9.2: וכאשר הגיע אל האסטו' וקרה ממנו צער ודיות זיעה הוא רמויילאר עם קיא ונפח ושנוי מראה ופלצות ושרפה ועצור בפי האסטו' ומחשך הראות הנה אז ראוי למהרו ברפואה ואם לא ימות מהר (If it reaches the stomach and it causes distress and transudation of sweat together with vomiting, flatulence, change in colour, shivering, burning, pressure in the heart[152] region and dimness of sight, he should be treated as soon as possible, otherwise he will die soon); II. Arab. مغص 'cramps'; cf. 10.1: הנה יקרה למי שנשכו אפעה בתחלת הענין שישוב מראהו לבן ויתנפח ממנו מקום הנשיכה והנה גבה הנפח הרבה ויעשה המקום אבעבועות עד שיהיה דומה לשרפת אש ויקרה לו עלוף רב וסבוב וזיעה קרה ועוצר השתן ועצור ויקיא מרה כרכומית ואם לא ימהרו ברפואתו יגיע הארס אל הלב וימות (The first thing that happens to someone who has been bitten by a viper is that his colour turns white and that the spot of the bite swells up. Sometimes it swells up very much and it becomes so blistered that it resembles a burn. Extreme feebleness, dizziness, cold sweat, dysuria, cramps, and vomiting of yellow bile befall him. If it is not immediately followed by treatment, the poison will reach the heart and the patient will die). Hebrew עִצּוּר only features in the current dictionaries in the sense of 'closing up (of the womb)', and 'obstruction of orifices'; cf. JD 1074. Arab. عصر is translated by Z as עצור as well, while N has סחיטה or עשוי (MA 10.9; 16.29; 23.6). Arab. مغص, Plur. أمغاص is translated by both N and Z as חליים (MA 13.52).

עצלה = Arab. رهل 'flabbiness'; cf. 15.2: והמורסא המתחדשת מליחה לבנה תקרא מורסא רפה ואותותיו לובן ורפיון וישאר מקום נעיצת האצבע עמוק ואין כאב עמו אבל לחות ועצלה (The tumour that arises from phlegm is called a 'soft swelling' [oedema]. It symptoms are whiteness and softness and the spot where one touches it with the fingers remains depressed, it is not accompanied by pain, but by moisture and flabbiness). Hebrew עצלה is mentioned in BM 4645 in the sense of 'laziness' only.

152 'heart region'; i.e. Arabic فؤاد.

ערבוב שכל: ערבוב = Arab. تخليط 'delirium'; cf. 13.2: והמקרים אשר יקרו למי שנשכו כלב שוטה אולם בהתחלה יחלום חלומות שאחריתם ערבוב שכל ופעמים יפחד תוך שנתו בעבור דבר שיפחידהו ויקרה לו בעת היקיצה כעס ויגון מבלתי סבה שתכעיסהו ואינו סובל לאדם שיביט אליו וירבה להביט סביבו (The symptoms that someone who has been bitten by a mad dog shows in the beginning [of the disease] are that he has dreams that are mostly[153] delirious and that sometimes during the sleep he is afraid of the scary things happening to him when he is awake, that he is distressed[154] for no evident reason, cannot bear someone looking at him, and often turns to look at what is around him). Hebrew ערבוב שכל is attested in BM 4707 in a quotation from Nathan ha-Me'ati's translation of Maimonides' *Medical Aphorisms*. In addition to this term N has בלבול (ה)שכל, while Z has בלבול) הדעת) and ערבוב) דעת) for Arab. العقل (اختلاط) (MA passim).

עשה = Arab. استعمل 'to apply' (medicines): cf. 9.3: והנה זכר גאליה ודיאשקורידוש רפואות יעשו בעת הפחד והיראה וינצל בלקיחתם מנזק הסמים הממיתים (Both Galen and Dioscurides have mentioned remedies that should be applied when someone is afraid [of being poisoned], because their ingestion protects him against the harm caused by lethal drugs). Hebrew עשה does not feature in this sense in the current dictionaries. Hillel has הרגיל or היה רגיל as a translation of Latin 'administrare' or 'uti' (to administer, to apply).

עשה הנגע:- = Arab. أقرح 'to ulcerate'; cf. 13.4: ואולם הרפואות אשר יעשו הנגע וירחיבוהו וימשכו הארס ממנו כמו שיקח שום ויכתוש אותו ויושם על המקום (As to drugs which make [the spot] ulcerate, widen it and attract the poison from it: Take for example garlic, pound it and put it on the spot). Hebrew עשה הנגע does not feature in this sense in the current dictionaries. Cf. entry נֶגַע.

הפסיק (פסק) = Arab. قطع 'to dissolve'; cf. 19.2: וראוי לרפאת המין הראשון מן הקובא בהוצאת הדם בהקזה אם עזר הזמן והשנים והמנהג ואחר כן בשלשול ברפואות אשר יפסיקו חומר השריפה (The first kind of eczema should be treated by bleeding through venesection, if the time [of the year], the age [of the patient] and [his] habits allow it. Then [it should be treated] with purgation, with remedies which dissolve the burning hot matter). In the sense of 'to dissolve' Hebrew הפסיק is a non-attested semantic borrowing from Arab. قطع. The same term is translated by N as חיתך and by Z as חתך (MA 7.23).

153 'mostly': translated after the Arabic أكثرها.

154 'distressed': translated after the Arabic ضجر.

פרוד: פרוד (ה)דבוק = I. Arab. انحلال الاتّصال 'the dissolution of continuity'; cf. 14.3: ואולם הכאב הנה הוא שנוי פתאום יהיה מן מזג חם או קר או מפרוד דבוק (Pain is [provoked by] a sudden change of a hot or cold temperament or by the dissolution of continuity). Hebrew פרוד דבוק does not feature in the current dictionaries. N translates the Arabic equivalent تفرّق الاتّصال as פרוק חבור and Z as הפרדת הדבקות (MA 7.6; 25.21), while Hillel translates the Latin equivalent 'solutio continuitatis' as התרת הדבקות; II. Arab. تفرّق الاتّصال; cf. 25.1: כשיתחדש פרוד הדבוק בעצם הנה הכונה ברפואתו הדביק העצם (If a dissolution of continuity occurs in a bone, the aim of its treatment is to cause the fracture to close up).

קבסא = Arab. غثيان 'nausea'; cf. 9.4: וזאת הרפואה כשישתה אותה ולא יקח אחריה סם המות תעמוד במקומה ואם ישתה אחריה סם ממית תחדש קבסא ויצטרך הסם הממית אשר שתה לצאת בקיא מכה[155] המרקחת (If one takes this remedy and does not take a lethal drug after it, it lingers in its place. And if one takes a lethal drug [after taking this remedy], it causes nausea so that the lethal drug one took is perforce thrown up together with the antidote). Aramaic קבסא features in SDA 1009 in the sense of 'vomit', while the Hebrew parallel קבסה is mentioned by Ben Yehuda (BM 5707) in the meaning of 'Brechdurchfall; cholerine'. N translates the same Arabic term as אסטנסות and חפץ קיא, while Z has קרבונקלי or קרבונקולו (MA 9.55; 13.54; 23.86, 87).

קִבּוּץ = Arab. قَبْض 'astringency'; cf. 26.2: וזאת ההרכבה נאותה לגופות הקשים כשיצטרכו מן הקבוץ אל שעור יותר נוסף (This compound is beneficial for hard bodies as they need [remedies] that are more astringent). Hebrew קִבּוּץ does not feature in this sense in the current dictionaries. N translates the Arabic قَبْض a.o. as קביצות and Z a.o. as קיבוץ/ קביצה/ קביצות (MA passim).

קִוּוּץ = I. Arab. تشنّج 'spasm'; cf. 9.2: וכאשר יקרה ממשוש מזון או משקה שרפה או תרדמה או קווץ בצפרנים או נפח לאצבע הנה ראוי להשמר ממנו כי בו סם המות (If someone who touched food or drink is affected by burning or numbness or spasm [i.e. shrivelling] of the nails, or by swelling in the fingers, he should take care, because he has been poisoned). Hebrew קִוּוּץ features in this sense in BM 5824 (see as well entry קויצה in BM 5826–7). N translates Arabic تشنّج as כויצה, Z as כווץ or התכווץ (MA passim). Hillel uses the same term קיווץ for the Latin equivalent 'spasmus'; cf. KZ 65; SG Kaf 21; Shem Tov (S), s.v. כווץ; II. Arab. فسخ 'disrupture'; cf. 14.3: ופעמים שיתחדש הכאב מסבות מחוץ ולא

155 מכה: Translated after the Arabic مع المعجون.

הרגיש בהם החולה והוא שיהיה כבר העמיד האבר ההוא אשר התחדש לו בו הכאב בעת נומו בתכונה בלתי ראויה או שעותו פתאום וכל שכן אם קרהו קור עד שיתחדש בו קווץ (Pain can also be caused by external causes while the patient does not notice it, as may be the case during one's sleep when that part of the body that is [subsequently] affected by the pain is in a wrong position or is twisted all of a sudden, especially if it is affected by cold, so that it suffers from a disrupture). Hebrew קִוּוּץ does not feature in this sense in the current dictionaries. Arabic فسخ is translated by N as רסוק and by Z as הפסד (MA 3.109); III. Arab. تقبُّض 'contraction'; cf. 17.2: ואם יתילד החולי הזה מפני שרפת מרה כרכומית הנה אותותיו כרכומית המראה ויובש החזה וסדיקת הידים והרגלים וקווץ ויבשות ויגלה מעט מעט בשעור מן הזמן (If this disease originates from the burning of yellow bile, its symptoms are: yellow complexion, dryness of chest, cracks in hands and feet, [their] contraction and aridity, the disease appears slowly slowly during a longer period). Hebrew קִוּוּץ does not feature in this sense in the current dictionaries.

קלוח, Plur. **קלוחים** = Arab. حقن 'clysters'; cf. 9.7: וכאשר נדע שהאסטו' כבר נקתה ולא ימצא בה מן הסם עקיצה ולא שרפה ולא צער אז נצוה לשלשל הטבע בקלוחים ממוצעי החום כדי שישלשלו מה שהגיע מן הסם אל המעים (And if we know [for sure] that the stomach is clean and that the poison does not have a biting or burning [effect] in it and does not cause distress in it, we order to relieve the bowels with clysters that are moderately hot so that the poison that has reached the intestines is purged). Hebrew קלוח is attested in this sense in BM 5940 in a quotation from Me'ir Aldabi's *Shevilei Emunah*. In Ibn Tibbon's translation of Maimonides' *Regimen of Health* (4:13),[156] *On Hemorroids* (4.6)[157] and *On Poisons* (cf. introduction above) we find the Romance קלישתירי/ קלישטרי. N translates Arab. حقنة as חוקן and Z as קרישטרי (MA 9.47,48; 13.35,37,40). S has פדלקון for Arab. محقن 'clyster'.

קליפה: קליפות = Arab. قشور 'scabs'; cf. 22.1: ואם יהיה עם ליחה לבנה יוליד נגעים לחים עם קליפות לבנות (If it [i.e. the blood] is accompanied by phlegm it produces moist ulcers that have white scabs). Hebrew קליפה in the sense of 'scab' is a non-attested counterpart to Aramaic קלפא, cf. JD 1381: '1. split parchment; 2. scaly surface, scab; 3. streak made by peeling'.

156 Forthcoming edition Gerrit Bos.

157 Forthcoming edition Gerrit Bos.

קשר: קשרים = I. Arab. عقد 'tumours'; cf. 23.1: וזכר גם כן כי פגי תאנים כשיבושלו ויעשה מהם תחבושת ירכך הקשרים והחזירים ויתיכם (He [i.e. Dioscurides] also relates that if one boils green figs and makes a poultice of them they soften and dissolve tumours and scrofula). Hebrew קשרים in the sense of 'tumours' is a non-attested semantic borrowing from the Arabic عقد. This last term is a semantic borrowing from the Greek σύστροφαι (cf. LS 1736); II. Arab. رباط 'bandage'; cf. 15.5: ואם התילדה המורסא מפני ליחה לבנה והיא אשר תקרא מורסא רפה הנה ראוי להשקות החולה הרפואות אשר יורידו ליחה לבנה ואחרי כן יושם עליה אספוג בלול במים שנתערב עמהם חומץ ויקשור האספוג בקשרים תהיה התחלתם מלמטה ותכליתם למעלה (If the tumour originates from phlegm which is the one called 'the soft swelling' [oedema], the patient should be given remedies which bring down [evacuate] the phlegm; then a sponge moistened with water that has been mixed with vinegar should be put on the [affected] spot, and the sponge should be fastened with a bandage beginning below and finishing above). Hebrew קשר does not feature in this sense in the current dictionaries. The same term is used by Hillel to render the Latin equivalent 'ligatura'.

ריר = Arab. لعاب 'mucilage'; cf. 8.5: ואם יצא ממנו דבר בפה ימשחהו בריר שיליום עם ריר זרע חבושים ומעט שמן ורדים (If any [pustules] come out in the mouth, rub it with mucilage of fleawort [*Plantago psyllium*] seed together with mucilage of quince seed and some rose oil). In the sense of 'mucilage' (from plants) the Hebrew term is attested in BM 6585 in a quotation from Nathan ha-Me'ati's translation of Ibn Sīnā's *K. al-Qānūn*.

רִסּוּק = Arab. وثء 'bruise'; cf. 25.4: ומזה רפואה תועיל מן השבר והרסוק (Such as [the following] remedy which is beneficial for a fracture and bruise). Hebrew רִסּוּק is attested in Rabbinic literature in the sense of 'crushing, lesion' and as ריסוקי איברים in the sense of 'lesion of vital organs, internal injury' (JD 1475; BM 6626). Hebrew רסוק is also used by Ibn Tibbon to translate Arabic رضّ (contusion, bruise), while for Arabic وثء he also uses סדק (cf. entry הקעה).

רִקּוּחַ = Arab. تأليف 'composition' (of a remedy); cf. 26.1: והנה זכר גליאה בספר תחבולות הבריאות כי זאת הרפואה תהיה רקוחה על שלשה מינים (Galen said in the work *De methodo medendi* that this remedy is composed in three [different] ways). Hebrew רִקּוּחַ is attested in Rabbinic literature in the sense of 'perfume' (JD 1477) and in modern literature in the sense of 'the composition of spices' (EM 1744). In addition to רִקּוּחַ Ibn Tibbon uses the common חבור.

שוטה : see **כלב**.

שטות = Arab. كَلَب 'rabies'; cf. 13.1: הכלב בטבעו קר ויבש גוברת עליו מרה שחורה ולשפעת הליחה הזאת השחורית בו והיותה גוברת עליו תתעפש ותכלול הפסדה כל גופו ויוציאהו זה אל השטות (A dog has a dry and cold nature which is dominated by black bile. When this melancholic humour becomes excessive and dominant it putrefies and the putrefaction pervades all parts of its body and [the dog] is affected by rabies). Hebrew שטות is not attested in this sense in the current dictionaries.

שלהבת = Arab. لهيب 'temperature' (cf. WKAS II,3, p. 1476); cf. 15.4: וכאשר שככה שלהבת האבר החולה נחבשהו קודם שישוב ירוק (When the temperature of the affected part subsides we apply a poultice before it turns livid). Hebrew שלהבת in the sense of 'temperature', a semantic borrowing of Arabic لهيب, only features as 'flame, flaming fire' in the current literature (cf. JD 1578).

שמירה = Arab. حمية 'diet'; cf. 17.5: והנה תועילהו גם כן הכויה ויתמיד השמירה ויעזוב התערובות במאכלים וכבר שאלו לגאליה מה היא הרפואה היותר גדולה? אמר המעצור (Cauterization may also be beneficial. They should adhere to a diet and avoid eating different kinds of food at the same time. Galen was asked: what the best [kind of] treatment? He answered: a diet). Hebrew שמירה is not attested in the sense of 'diet' in the current dictionaries. Hebrew שמירה is also used by both N and Z for Arabic حمية 'abstinence' (MA 8.8), while Hillel uses or הנהגת השמירה for Latin dieta 'diet'. Cf. entry מעצור.

תכונה = I. Arab. قوام 'consistency'; cf. 15.7: תואר אספלנית למורסא אשר אין לה ראש והיה צורך לפתחה והוא מנוסה: יקח זרע פשתן וזבל יונים ופניגריג מזרחי מ"א חמשה שקלים שישמאן שרוף עשרים שקלים יודק השישמאן עד שיהיו כמוח ויולשו בו הסמים בעלי עד שישתוה תכונתו (Another [compound remedy] is a salve for a tumour that has not come to a head[158] and which is intended to make it burst and which has been tried. Its composition is: Take five *mithqāl*s each of linseed, pigeon droppings and Syrian fenugreek; twenty *mithqāl*s of burned sesame; pound the sesame until it becomes like marrow and knead the [other] ingredients with it in a mortar until it assumes an equal consistency). Hebrew תכונה does not feature in this sense in the current dictionaries; cf. BM 7743–6; KT 4:191–6; II. Arab. سحنة 'external appearance'; cf. 17.3: ואות המותר כאשר הוא

158 I.e. that has not matured, suppurated.

חוץ מן העורקים שתפסד תכונת החולה ויפתחו ידיו ויקרה לו נגעים בעלי מוגלא ומורסות (When the superfluity is outside the vessels, it is indicated by the fact that the external appearance of the patient is corrupted, that his[159] body swells up, that he is befallen by purulent ulcers and tumours). Hebrew תכונה does not feature in this sense in the current dictionaries. N translates Arab. سحنة as פנים or תואר, while Z has זיו or מראה (MA 12.3; 23.47).

תכלית = Arab. منتهى 'climax'; cf. 15.3: ובתכלית המורסא ישתמש באלו הרפואות אשר זכרנו ממה שיתיך (When the tumour reaches its climax, one should apply next to those remedies we [just] mentioned, [remedies] which have a dissolving [reducing] effect). Hebrew תכלית is mentioned in the more general sense of שעור שאין למעלה ממנו (maximum) in EM 1936 and KT 4:200. The same Arabic term is translated by N as העמדה/ תכלית/ תכלית העמדה and by Z as עמידה (MA passim).

התמיד (תמד) = Arab. ألزم 'to apply' (cf. WKAS II,1, 560); cf. 12.1: או יקח קישואים ותבושל ותכתוש אותה ויתמידה על המקום (Or take cucumber [*Cucumis sativus*], boil and pound it and apply it to the spot [of the stings by wasps and bees]). Hebrew התמיד in the sense of 'to apply' is a non-attested semantic borrowing from the Arabic ألزم.

תרדמה = Arab. خدر 'numbness'; cf. 8.2: וכאשר יקרה ממשוש מזון או משקה שרפה או תרדמה או קווץ בצפרנים או נפח לאצבע (If someone who touched food or drink is affected by burning or numbness or shrivelling of the nails, and by swelling in the fingers). Hebrew תרדמה does not feature in this sense in the current dictionaries. Cf. next entry.

תרדמת האברים:- = I. Arab. تخدير 'numbness'; cf. 17.1: ומסגולת הליחה הלבנה תרדמת האברים (the specific activity of the phlegm is the numbness). Hebrew תרדמת האברים features in BM 7902, a.o. in an attestation from Nathan ha-Me'ati's Hebrew translation of Maimonides' *Medical Aphorisms*. In addition to תרדמת האברים N translates the Arab. خدر as תרדמת החוש while Z has ביטול and הביטול הנקרא בערבי כדר ברפה הכף (MA 7.66; 22.38,43; 23.22, 23); II. Arab. خدر 'numbness'; cf. 17.2: ואם התילד החולי הזה מפני עפוש ליחה לבנה ושריפתה הנה אותותיו לחות הגוף וריבוי הגרנדולש ורפיון ורבוי הגרת העינים ולובן המראה ותרדמת האיברים (If this disease originates from the putrefaction and burning of the phlegm, its

159 'that his body swells up': translated according to Arab. وينتفخ بدنه.

symptoms are: moisture of the body, appearance[160] of glandular swellings, feebleness, very watery eyes, whiteness of complexion, numbness).

Materia Medica

דם שני האחים = Arab. دم الأخوين lit. 'the blood of the two brothers', is a red resin derived from diverse Liliacea; in the Orient the Dracaena Draco Willd. and in the West the Dragon-tree (Dracaena Draco L.). It is also known under the name *dam at-tinnīn* or *dam at̲-t̲u'bān* 'dragonblood' (DT 4:79; R 96; LF 2:198ff.); cf. 26.3. Hebrew דם שני האחים, a loan-translation of the Arabic دم الأخوين, is not attested in the current dictionaries and secondary literature. Arabic دم الأخوين is translated both by N and Z as: דם תנין (MA 21.83). Cf. SG Dalet 2.

זרעון = Arab. حمّص 'chickpeas' (*Cicer arietinum* and var.); cf. 16.3: ואמר דיאסקורידוס כי יאמרו אנשים כי הזרעונים יבריאו מן היבלות הקשות כשיקח מהזרעונים וישים אחד אחד מהם על אחת אחת מן היבלות וזה יעשה ביום הראשון מן החודש ואחר כן יקבץ הזרעונים ויקשרם בצרור בגד וישליך אותם לאחוריו (Dioscurides relates that some people say that chickpeas cure hard warts if one takes some chickpeas and puts them one by one on every single wart on the first day of the month, then collects them and binds them in a cloth and throws them behind him). Hebrew זרעונים only features in the current dictionaries in the sense of 'vegetables'; cf. BM 1407–8; see as well SG Zayin 19. Hebrew זרעונים in the sense of 'chickpeas' for Arabic حمّص also features in Z, while N has אפונים (MA 21.72).

מיץ: מיץ חלב = Arab. ماء الجبن 'whey'; cf. 9.7: וישתה אחר זה החלב שנחלב מיד כי תועלתו גדולה מאד או ישתה מיץ חלב או יין מבושל ישן (Then we let him drink fresh milk because it is very beneficial. One may also let him drink whey or a [drink] of old wine). Hebrew מיץ חלב features in BM 2978 in an attestation from Meir Aldabi's *Shevilei Emunah*. The Rabbinic term for 'whey' is נסיובי (דחלבא); cf. JD 916. Arabic. ماء الجبن is translated by N as מי הגבינה and by Z as מי הגבינה or מי חלב (MA 9.108; 21.29).

עדשה: עדשי המים = Arab. طحلب 'duckweed' (Lemna L.); cf. 15.4. The Hebrew term features as עדש המים in SG 'Ayin 2. N transcribes and translates the

160 'appearance of glandular swellings': translated after the Arabic والتغدّد.

Arab. طحلب as טחלב/ עדשי המים, while Z has טחלב/ הירוקה שעל פני המים (MA 9.106; 21.79; 25.54).

עפר: עפר ספרד = Arab. قيموليا 'Cimolian earth'; cf. 28.2. The Hebrew term is not attested in secondary literature. For other kinds of earth cf. R 172.

קלפה: קלפת נחשת = Arab. قشور النحاس 'copper filings'; cf. 16.2. The Hebrew term which is not attested in the current dictionaries features as קליפי הנחשת הם הקליפות הנופלות בעת הכאת החרש בפטיש in SG Quf 43 (QLYPY HNḤŠT, these are filings which fall down during the craftsman's striking with the hammer).

קצף: קצף הים = Arab. زبد البحر sepiolite (*Spuma maris*); cf. 16.3. The Hebrew features in BM 6106 in an attestation from Nathan ha-Me'ati's translation of Ibn Sīnā's *K. al-Qānūn*.

3. Shem Tov Ben Isaac, *Sefer ha-Shimmush*

Introduction

While in Marseilles Shem Tov translated the famous medical encyclopaedia entitled *Kitāb al-taṣrīf li-man 'ajiza 'an al-ta'līf* (The Arrangement of Medical Knowledge for One Who is Not Abel to Compile a Book for Himself), which was composed in the tenth century by the Andalusian physician Abū l-Qāsim Khalaf ibn 'Abbās al-Zahrāwī, known in the western world as Abulcasis.[161] In addition to the *Kitāb al-taṣrīf*, Shem Tov translated Abū Walīd Muḥammad ibn Rushd's *Middle Commentary on Aristotle's* De Anima,[162] Abū Bakr Muḥammad ibn Zakariyya al-Rāzī's medical encyclopaedia *K. al-Manṣūrī*,[163] and Hippocrates' *Aphorisms* with Palladius' commentary.[164] Shem Tov started his translation of the *Kitāb al-taṣrīf*, which he called Sefer ha-Shimmush, in 1254 and completed it at an unknown date. Instead of translating Zahrawī's glossary of medical terms in book 29, Shem Tov compiled two independent lists of medical synonyms, the first in Hebrew-Arabic-Romance and the second in Romance-Arabic and sometimes Hebrew. These lists are being edited, translated and annotated as part of a project initiated by Gerrit Bos and Guido Mensching.[165] A striking feature of Shem Tov's translation technique is

161 For Shem Tov's life and works see Bos, 'The Creation and Innovation of Medieval Hebrew medical terminology: Shem Tov Ben Isaac, Sefer ha-Shimmush', in Anna Akasoy and Wim Raven (eds), *Islamic Thought in the Middle Ages: Studies in Text, Transmission and Translation, in Honour of Hans Daiber*. (Leiden-Boston 2008), 195–218.

162 Cf. Steinschneider, *Die hebräischen Übersetzungen*, 148; Averroës. *Middle Commentary on Aristotle's* De Anima. A Critical Edition of the Arabic Text with English Translation, Notes, and Introduction by Alfred L. Ivry. (Provo, Utah 2002), xxviii–xxix, 150. n. 69.

163 Cf. Steinschneider, *Die hebräischen Übersetzungen*, 725–6.

164 His commentary is no longer extant in Greek, but it has recently been rediscovered by Hinrich Biesterfeldt and Y. Tzvi Langermann, who hope to publish soon a preliminary study of Palladius' commentary, to be followed by a full edition and analysis.

165 The project is dedicated to the edition and the analysis of various unedited scientific texts written in Middle Hebrew that belong to the field of medico-botanical literature. Within this project the Cologne group consisting of Gerrit Bos and Martina Hussein is responsible for the Hebrew-Arabic linguistic material, while the Berlin group, consisting of Guido Mensching and Frank Savelsberg, is in charge of the Latin-Romance material. First results of the research carried out in the context of the project are: Bos-Mensching, 'Shem Tov Ben Isaac, Glossary of Botanical Terms, nrs 1–18', *Jewish Quarterly Review*, vol. XCII (July-October 2001), 1–20; Bos-Mensching, 'Hebrew Medical Synonym Literature: Romance and

that in several cases he created a novel[166] Hebrew medical terminology which was, in some cases adopted by subsequent authors such as Nathan ha-Me'ati and Zeraḥyah Ḥen. An example is entry He 11 in our edition of the first glossary: המעדת המעים ב''ה זלק אלאמעא. The Hebrew *HM'DT HM'YM*, which is not attested in secondary literature, may have been coined by Shem Tov as a Hebrew loan translation of the Arabic *zalaq al-am'ā'* 'Dysenteria spuria'. The same Hebrew term features subsequently in Nathan's and Zeraḥyah's Hebrew translations of Maimonides' *Medical Aphorisms* (XXII, 36; XXIII, 80, 90, 93, 94). However, since these glossaries do not cover all the technical terms featuring in the *Sefer ha-Shimmush*, and since they do not give these terms in a specific context, further analysis and discussion of the novel medical terminology employed by the author is necessary to facilitate the reading of his translations in general, to ensure recognition of his technical terminology in future dictionaries of the Hebrew language, and to properly define his technical vocabulary. With this end in view the following study is devoted to an analysis of a selection of the technical terminology of book 30, which deals with surgery, and was by far the most popular and most influential part of this vast medical encyclopaedia. Translated into Latin by Gerard de Cremona in Toledo in the second half of the twelfth century and into Occitan in the fourteenth century, it was a major source for the European treatises on surgery composed subsequently, foremost that by Guy de Chauliac (d. 1368) who quotes it not less 157 times. Thus it played a significant role in the development of the art of surgery in Europe.[167] While the original Arabic text of book 30 has been published in a critical edition and English translation by

Latin Terms and their Identification', *Aleph*, Historical Studies in Science & Judaism, vol. 5 (2005), 11–53; Bos-Mensching, 'A 15th Century medico-botanical synonym list (Ibero-Romance-Arabic) in Hebrew characters', in: *Panace@*), vol. VII, no. 24 (December 2006); see:http://www.medtrad.org/panacea/IndiceGeneral/n24_tribunahistoricabos.mensching.pdf; Bos, *The Creation and Innovation of Medieval Hebrew medical terminology*.

166 With novel terms I mean either one of three things: 1. terms that do not feature in the current dictionaries at all; 2. terms which can be found in current dictionaries but not in the sense they have in our text; 3. terms which can be found in current dictionaries but are not registered as medieval.

167 Cf. D. Jacquart and F. Micheau, *La médicine arabe et l'occident médiéval* (Paris 1990), 150–1.

Spink-Lewis[168] and the Occitan translation has been edited by Grimaud-Lafont,[169] the Hebrew text is still unedited.

The analysis of the technical medical terminology of the Hebrew text is based on MS Paris, BN héb. 1163 which is the only manuscript to have preserved book 30 and which was copied in a sephardic script in the fourteenth century.[170] The text appears in double columns on fols. 201a–239a and has been illustrated with many drawings of the surgical instruments recommended by the author, copied from an Arabic Vorlage. In my study the terms, alphabetically arranged, are compared throughout with those of the Arabic edition and English translation by Spink-Lewis. I will refer to parallel terminology used by other major translators, namely Nathan ha-Me'ati, Zeraḥyah Ḥen, and Moses Ibn Tibbon. Of these translators both Nathan and Zeraḥyah were active at a later date than Shem Tov Ben Isaac; Nathan worked in Rome between 1279 and 1283 and Zeraḥyah worked in the same city between 1279 and 1291. It is possible that both used part of the novel terminology invented by Shem Tov Ben Isaac. In the case of Moses Ibn Tibbon, however, it is hard to determine who influenced whom, as he was active as a translator between 1240 and 1283 and some of his translations are earlier than those by Shem Tov.[171]

The sources consulted for these comparisons are the translations of Maimonides' medical works which are being published as part of the project 'Maimonides' Medical Works' mentioned above. I also consulted Moses Ibn Tibbon, *Sefer Ẓedat ha-Derakhim*. Of the many manuscripts testifying to its popularity in Jewish circles I consulted MS Munich 19 which was copied in 1552.[172]

---

168 M.S. Spink and G. Lewis, *Albucasis. On Surgery and Instruments*. A definitive edition of the Arabic text with English translation and commentary (Publications of the Wellcome Institute for the History of Medicine. New Series. Volume XII, London 1973).

169 J. Grimaud and R. Lafont, *La chirurgie d'Albucasis*, texte occitan du XIVe siecle, (Montpellier 1988).

170 For the manuscript cf. Zotenberg (ed.), *Catalogues des Manuscrits*.

171 For an extensive discussion of the question of the authors consulted by Shem Tov and the authors influenced by him see G. Bos, *The Creation and Innovation of Medieval Hebrew medical terminology: Shem Tov Ben Isaac, Sefer ha-Shimmush*.

172 See M. Steinschneider, *Die hebräischen Handschriften der K. Hof- und Staats-bibliothek in München*^{2} (Munich 1895).

A final introductory note concerns the faithfulness of the translator in adhering to the original text. Hebrew translations of medical texts in general closely follow the original text. Only rarely does one find additions of a personal nature. A remarkable example of such a personal addition and witness to the religious identity of the translator can be found in Book 1, ch. 47 where Shem Tov translates the Arabic عند نهاية الشعر (about the hairline) as במקום הנחת תפלין (where where one places the Tefillin).[173]

List of Terms

אבר: האבר המושל = Arab. العضو الرئيس: 'the major organ'; cf. II:40 (SP fol. 215a; SL 321,13): ויהיה הצמח לפעמים קרוב מאבר מושל שהמאחר לדקרו וממתין עד שיתבשל יזיק לאותו האבר המושל (Or if the tumour be near a major organ, if you delay the opening of it until it ripens you will damage that major organ).[174] In addition to האבר המושל, Shem Tov has האבר הראשי (II:86; SP fol. 225a; SL 555, 24), and אחד מן האיברין השרים (for عضو رئيس; SP fol. 225b; SL 557, l. 52). N translates Arabic العضو الرئيس as האבר הראשי and Z as האבר השרי (MA 25:70). M (BIZ 9:8) translates the plural الأعضاء الرئيسة as האברים הראשים.

אגודה: אגודות. This term features with the following meanings: 1. Arab. عقد: 'nodules'; cf. II:27 (SP fol. 202b; SL 269, 1): בהוצאת האגודות אשר תקרנה בשפתים (on the extraction of nodules occurring on the lip). The same Arabic term is translated as קשרים by M (BIZ 23:1); 2. Arab. تعقّد : 'callus'; cf. III:20 (SP fol. 236b; SL 781,1): ברפואת האגודות המתהוות בעקבות קצת השברים (On the treatment of the callus that remains from a fracture); 3. Arab. غدد: 'buboes'; cf. L 2231, s.v. غدّة: 'A ganglion; i.e. any hard lump in the tendinous parts'; cf. II:36 (SP fol. 214a; SL 301, 3): לפעמים תקרנה בגרון אגודות דומות אל האגודות אשר תקרנה מחוץ (Sometimes there occur in the throat buboes [called 'tonsils'], which resemble the buboes occurring externally. The Arabic غدد is translated by N as גדרים or גידים and by Z as גלנדולי or גרנגולי (MA 1:8); 4. Arab. سلع: 'cysts' (= אגודות הבשר); cf. II:41 (SP fol. 215a; SL 329, 3): יקרו בעור הראש צמחים קטנים והם ממיני האגודות יקיפום קרומות הם להם נאדות דומים לזפק התרנגולת (Small swellings form in the scalp, which are of the various kinds of cyst, contained within membranes which form a capsule to them like the crop of a chicken); see SG Alef 38.

---

173 See below s.v. חלל העורף.

174 The English translation is that by Spink-Lewis unless indicated otherwise.

אגודות הבשר :- = Arab. سلع : 'cysts'; cf. 2:45 (SP fol. 216a; SL 343, 1): שער מ"ה בבקיעה על מיני אגודות הבשר (Chapter forty-five. On incision for various kinds of cyst). Cf. SG Alef 38 and below s.v. תלולית.

איכול: אִכּוּל = I. Arab. آكلة: 'gangrene' (cf. D 1:31, s.v. أكلة: 'gangrène, chancre, ulcère'; cf. I:52 (SP fol. 208a; SL 155, 2–3): האיכול אמנם הוא הפסד מתפשט באבר ויאכלנו כאכילת האש העצים היבשים (Gangrene is a creeping corruption of a limb, consuming it as fire consumes dry wood); II. Arab. أكال 'irritation'; cf. II:96 (SP fol. 231a; SL 657, 20): ומהם מי שימצא חכוך בפניו ובמצחו וחשיכות ואיכול בעיניו (some have an itching in their face and forehead and a dimness and irritation in their eyes). Hebrew איכול is only attested in Ben Yehuda (BM 205) as occurring in medieval literature in the sense of 'itching'. It features in N for Arab. أكلة (corrosion/ canker/ cankerous sore), whereas Z has אוכלת or חולי (MA 3:109; 7:60; 9:105; 12:32; 16:7). See as well MD 188, s.v. 'corrosion'.

אליה = Arab. ألية : 'buttock'; cf. 4:14 (SP fol. 235b; SL 757, 14–16): אך הדוקו ראוי להיותו על זה התאר והוא לכרוך על השבר במצנפת גסה שלש כריכות או ארבע ולהעדיף ממנה מותר ואחר כך לקפול השוק עד שוב העקב אצל שרש האליה (As to the bandaging, you should wrap a firm broad sash three or four times [two or three times SL] round the fracture [of the femur], leaving some over; then bind the leg up so that the heel is brought to reach the root of the buttock). Hebrew אליה, i.e. fat tail (BM 241) in the sense of 'buttock' is a non-attested semantic borrowing from the Arab. ألية which has both meanings (cf. L 87).

אומץ המעים: אֹמֶץ = Arab. اعتقال الطبع: 'constipation'; cf. II:81 (SP fol. 223b; SL 515, 31–2): והפלחים יקרו הרבה מצד נגוב הצואה ואומץ המעים (Fissures often arise from dryness of the faeces and from constipation). Hebrew אומץ המעים is a non-attested term derived from לאמץ את המעים (to constipate) which is attested in Maimonides, *Hilkhot De'ot* 6:4; cf. BM 287–8. N and Z translate the Arabic synonym احتباس البطن as עוצר הבטן (MA 9:55). M translates the Arabic synonym احتباس الطبيعة as עוצר הטבע (MZ fol. 91b).

אִסָּר or **אֱסָר** = Arab. رباط: 'ligament'; cf. II:88 (SP fol. 226b; SL 583, 2–5): כשנתחדש צמח במקצת האיברין הבשריים וארך זמנו עד שקבץ מוגלא ואחר נתבקע או שדקרוהו ויצא כל מה שהיה בו מן המוגלא ונשאר המקום ריקן ככיס והעור אשר עליו כבגד שכבר נתדקדק ולא הגיע אל ההפסד לגמרי לעשות רושם בעצם ולא בעצב ולא באסר (When an abscess occurs in any of the fleshy parts and becomes chronic and eventually collects pus, and then it breaks open or is perforated, and all the contained matter comes out and the site is left hollow, like a vessel, and the overlying skin thinned like a rag, but the suppuration has not gone so far as to involve bone or tendon or ligament). Hebrew or Aramaic אסר is only attested in Rabbinic literature in the sense of 'band, chain, vow of abstinence'; cf. JD 57, and DA 32 for the Aramaic term). In addition to אסר Shem Tov uses קשירה for رباط; cf. II:86 (SP fol. 225b; SL 563, 103). N and Z translate Arab. رباط as קשור, קשורים, קשירה (MA 1:8, 9–11; 3:21, 52; 7:33; 15:29, 40, 47, 66, 69, 70; 23:18; 25:36, 51, and M as קשרים (BIZ 15:5).

אפר: אפר העינים = Arab. رمد: 'ophthalmia'; cf. II:95 (SP fol. 228b; SL 629, 34–6): והשני ורידין אשר בשתי הרקות תועלת הקזתם לכאב הצלחתא הישנה והכאב הקשה ואל אפר העינים המתמיד והגרת המותרות הנשפכות החדות אל העינים (The section of the two arteries in the temples gives relief for chronic migraine and severe headache and constant ophthalmia and the flow of acrid superfluities into the eyes). Hebrew אפר העינים, a loan translation of the Arab. رمد, is not attested in the current dictionaries. Both N and Z did not have a Hebrew equivalent for the Arabic term, as N transcribed it as רמד, and Z used both רמד and the Romance equivalent לגניא or לַגְנַיֵּיא (MA 9:31; 12:22; 19:16; 22:39; 23:70; 24:20). See as well KS 114–15.

אצבע: אצבע קטנה = Arab. خنصر: I. 'little finger'; cf. III:12 (SP fol. 235a: SL 747, 13–14): ולהיות האצבע הקטנה למטה מכל האצבעות (and the little finger downmost); II. 'little toe'; cf. II:95 (SP fol. 230b; SL 655, 284–5): ואם לא ימצא ולא יראה לחוש כלל ראוי להקיז קצת סעיפיו והם הנראים בגב הרגל בין אצבע קטנה והשני לו (and if you do not find it [i.e. the sciatic vein] or it is in no way palpable, then venesect one of its branches, which will be seen on the surface of the foot between[175] the little toe and the fourth toe). Hebrew אצבע קטנה is not attested in the current dictionaries.

אצילה = Arab. إبط: 'axilla'; cf. I:25 (SP fol. 205b; SL 77, 1): שער כה' בכוית האצילה (Chapter twenty-five. On cauterization of the axilla). The Hebrew term features in the Bible in the sense of 1. joint and 2. cubit (cf. KB 81–2). Ben Yehuda also gives several references to its occurrence in medieval literature in the last sense only (BM 368). N translates the Arabic إبطان as אצילים and Z as שחי (MA 7:21; 10:15). M (MZ fol. 90a) translates Arabic إبطان (BZ 147, l. 678) as השחיים.

175 'between the little toe and the fourth toe': 'towards the fourth toe and the little toe' SL.

אצילי = Arab. إبطي: 'axillary'; cf. II:95 (SP fol. 228b; SL 627,13–14): והבאסליק הוא בזרוע למטה מן הגיד האמצעי לעמת הלב ויקרא גם כן האצילי ויקראוהו עם הארץ גיד הבטן (then the basilic vein; this is the one situated on the inner side and is termed also the axillary vein, but popularly it is called the 'belly-vein'). Hebrew אצילי is attested in BM 369 as featuring in Nathan's translation of Ibn Sīnā's *K. al-Qānūn*.

אשך: האשך הבשרי = Arab. الأدرة اللحميّة: 'a fleshy hernia'; II:63 (SP fol. 219b; SL 435, 1): שער ס"ג בבקוע על האשך הבשרי ורפואתו (Chapter sixty-three. On cutting for a fleshy hernia and its treatment).

-: האשך הזמורי = Arab. الأدرة التي مع دالية: 'hernia with varix'; II:64 (SP fol. 220a; SL 439,1): שער ס"ד ברפואת האשך הזמורי ר"ל אשר יהיה עם זמורה (Chapter sixty-four. On the treatment of hernia with varix). Cf. entry זמורה below.

-: האשך המימי = Arab. الأدرة المائية: 'a watery hernia'; cf. II:62 (SP fol. 219a; SL 425, 2).

-: האשך המעיי = Arab. الأدرة المعائيّة: 'intestinal hernia'; II:65 (SP fol. 220a; SL 441,1).

-: האשך הרוחיי = Arab. الأدرة الريحيّة: 'flatulent hernia'; II:66 (SP fol. 220a; SL 447,1).

The term אשך only features in the current dictionaries in the sense of 'testicle'; cf. BM 416. Another term for 'hernia' used by Shem Tov is פיתקא (see below). Both N and Z have בקיעה for Arabic أدرة (MA 9:123). Masie (MD 351) mentions the following synonyms for 'hernia': שבר, שברון, פרץ, בקיע.

בדק: בדק עצמו = Arab. تبرّز: 'to open one's bowel'; i.e. to defecate; cf. II:81 (SP fol. 2223a; SL 513, 9–11): ורפואת הטחורים אשר יהיו מבפנים לצוות אל החולה לבדוק עצמו ולהרגיל העיצום עד שיבלוט פי הטבעת ויראו היבלות (The treatment of internal piles: bid the patient open his bowel and bear down until the anus opens out and the swellings are disclosed to you). בדק עצמו is a non-attested Hebrew term coined after the Aramaic בדיק נפשיה; cf. SD 187. N translates Arab. تبرّز as הוציא בציאה and Z as יצא מנקב פי הטבעת (MA 9:64).

בית: בית הפרשות = Arab. فضاء: 'perineum'; cf. II:80 (SP fol. 220a; SL 503, 8–9): ולפעמים יהיה מהם טחורים כשיהיו בבית הפרשות מפולשים אל כיס מקוה המים ואל מעבר השתן (Sometimes also there are fistulae occurring in the perineum which penetrate to the urinary bladder and to the urethra). Hebrew בית הפרשות is not mentioned in the current dictionaries. It is attested in BIR in a quotation from *Sefer ha-Orah* (Part 2, [67], Din Niqqur, beginning with: Heshiv R. (ed. S. Buber, 1905): בית הפרשות שלו שקוראים קודי"ל (Its perineum, that is its QWDYL).[176] In addition to this term Shem Tov uses ריקות to render Arab. فضاء; cf. below.

בליטה = Arab. نتو: 'protuberance'; cf. II:16 (SP fol. 211b; SL 233, 31–3): אמנם בליטת בשר ראש העין אם תהיה הבליטה מזקת העין נזק מכוער ראוי לתלות הבליטה ההיא בחכה ולחתוך ממנה קצתה מבלי רבוי חתוך פן תתחדש הגרת הדמעות (As for a protuberance of flesh in the angle [of the eye], if it causes great hurt pick it up with a hook and cut part of it away, with not too big an incision lest there be a flux of tears). Hebrew בליטה only features in a medical sense in BM 549 in a quotation from Meir Aldabi, *Shevilei Emunah* which was completed in 1360.

בעבע: נתבעבע הצמח = Arab. تقرّح: 'to break out in open ulceration'; cf. Introduction (SP fol. 201b; SL 5, 32–3): וראיתי רופא אחר דקר צמח סרטני ונתבעבע הצמח אחר ימים (And I saw another doctor incise a malignant tumour; after some days the place broke out in open ulceration). The root בעבע only features in the dictionaries in the sense of 'to bubble'; cf. BM 569. N translates Arabic تقرّح as התחבל or השחין and Z as התחבל, חבל or התנגע (MA 6:72; 23:46); M (BIZ 13:3) translates the Arabic أقرح (to ulcerate) as לנגע. See also צמח below.

בֶּתֶק = Arab. فتق: 'opening; rupture'; cf. II:65 (SP fol. 220a; SL 441, 2–4): שער ס"ה ברפואת האשך המעיי. התחדש זה האשך יהיה מבקוע יקרה בקרום הנמתח על הבטן לעמת עיקרי הירכים וישפך המעי מן הבתק ההוא אל אחד מן הבצים (Chapter sixty-five. On the treatment of intestinal hernia. This hernia is due to a split occurring in the membrane stretched from the hypogastrium over the belly in the region of the groin. Through this opening the bowel descends upon one of the testes). Hebrew בֶּתֶק is only attested in Ma'agarim (שמעון/סליחות: אלה ברכב, סליחה <שו' 30> / מסירה). N translates Arab. فتق in the sense of 'hernia' as בקיעה and Z as בקיעה בלטין קְרְפַּטוּרָא (MA 9:123). M also has בקיעה (MZ fol. 86a).

176 'QWDYL', derived from Latin cauda is old French 'coueril': 'région où commence la queue' (FEW 2-1:523a).

גְזֵרָה = Arab. قَطْع: 'incision'; cf. II:95 (SP fol. 228b; SL 627, 29–31): ואחר להרים היד בגיד ובעור כלפי מעלה ולגזור הגיד עם העור לשנים ולהיות הגזרה שתי אצבעות מצומצמות (then lifting with your hand both vessel and skin make an incision dividing both skin and vein; the length of the incision should be about two fingers side by side). Hebrew גזרה is not attested in the sense of 'incision' in the current dictionaries; cf. BM 744: 'form, figure; balcony; derivation'. N translates Arab. قَطْع as חתך, לחתוך, חתיכה and Z as חיתוך, לחתוך (MA 15:10, 13, 14, 19, 25, 36, 40, 48; 24:54; 25:72), and M as לחתוך (BIZ 10:2).

גיד (fol. 203a1; 206b1) = 1. Arab. عرق: 'vessel' or 'vein'; cf.I:35 (SP fol. 206b; SL 103, 4): הגיד אשר יגר ממנו הדם (the vessel whence the blood comes), and II:95 (SP fol. 228b; SL 625,1): הקזת הגידים (venesection). 2. Arab. شريان 'artery'; cf. II:42 (SP fol. 215b; SL 333,10). Next to גיד Shem Tov uses הגיד הנח for Arab. وريد: 'vein' (II:52; SP fol. 217a; SL 377,16) and וריד for Arab. شريان 'artery' (see below). And cf. the introduction (SP fol. 201a; SL 3,14) where Shem Tov uses הגידים הדופקים והנחים for Arab. العروق النوابض والسواكن 'arteries and veins'. The term גיד is subsequently used by Z for Arab. عرق 'vessel, vein, artery', while N uses עורק (MA passim), just like M (26:2). See as well SG Gimmel 28. 3. Arab. قضيب 'penis'; cf. II:70 (SP fol. 220b; SL 454, 5–7): אמנם בנשים הוא מין אחד ויהיו למעלה מן הקיבה על הזקן התחתון כבצי אדם קטנים בולטים לחוץ האחד מהם כגיד האדם והבצים כבציו (There is also one kind [i.e. of hermaphrodites] among women, in which there is, above the female pudenda, on the pubes, what resembles the male organs. These are small indeed, but protuberant, one being like the penis and the two others like testicles); for its meaning of 'penis' in Rabbinic literature; cf. DA 76; JD 234. For a summary account of all its meanings see E. Lieber, *Asaf's Book of Medicines*, 238, n. 42.[177]

177 E. Lieber, 'Asaf's Book of Medicines: A Hebrew Encyclopaedia of Greek and Jewish Medicine, Possibly Compiled in Byzantium on an Indian Model', in J. Scarborough (ed.), *Symposium on Byzantine Medicine* (Dumbarton Oaks Papers. Number 38, 1984, Washington 1985), 233–49.

-: הגיד המדני = Arab. العرق المدني: ‘the Medina vein’ = dracunculus medinensis; cf. II:91 (SP fol. 227b; SL 601, 1): בהוצאת הגיד המדני (On the extraction of the Medina vein).[178] MD 233 has: דרקונית מדינה.

-: גיד הראש = Arab. القيفال: ‘the cephalic vein’; cf. II:95 (SP fol. 229a; SL 633, 84–5): ושני הגידים אשר תחת הלשון תועלת הקזתם אחר הקזת גיד הראש אל החניקה אשר תהיה בגרון וחלי ערלתו ותחלאי הפה (The two veins under the tongue: their venesection is, after section of the cephalic, of good effect in the quincy arising in the throat from disease of the uvula, and diseases of the mouth). Hebrew גיד הראש is not attested in the current dictionaries. N transcribes the Arab. قيفال as קיפל or translates it as Latin ספליקא, and Z has Latin ציפליקה or גיד הראש הנקרא ציפאליקה (MA 12:23, 33, 36; 25:11).

גלגל = Arab. لولب: ‘speculum’ (see WKAS 1795: ‘a surgical instrument’); cf II:77 (SP 222a; SL 484, 3): זאת צורת גלגל לפתוח בו הרחם (Speculum for opening the entrance of the womb). Hebrew גלגל is not attested as a medical instrument in the current dictionaries; cf. BM 763–5.

גלד: הגלד הענבי = Arab. الطبقة العنبية: ‘uveal membrane’; cf 2:21 (SP 212a; SL 249, 2): כשתקרה בליטה (= בקיעה) בגלד הענבי (When a rupture befalls the uveal membrane). Hebrew גלד features in the Bible in the sense of ‘skin’ (KB 1:191); in Rabbinic literature as ‘coating, skin; thickness’ (JD 1:245), and in medieval literature as ‘peel’ (for instance of an onion) (BM 770). In the sense of membrane it is not attested in the current dictionaries; however, Kaufmann (KS 86) refers to a passage in *Tiqqunei ha-Zohar* fol. 15b, where we find the same term as גלידי. For an extensive discussion of the different terms used for the membrane(s) of the eye cf. Kaufmann, ibid., 85–7. For Hebrew ענבי ‘grapelike’ cf. BM 4575; Kaufmann, ibid., 90–2. N translates Arab. الطبقة العنبية as הכתנת הענבית and Z as הכת<נת> השכבית, הכת<נת> הענבי, הקרום הענבי.

גלידה = Arab. التحام ‘adhesion’; cf. II:63 (SP fol. 219b–220a; SL 435, 17–19): ואם תהיה הגלידה בין כלום מן הקרומות או במה שיש בין הכיסים ראוי להפריד כל הגלידה ההיא ולחתכה חתיכות חתיכות עגולות (But should the adhesion have formed somewhere inside the membranes or in the space between the vessels, then

178 For this disease cf. the extensive discussion in Gerrit Bos, *Qūsṭā ibn Lūqā's Medical Regimen for the Pilgrims to Mecca*. Edited with Translation and Commentary. (Leiden 1992), ch. 14.

you must free the adhesion as a whole and cut it away with a circular incision). Hebrew גלידה is not mentioned in this sense in the current dictionaries. In the sense of a bodily defect it is attested in BIR in a quotation from *Sefer ha-Ittur* (*Sha'ar sheni*, *hilkhot sheḥitah*, *daf* 30, *'ammud* 2) composed by Isaac b. Abba Mari of Marseilles (1120?–1190?). In the Enẓyklopediah Talmudit (vol. 6, cols. 68–71) we find גלודה defined as a defect (spec., missing skin, whether due to abbrasion, injury or disease) that renders an animal terefah (ritually unclean). In Rabbinic literature we find Aram. סירכא in the sense of 'adhesion, cohesion', esp. of the lobes of the lung; cf. JD 1028.

גְּנוּחַ = Arab. ربو 'asthma' cf. II:96 (SP fol. 231a-; SL 659, 35–6): אמנם נתינת הרבידות על המקום הנקרא אל כאהל והוא אמצע הצואר הוא תמורת הקזת הגיד הנקרא אל אכחל...והקזת הבאסליק ולפיכך יועילו מן הגנוח וצרות הנשימה וקריעת כלי הנשימה והשעול והמלוי (Now as to the application of cupping-vessels to the interscapular region: it is instead of venesection of the median and basilic veins; so it is effective for asthma and dyspnoea and for rupture of the organ of respiration, and for cough and pletora). Hebrew גְּנוּחַ, derived from גנח 'to groan, esp. 1. to sigh heavily under an attack of angina pectoris; 2. to cough and spit blood' (JD 259), is not attested in the current dictionaries. N translates Arab. ربو as גניחה and Z as שעול or הרימפלי הנקרא בערבי רבו ובלעז אַסְמוֹ (MA 2:25; 8:19; 22:30; 23:78).

גרב = Arab. جرب 'granular conjunctiva; i.e. trachoma'; cf. II:95 (SP fol. 229a; SL 631, 54–5): ושני הגידים אשר בראשי העינים תועלת הקזתם לתחלאי העינים מן הגרב והאדימות והגידים המסתבכים האדומים הנקראים בלשונם סבל (Venesection of the two lachrymal veins gives relief in diseases of the eyes such as granular conjunctiva and inflammation and pannus). גרב features in BM 830 as 1. scabies, and 2. an affection of the eye in a quotation from Nathan ha-Me'ati's translation of Ibn Sīnā's *K. al-Qānūn*. N and Z also translate or transcribe Arab. جرب as גרב (MA 15:24).

גרגורים: גרגור = Arab. غراغر: 'gargles'; cf. I:6 (SP fol. 204a; SL 31, 5): כשירפא הרופא זה המין מן הנטייה במיני הג'ירא פיקרא והעיטושים והגרגורים (When this kind of deformity [i.e. twisted mouth] has been treated with electuaries, errhines, and gargles) (see as well below s.v. הטפה). BM 831 refers to the term גרגורים as featuring in the Hebrew translation of Ibn Sīnā's *K. al-Qānūn fī al-ṭibb,* by

Nathan ha-Me'ati. In addition to this term, Nathan uses ערעורים while Z has the Romance גרגריזמו (MA 3:11, 87); cf. SG Gimmel 14. MD 317 refers to the term גרגור as featuring in *Sefer ha-Refu'ot* by Asaph ha-Rofe.

גרגתני = Arab. ناصور: 'fistula'; cf. I:17 (SP fol. 205a; SL 56,1): שער י"ז בכוית הגרגתני אשר יקרה בראש העין (On cauterization of a fistula in the angle of the eye). Hebrew גרגתני originally means 'a wicker or network in the wine or oil press' and has a secondary meaning of 'the scarry and lifeless surface of a healed up wound, eschar' (JD 264; cf. Low XLV: 'keloidosis'). N transcribes Arab. ناصور as נאצור and Z translates it as Romance פישטולא (MA 15:29, 44). Cf. SG Gimmel 19.

גרד = Arab. جرد: 'to strip'; cf. I:17 (SP fol. 205a; SL 59,17–18): ואם עברו עליו ארבעים יום ולא נרפא ראוי לתת עליו הסם החד האוכל עד שיתגלה העצם ולגרדו על מה שיבא זכרו מן המלאכה במקומו (And should forty days have passed and it does not heal, apply a sharp corrosive ointment so as to expose the bone, and strip it as will be explained in the appropriate chapter). The Hebrew term normally means to 'scratch, shave', cf. BM 834. In the sense of 'to strip, to lay bare', a semantic borrowing from the Arabic cognate, the Hebrew term is not attested in secondary literature.

גרה = Arab. ترقوة: 'collar-bone'; cf. III:5 (SP fol. 235a; SL 721,1): בחבוש הגרה כשתשתבר (On the repair of a broken collar-bone). The Hebrew term is the general name of that part of the body which extends from the neck to the chest (JD 266; BM 836) and features in Rabbinic literature; cf. SG Gimmel 27. The Arabic term is transcribed by N as תרקוה and translated by Z as קטולה, קטיולה (MA 6:55, 57; 7:54; 12:27; 15:62). According to Goyanes (*Medieval Hebrew anatomical names*, pp. 197–8) there was no traditional name for the clavicle in Hebrew and the Academy of the Hebrew Language chose the name בריח 'bolt', translation of the Greek κλείς. He adds that Razi (i.e. Shem Tov Ben Isaac, the translator of the *K. al-Manṣūrī*) has the term עצם הגרה 'neck bone'; see as well SR 20, n. 104, 107.

גרירה = Arab. نَشْر: 'saw-cut'; cf. II:86 (SP 225b; SL 562, 108–10): וראוי להיות הגרירה במגרה למעלה ממקום ההפסד מעט פן יהיה בתוך העצם הפסד ולא יראה מחוץ לחוש ויביא הצורך לגררו במגרה פעם שנית (The saw-cut should be made a little above the site of the disease in case there should be disease in the cavity of the bone that is not apparent on the surface, which might compel you to carry out the sawing a second time). Hebrew גרירה is only attested in Rabbinic literature in the sense of '1. scraping off; 2. dragging, pulling, moving an object without lifting; 3. carrying with, involving' (JD 269).

גָּרָע = Arab. فاصد: 'one who carries out venesection'; cf. II:95 (SP 229b; SL 637, 105–6): וצריך הגרע להיותו נזהר בעת הקזתו כי יש תחתיו וריד ואם פשע ויוסיף בתחיבת המסמר ויחתוך הוריד ההוא תתחדש ממנו רעיפת דם (When one venesects it [i.e. the basilic vein] one must be careful and wary of it, for beneath the vein is an artery, so that if one is inaccurate and sticks the scalpel in too far one will cut the artery and cause a haemorrhage). Hebrew גָּרָע is attested in Rabbinic literature in the sense of 'scraper, barber, in gen. low class surgeon, bloodletter' (JD 271).

גרר: גרר במגרה = Arab. نشر: 'to saw'; cf. II: 86 (SP fol. 225b; SL 561, 91–2): ואחר כך שבתי וגליתי העצם שנית למעלה מן הגלוי הראשון ומצאתי ההפסד הגיע אל העצם וגררתי במגרה מה שנראה לו גם כן מן ההפסד ההוא (Then I again uncovered the bone, above the first opening, and found the corruption co-extensive with the bone. So again I sawed away as much of the corruption as I could see). Hebrew גרר is only attested in the sense of 'to saw' in Rabbinic literature; cf. JD 272. See as well Ma'agarim, s.v. גרר.

דבשת = Arab. حدبة (SP fol. 202b; SL 129, 1): 'hunchback'; cf. I:43 (SP fol. 202b; SL 129,1): בכוית התחלת הדבשת (on cauterization of early hunchback). The Hebrew term is a hapaxlegomenon featuring in Isa. 30:6 meaning 'hump' (of a camel); cf. KB 1:213.

דליות = Arab. دوالي: 'varices' (cf. UW 346-347, s.v. κιρσός); cf. II:90 (SP fol. 227a; SL 595, 2): הדליות הם גידים נפתלים עבים מלאים מהעדפות שחוריות מתחדשות ברוב איברי הגוף (Varices are thick twisted veins filled with melancholic superfluities); the same Hebrew term features in M (BIZ 22:1): נגעים נקראים דליות (swellings called 'varicose veins'). BM 944–5 only refers to this term in the singular form דָּלִיּוּת as featuring in Nathan ha-Me'ati's translation of Ibn Sīnā's *K. al-Qānūn*; MD 761 also refers to a singular דלית. See as well זמורה below.

דרדני = Arab. لثة: 'gums'; cf. II:95 (SP 229a; SL 633, 77): וגידי השפה והפסד הדרדני והשחין הרע (and rotting of the gums). דרדני (= Persian *darîdanî* meaning 'fragments', derived from the Persian verb *darîdan*? [VL 1:844]). is not attested in the current dictionaries. Cf. SG Dalet 11. N translates Arab. لثّة as לסתות and Z as חניכים (MA 9:123).

הברה = Arab. قرقرة: 'borborygmi' (cf. UW 239, s.v. ἐμπνευμάτωσις: 'Blähung, Aufblähung'); cf. II:90 (SP fol. 220a; SL 441, 12–14): ולפעמים הלך במעי הצואה ותתעכב שמה ויהיה ממנה אבדת החולה שהיא תחדש כאב קשה והברה וכל שכן בעת הסחיטה עליו (Sometimes also the excrement comes down with the bowel and gets held up there, and this involves the patient's death, for thence arises an intractable pain and borborygmi, specially when pressed down). Hebrew הברה is not attested in a medical context in the current dictionaries. N translates Arab. قرقرة as קרקור or קרקורים בבטן and Z as קולות or רעם (MA 6:52; 7:55).

הגלדה = I. Arab. اندمال: 'healing'; i.e. of a wound; cf. II:89 (SP fol. 227a; SL 593, 34–5): והדבקות אשר יקרה אל האצבעות קצתם בקצתם יתכן היותו מזמן היצירה או מהגלדת חבורה או משרפת אש וזולתם (As for webbing of the fingers one to another, that occurs very frequently. It may be either congenital or from the healing of a wound or burn or the like); II. Arab. التحم 'to mend'; cf. III:1 (SP fol. 232a; SL 679, 18–681, 20): וידוע שהעצמות הנשברות כשתהיינה באנשים כחושים וזקנים לא יתכן חבורם והגלדתם על טבעם הראשון לעולם לנגוב עצמותם וקשים (You should know that fractures occurring in mature (Shem Tov, 'skinny') and old people cannot join and mend into the original condition, on account of the dryness and hardness of their bones). Hebrew הגלדה is only mentioned as a modern term in EM 343. N translates Arab. اندمال as הבראה and Z as חיות (MA 23:44). Arab. التحم is translated by N as דבק or התדבק and by Z as התרקם or עלה בשר or התרקם בשר (MA 15:46, 56, 62; 25:17).

הִדּוּק = Arab. شدّ: 'ligature'; cf. I:56 (SP fol. 208a–b; SL 165, 18–20): והמתעסק בהפסקתו בקשירה או בהדוק בבגדים או בתת הדברים השורפים וכיוצא בהם לשוא יטרח כי לא יועילנו כלל אלא במקרה (But those who try to stop bleeding with ligatures or cloths, or by the application of caustics and the like, never stanch it by these means, or at least very rarely). Hebrew הִדּוּק features in both Jastrow and Ben Yehuda as a synonym of חִדּוּק in the sense of 'that which is squeezed in to fill a gap, repair, insertion' (JD 451, BM 1042). Even-Shoshan mentions it in the sense of 'a strong binding, connection' (EM 346) (trans. Bos).

הזלה: הזלות הראש = Arab. نظلات: 'catarrhs'; cf. II:95 (SP fol. 228b; SL 627, 22–3): אמנם שני הגידים אשר אחורי האזנים תועלת הקזתם מהזלות הראש הישנות ומכאב

הצילחתא ומן השחין הנקרא בלשונם אל סעפה ומן השחין הרחב הישן אשר יהיה בראש (Venesection of the two veins behind the ears. Bleeding from both of these will give relief in cases of chronic catarrh, migraine, chronic foul pustules and scabs of the head). Hebrew הזלה is attested in BM 1065 as featuring in Meir Aldabi, *Shevilei Emunah* which was completed in 1360; the term features as הזלת החוטם for Arabic زكمة 'rheum' in Moses Ibn Tibbon's Hebrew translation of Maimonides' *Regimen of Health* (BMR 4:21). N translates Arab. نزلة as נזילה, נזל, נזלים and Z as נזילה, נזל, ריומא (MA 3:66; 6:41; 8:38; 9:7; 13:13; 16:30).

הזרה = Arab. ذرور: 'powder'; cf. II:17 (SP fol. 211b; SL 235,11–12): וכשישלם החתוך ויכלה כל הבשר ראוי למלא העין במלח שחוק או להטיף בו מן ההזרה האדומה (And when you have finished your incision and removed all the chemosis, fill the eye with powdered salt or instil the red powder…). The Hebrew term is a non-attested verbal noun from the root זרה, to winnow, disperse (BM 1395–6). M translates the Arabic ذرور as אבק (BIZ 26:4): אבק ידביק החתוך מן הסכין והסיף (A powder which heals a cut of a sword or knife).

הטפות: הטפה = Arab. تنطيلات: 'embrocations'; cf. II:37 (SP 214b; SL 309, 30–1): ואחר כך לגמע במים קרים ולרפא מחוץ בהטפות ומבית בגרגורים עד שיבריא (Then let him rinse his mouth with cold water and do you treat with external embrocations and gargles within, till he is well). Hebrew הטפה is not attested in this sense in the current dictionaries, cf. BM 1070. N translates Arab. تنطيل as יציקה and Z as נטילות (MA 13:38). M (MZ fol. 100b) translates the Arab. نطولات (fomentations) (BZ 225, l. 1394) as טבילות.

הטפחה = Arab. نطول: 'fomentation'; cf. III:26 (SP fol. 237a; SL 797, 19–797, 21): ואם לא ישוב במה שזכרתי ותהיה לשמיטה מעת שנתחדשה ימים רבים ראוי להשיב החולה במים חמין במרחץ ולהרגיל ההטפחה המרפה והמרככה (If it [i.e. the dislocation of the humerus] is not reduced by the means we have stated, being a dislocation of many days' standing, the patient should take a hot bath and use relaxing and softening fomentations). Hebrew הטפחה is not attested in a medical context in the current dictionaries. Ben Yehuda (BM 1070) adduces the term in the sense of 'moistening' in a quotation from Kalonymus b. Kalonymus' ס' הצמחים; i.e. the Hebrew translation of Nicolaus Damacenus'

De plantis which Kalonymus completed in the year 1314.[179] N translates the Arab. نطولات as יציקות and Z as טיבולים (MA :2, 42; 21:63), while M (MZ fol. 100b) has טבילות. See as well entry הטפיה.

המעדה = Arab. إزلاق: 'fomentation'; cf. III:27 (SP fol. 237b; SL 805, 19: המעדת הפרק (the lubrication of the joint). Hebrew המעדה is not attested in this sense in the current dictionaries, cf. BM 1117. Cf. the disease called زلق or زلق الأمعاء; i.e. lientery, which is translated by N as המעדת המעיים or מעידת המעיים, and by Z as המעדת המעיים or חלקות המעיים (MA 22:36; 23:80, 90, 93, 94), while M translates the Arabic as הגרת המעים (BMR 4:22). Cf. SG He 11.

העדפה: העדפות = Arab. فضول: 'superfluities'; cf. Introduction (SP fol. 202a; SL13, 41): ומה שיזדמן בגופו מהתקבץ ההעדפות בו (and from the formation of a mass of superfluities in the body). The Hebrew term is attested in Ben Yehuda (BM 1143), referring to Nathan ha-Me'ati's Hebrew translation of Ibn Sīnā's *K. al-Qānūn*. The same Arabic term is translated by N as מותרים/מותרות and by Z as ליחות (MA passim); M (BIZ 17:4) translates the Arab. term as מותרות.

השבה: השבת השברים = Arab. جَبْر: 'setting of bones'; cf. Introduction (SP 201a; SL 7, 50). The Hebrew term is not attested in the current dictionaries. In addition to this term Shem Tov uses the term לחבש; see entry חבש.

התלבדות = Arab. تَلَبُّد: 'granulation'; cf. II:86 (SP fol. 225b; SL 555, 39–557, 42): והיא להסתכל ואם יהיה הגרגתני נכר קרוב ובמקום בטוח רחוק מפרק או מעצב או מוריד או מגיד נח או אחד מן המקומות אשר זכרתי ראוי לבקעו על מה שקדם מן המלאכה ולהסיר מה שיש בו מן ההתלבדות[180] (See if the fistula is obvious and accessible, or in a harmless situation far removed from a joint[181] or nerve or artery or vein or any of the other places I have mentioned to you. Then lay open the fistula by the method I have described and fetch out of it all the granulations…). Hebrew התלבדות is not attested in the current dictionaries. See לבד below.

---

179 On this work traditionally ascribed to Aristotle cf. H.J. Drossaart-Lulofs and E.L.J. Poortman, *Nicolaus Damascenus. De plantis. Five translations* (Amsterdam 1989).

180 ההתלבדות: emendation editor ההתלבדוד MS.

181 'joint or nerve or artery or vein': translation Bos. SL translate: 'joint or vein or artery or tendon'.

התלהבות = Arab. التهاب: 'inflammation'; cf. II:74 (SP 221a; SL 465, 8–10): ראוי להתבונן ואם יהיה כאב הצמח בתחלתו חם עם דפיקה והתלהבות וקדחת ויהיה אדום אין ראוי למהר לדקרו (You should inspect it, and if the pain of the tumour is acute from the outset, with pulsation and inflammation and fever, and it is red, then do not be in a hurry to open). As 'inflammation', a semantic borrowing from the Arabic التهاب, the Hebrew term is not attested in the current dictionaries; cf. MD 1232: 'enthousiasm'. N translates Arab. ملتهب as נלהב and Z as מתלהב (MA 6:47). M translates Arab. التهاب as התלהבות (BIZ 12:1).

התפוצצות = Arab. تفتّت: 'shattering'; cf. III:15 (SP 235b; SL 761, 2–3): פלך הארכובה לא יקרה בו שבר אלא על המעט אבל יקרה לו הריסוק ואם יקרה לו שבר אולם יהיה בקוע או התפוצצות (You should know that the patella is rarely fractured, but crushing often occurs. If a fracture does happen to it, it will be either a splitting or a shattering). Hebrew התפוצצות is attested as modern in EM 438 in the sense of 'explosion'.

וריד = Arab. شريان: 'artery'; cf. I:4 (SP 204a; SL 27, 11–12): ועתיד אני עוד להביא זכרון הנהגת הרעיפה אשר תקרה מן הוריד (We shall later on mention a treatment for accidental haemorrhage of the artery). The term וריד is attested as 'jugular vein' in Rabbinic literature and as a synonym of גיד in Nathan ha-Me'ati's Hebrew translation of Ibn Sīnā's *K. al-Qānūn* (BM 1272). See גיד above.

זיכום = Arab. زكام: 'defluxion'. Cf. II:86 (SP fol. 225a; SL 553, 2–4): ידוע שכל חבורה או מורסא כשתתישן וארך זמנה ושבה שחין ולא הגלידה והיה יוצא ממנה מוגלא תמיד בלי הפסד תקרא על הכלל גרגתני באיזה אבר שתהיה ואני קראתיה זיכום (You should know that any wound or tumour, when it becomes old and chronic, and turns into an ulcer, and does not heal over, but discharges pus chronically and constantly, is generally called a fistula, in whatever part of the body it may be; but we call it a defluxion). Hebrew זיכום is a hebraised form not attested elsewhere. N transcribes the Arab. term as זכאם and Z translates it as Romance קטרא and ריומא (MA 19:35); cf. SG Zayin 5.

זמורה = Arab. دالية: 'varix' (see UW 346–7, s.v. κιρσός: 'Krampfader, Varize'); cf. II:64 (SP fol. 220a; SL 439, 2–3): הזמורה היא צמח נפתל קצת פיתול דומה לאשכול עם רפיון הבצים ותקשה על החולה התנועה והטיול וההליכה (A varix is a twisted tumour resembling a cluster of grapes, with relaxation of the testicles, which makes movement and exercise and walking difficult for the patient). Hebrew

זמורה is not attested in this sense in the current dictionaries, cf. BM 1349–51. See entry דליות above.

זנב: זנב העין = Arab. ذنب العين: 'the outer corner of the eye'; cf. I:13 (SP fol. 204b; SL 45, 6–7): והרוצה להוסיף יוכל לכוות כויה אחת בכל צד מזנב העין על קצות גב העין במכוה קטן (and, if you are compelled to add more, one cauterization on the side of the outer corner of the eye at the end of the eyebrow, with a small cautery). The Hebrew term is not mentioned in the current dictionaries, but features in BIR as זנב עינו in an attestation from Maimonides, *Mishneh Torah*, Hilkhot Bi'at ha-Mikdash, Ch. 8, Halakhah 6. In SG Zayin 8 the same Hebrew term features for Arab. الماق الصغير i.e. 'the outer angle of the eye'. See as well ראש העין below.

זקן: הזקן התחתון = Arab. العانة: 'pubes'; cf. II:54 (SP fol. 217b; SL 383, 14, 385, 1–2): ואחר כך להסתכל ואם יהיה התילד השקוי מצד המעי ראוי להרחיק הביקוע מן הטיבור שעור שלש אצבעות מלמטה עד למעלה מן הזקן התחתון (Then consider; and if the dropsy arises from the region of the intestines then you should make an incision three fingers' breath directly below the umbilicus, above the pubes). For the Hebrew term meaning 'pubic hair' and attested in Rabbinic literature see BM 1383; N translates the Arab. عانة as ערוה or גב הערוה and Z as ערוה or עצם הערוה (MA 1:67; 3:2, 76; 16:12); see as well SG Zayin 11, and below s.v. חומש and קיבה.

חִבּוּשׁ = I. Arab. جَبْر: 'setting (of a fracture)'; cf. III:0 (SP fol. 232a; SL 677, 1–2): זה החלק גם כן גדול הצורך והתועלת במלאכה והוא חבוש השבר והשמיטה המתחדשים בעצמות (This [third] part of the book, too, is an essential necessity in the practice of medicine; it concerns the setting of the fracture or dislocation occurring in bones); II. Arab. علاج: 'treatment'; cf. III:2 (SP fol. 233a; SL 701, 22): וחבוש השבר הוא להסתכל בתחלה אל מקרי החולה (As to the treatment of the fracture: begin by paying attention to the patient's symptoms). חִבּוּשׁ is only attested as modern in EM 495 in the sense of 'binding, bandaging'.

חבל: חבל הזרוע = Arab. حبل لذراع: 'cord of the arm'; i.e. the vena cephalica pollicis and the vena cephalica antibrachii (cf. DKT 816) cf. II:95 (SP fol. 230a; SL 651, 244–5): והקזת חבל הזרוע יוקז תמורת גיד האכחל והבאסליק כשלא ימצאו או כשיהיו נעלמים כי הוא מורכב מהם (Section of the cord of the arm: this is cut in place of the median and basilic veins when these are not to be found or hidden; for this vein is composed of those two). Hebrew חבל הזרוע, a loan-translation of the Arab. حبل لذراع, is not attested in the current dictionaries.

חבש: חִבֵּשׁ = Arab. جَبْر: 'repair'; cf. I:13 (SP fol. 232b; SL 693, 129–30): וזאת התחבושת אין בה כח לחבש (Now this plaster has no power of repair), and ibid. (SL 693, 132): תאר תחבושת מחבשת העצמים הנשברים (Description of a plaster for the repair of a broken bone). Hebrew חִבֵּשׁ is not attested in this sense in the current dictionaries. In the Bible we find the term in the sense of 'to bind up (wound)'; cf. KB 289; BM 1439. See as well entries מחבש and השבה.

-: **התחבש** = Arab. انجبر: 'to mend'; cf. III:12 (SP fol. 235b; SL 751, 45–6): וידוע ששבר הזרוע יתחבש בשלשים יום או בשנים ושלשים על הרוב ואפשר שיחבש לפעמים בשמנה ועשרים יום (You should know that this fracture of the arm mends in thirty or thirty-two days, and sometimes in twenty-eight). Hebrew התחבש is not attested in this sense in the current dictionaries.

-: **נחבש**: see previous entry.

חוט: החוטים הנתלים = Arab. معلاق: 'suspensor' (see DKT 828: 'suspenseur, Canal déférent', however, according to SL 426, n. 1 it is rather the spermatic cord); cf. II:63 (SP fol. 219b; SL 434, 12–16): וזה המין לפעמים יתכן לבקע עליו ועל יתר מיני הבשר והוא לבקע עור הבצים ואחר כך למשוך הביצה למעלה ולהוציאה מן הקרום הלבן ולהפריד החוטין הנתלין מן הכיסים ולקשור הכיסים ולחתך החוטין אחר הפרדם מכל צד מצדי הביצה (It is sometimes possible to cut down on this kind and also on the other fleshy tumours thus: make an incision in the skin of the testicles; then draw the testicle upward and out of the tunica albuginea, and free the suspensor from the vessels). See as well II:69 (SP fol. 220b; SL 453, 11): החוטין הנתלין הבצים מהם (the spermatic cord). The Hebrew term does not feature in the current dictionaries.

חומש = Arab. خاصرة: 'hypochondrium' (cf. L. 748: 'flank, i.e. each of the ilea'); cf. I:33 (SP fol. 206a; SL 99, 7–8): ואם תראינה הלחויות רבות והחולה סובל הכויה ראוי לכוותו על הזקן התחתון כויה אחת וכויה אחרת על כל חומש (And if you see that the humidities are superabundant, and the patient fit to tolerate it, then make one cauterization over the groin and one over the hypochondrium). The Hebrew term חומש features in the Bible (KB 331) in the sense of 'abdomen, belly'. In medieval medical literature we find the Arabic خاصرتان, i.e. 'both the flanks', translated as שני הכסלים by N and as שתי החלצים by Z (MA 24:29).

The *Ma'aseh Tuviyyah* by Tobias Ben Moses Cohn (1652–1729) has ירכתי הבטן for the same bodily part (following MD 370).

חָח = Arab. صنّارة: 'hook' (see UD 67 s.v. ἄγκιστρον (cf. LS 10: 'fish-hook; hook of a spindle; surgical instrument'): 'Angelhaken'; cf. II:6 (SP fol. 209b; SL 193, 11–12): ואם יצא החצץ במלקחים טוב ואם לא צריך להשתדל להוציאו בחח דק כפוף מעט (If it [i.e. something that has fallen in the ear] comes out with the tweezers, good. But if not, try to extract it with a fine hook slightly curved). Hebrew חָח is attested in the Bible as 1. thorn, hook (through nose or cheek of animals or captives to lead them away); 2. fibula. For its occurrence in Rabbinic literature in the same meaning(s) see Ma'agarim. It is not attested in the sense of 'hook' as a surgical instrument.

חטה: שני החטים = Arab. اللوزتان: 'tonsils'; cf. II:43 (SP fol. 215b; SL 337, 6–7): אבל אשר יש להם צמח חם בפה או בגרון או בשני החטים כשלא יהיה חולי בקנה מחייב לבקע השפוי כובע פחד החניקה (But in those with an abscess in the mouth, throat, or tonsils, and when there is no disease in the windpipe itself, you must employ laryngotomy to avoid the mischief of suffocation).The unattested Hebrew term חטים corresponds to Aramaic חיטי, Sing. חיטתא, the meaning of which is uncertain, but which is traditionally explained as 'a cartilage on the trachea'; cf. SDA 453. The regular Hebrew term for 'tonsils' is שקדים (see II:36; SP fol. 214a; SL 301, 4).

חיק: חיק העין = Arab. شحمة العين: 'orbit'; cf. II:93 (SP fol. 228a; SL 613, 42–3): והוצאתי חץ אחר ליהורי שכבר נפל לו בחיק עינו תחת העפעף השפל (Also I extracted from a Jew another arrow that had pierced the orbit beneath the lower eyelid). Hebrew חיק העין is not attested in the current dictionaries.

חלב: החלב המכסה את הקרב (fol. 207b) or **החלב אשר על הקרב** (fol. 217a) = Arab. ثرب (SL 135, 2; 377, 3): 'omentum'; cf. I:45 (SP fol. 207b; SL 135, 2: כשיקרה בתק בעקרי הירכים ויתגללו קצת המעים או החלב המכסה את הקרב אל האשכים (When a rupture occurs in the groin, and part of the intestine and omentum comes down into the scrotum). The Hebrew term is not attested in the current dictionaries. Both N and Z translate the Arabic ثرب as חלב (MA 1:54, 55, 60; 9:102).

חלוקה = Arab. لزوجة: 'glutinous property'; cf. III:1 (SP fol. 232a; SL 679, 15): וכשיתחיל העצם הנשבר להרפא ראוי ליזון במזונות זנין מזון עב שיש בו חלוקה (When the broken bone has begun to mend, the patient should be nourished with very nourishing food, fat, strong, having some glutinous property). Hebrew חלוקה is not attested in this sense in the current dictionaries. N translates Arab. لزوجة as דבקות and Z as דבקות or דבקות בלעז וויסקוזיטט (MA 6:44; 7:13, 19; 9:75; 10:6, 23; 13:6; 15:52). M (BIZ 20:2) likewise has דבקות.

חלחל: מתחלחל = Arab. متخلخل: 'porous'; cf. II:96 (97 MS Paris BN héb. 1163) (SP fol. 231a; SL 663, 68–70): כי מי שיהיה רך הבשר מתחלחל הנקבים ראוי לשרטו שריטה אחת לא יותר פן יתבעבע המקום (The person who is tender of flesh and porous of skin you should scarify once only, not more, lest the place ulcerate). Hebrew התחלחל is attested in JD 466 in the sense of 1. to be perforated, to be open, esp. to be permeated by poison; 2. to tremble. N translates Arab. الأجسام المتخلخلة (porous bodies) as הגשמים הרפים והרכים and Z as הגופות הרכות והנרפות (MA 3:6). Arab. تخلخل (to become porous) is translated by N as היה מחולחל and by Z as ספג (MA 7:12).

חלל: חלל הזנב = Arab. عجز الذنب: 'the last vertebra of the tail' (cf. DKT 821, s.v. عاجز: 'sacrum'); cf. I:47 (SP fol. 208a; SL 143, 11–14): אמנם אם הגדמות כבר נתפרסם על החולה ויראה ראייה מבוארת ראוי אז לכוותו אלו הכויות הנזכרות בראש...וכויה אחת גדולה על העצה אצל חלל הזנב (If the elephantiasis be widespread over the patient and appears obvious, you should give him, as well as the cauterizations described for the head...a great one over the coccyx by the last vertebra of the tail). The Hebrew term is not attested in the current dictionaries.

חלצים: תחת החלציים = Arab. تحت الشراسيف: 'beneath the false ribs, i.e. hypochondria'; II:76 (SP fol. 221b; SL 477, 13–14). The Hebrew term is not attested in the current dictionaries. N translates the Arab. ما دون الشراسيف as מה שלמטה מצדי הכסלים or תחת צדי הכסלים or מה שתחת הכסלים or למטה מן הכסלים and Z as מה מתחת הצלעות or מתחת הצלעות or מתחת החלצים or למטה מהחלצים (MA passim).

חלל: חלל העורף = Arab. نقرة القفا: 'nape of the neck'; cf. I:47 (SP fol. 208a; SL 143, 3–8): והרוצה לכוותו צריך להתבונן אם בתחלת הגדמות רפאוה במה שזכרתי במאמר החלוקה ולא כהה הנגע ויש חשש על החולה שמא ישלוט ההפסד על כל מזגו ראוי לכוותו על הראש חמש כויות האחת באמצע הראש המפורסמת והשנית למטה ממנה לעמת המצח במקום[182] הנחת תפלין ושתי כויות על שני הקרנים ואחת מאחוריו בחלל העורף (When you

182 במקום הנחת תפלין: عند نهاية الشعر SL (Arabic text).

wish to use the cautery, first look, and if the elephantiasis be in the early stage and you treat it with those remedies advised in the section but it does not abate and is not arrested, and you fear lest the corruption spread over the patient's whole constitution, then give him five cauterizations on the head: the well-known one in the middle of the head; the second one lower than that, toward the forehead, where one places the Tefillin,[183] and two at the temples; and one behind, on the nape of the neck). The Hebrew term does not feature in the current dictionaries; Cf. the Aramaic חללא דבי צואר below s.v. פרק הצואר.

חללות = Arab. تقعير: 'concavity'; cf. III:31 (SP fol. 238b; SL 821, 2–3): פרק כף הירך ופרק השכם אמנם תקרה להם השמיטה בלבד ולא יקרה להם מה שיקרה ליתר הפרקים מן ההסרה המעוטה וההחללות (A complete dislocation alone is sustained by the hip and shoulder joints; they do not sustain the lesser displacements with concavity [as do the other joints]). Hebrew חללות features as modern in EM 544 in the sense of 'emptyness, hollowness'. The common medieval term for 'concavity' was קערירות (cf. BM 6051), while the term חללות was also used by Z; thus he translates مقعّر الكبد (the concave side of the liver) as חללות הכבד, while N translates it as מקוער הכבד or קערירות הכבד or קערורית הכבד (MA 6. 57; 9. 70, 75; 10. 48; 11. 14; 25. 12).

חניקה = Arab. خوانيق: 'quinsy' (cf. UW 373, s.v. κυνάγχη: 'Halsentzündung, Bräune'; ibid., p. 654, s.v. συνάγχη: 'Halsentzündung, Diphtherie'); cf. II:95 (SP fol. 229a; SL 633, 84–5): ושני הגידים אשר תחת הלשון תועלת הקזתם אחר הקזת גיד הראש אל החניקה אשר תהיה בגרון וחלי ערלתו ותחלאי הפה (The two veins under the tongue: their venesection is, after section of the cephalic, of good effect in the quincy arising in the throat from disease of the uvula, and diseases of the mouth). Hebrew חניקה is not attested in a medical sense in the current dictionaries; cf. BM 1652. Arab. خوانيق is translated as מחנקים by N and as אסקיננציאה, חנק, חנק הנקרא אשכווינננציאה by Z (MA 12:33; 22:20; 25:11).

חֲרִיכוּת = Arab. حرقة: 'burning'; cf. II:87 (SP fol. 226b; SL 579, 31–2): ואני מודיע בדמיון שקרה לאדם ברגלו זה המקרה בעצמו אשר אגיד וזה כי נתחדש ברגלו שחרות עם חריכות דומה לשרפת האש (Now I shall relate to you an example; what I am going to tell you is exactly what happened to a certain man's foot. He had a blackening of the foot, with a burning like that of fire). Hebrew חֲרִיכוּת is

183 The Arabic reads: عند نهاية الشعر (about the hairline).

only attested once in Ma'agarim, namely in a Yoẓer by Khalaf Ibn Saʿīd (<29 ש> יוצרות לשבתות השנה: אדוניה וקרוא').

טיחה = I. Arab. لطوخ: 'poultice' (see WKAS II, 691–2): 'medicine to be rubbed in, oitment, paste, unguent, salve'; cf. II:20 (SP fol. 211b; SL 247, 4): ואחר לתת על העין טיחה עשויה מאקקיא ואילווא ולבונה וכרכום (then put to the eyes a poultice made of acacia and aloes and olibanum and saffron);[184] II. Arab. طلاء 'liniment'; cf. III:1 (SP fol. 232b; SL 685, 72). The Hebrew term טיחה features as 'plastering' in the current dictionaries, cf. JD 530; BM 1868. In SG Tet 6 it is mentioned as a synonym of Arabic طلاء. N translates Arabic لطوخ as יציקה, Z as מישרה (MA 9:18), and M as טיחה; cf. BIZ 18:4: והנה אמר גליאה שתתרפא הבהרת אחר נקיון הגוף בשיטוח המקום בסיד ויושם עליו אחר זה טיחה נעשית באנאקירד הוא בלאדור וקבשיא ואלואי ואקסייא וליטרגום וחומץ (Galen has ordered to treat *baraṣ* once the body has been cleansed by smearing quicklime on the spot. Then one should apply a liniment that has been prepared from marsh-nut, pepperwort, aloe, acacia, litharge and vinegar).

טפח: הטפיח = Arab. نطل: 'to foment'; cf. II:1 (SP fol. 209a; SL 173, 18–19): ואחר הבקיעה ראוי להוציא הלחות כלו ולהדק הבקיעות בבגדים וכלונסות ואחר להטפיחם ממעלה ביין ושמן עד היום החמישי (After incising, draw out all the humidity; then bind up the incisions with pads and bandages; and over the bandages foment with wine and oil till the fifth day). Hebrew הטפיח is mentioned in the current dictionaries as featuring in Rabbinic literature in the sense of 'to moisten, to wet' (cf. JD 546; BM 1906). It is not attested in a medical context in the sense of to 'foment' a part of the body. N translates Arab. نطل as יצק, Z as טבל or משח (MA 9:6; 15:17), and M (MZ fol. 98a) as טבל. See as well entry הטפחה.

טרפשה = Arab. حجاب: 'pleura' (see DKT 816: 'diaphragme'); cf. II:92 (SP fol. 228a; SL 611, 26–7): ואם יפול החץ על הטרפשה אשר בחזה יהיה קרוב מן הצלעות הקטנות (But if the arrow strike the pleura then it will be close to the small ribs). טרפשה, Hebrew parallel to Aramaic טרפשא (cf. SDA 519: 'membrane'; Low LIV: 'diaphragma'), or to Hebrew טרפש (BM 1935) does not feature in the current dictionaries. It is attested in BIR as featuring for the first time in the *Teshuvot* (Part 2, Yoreh Deʿah, Siman Ḥet, starting with: Katav ha-Ṭur) of Isaiah Ben Mali Di Trani (*c.* 1200–before 1260). N translates حجاب as

184 The Arabic reads: عنزروت (sarcocolla).

המסך המבדיל הנקרא דיאפרמה, אל חגאב הוא , Z as טרפש, טרפשא, טרפשה,טרפשות, מסך דיאפרמא, מסך (MA 1:2, 28–30; 3:40, 55, 98; 6:53; 9:85; 10:60; 12:29; 16:15, 16; 23:9a, 67; 24: 7), and M as המסך המבדיל (MZ fol. 86a).

התישן :ישן = Arab. أزمن: 'to become chronic'; cf. II:81 (SP fol. 223b; SL 515, 31–2): והפלחים יקרו הרבה מצד נגוב הצואה ואומץ המעים וכשיתישנו ולא יועיל בהם סם ראוי לגרדם בפי המסמר גרע (Fissures often arise from dryness of the faeces and from constipation. If they become chronic, and medical treatment is unavailing, you should scrape them with the edge of a scalpel). Hebrew התישן is only attested in Rabbinic literature in the sense of 'to be chronic'; cf. BM 2188. N translates Arab. أزمن as ישן, and Z as האריך (MA 9:123).

כד = Arab. أفطس 'blunt'; cf. II:85 (SP fol. 224b; SL 539, 23–6): וזאת צורת הכלי יהיה קצהו האחד הכפוף חד והקצה האחר בלתי חד והקצה הדק לא יהיה בדקות מסמר הגרע אבל יהיה כד מעט (This is the form of the instrument. The curved side should be sharpened, but not the other; the slender extremity should not be as slender as a scalpel, but rather blunt). Hebrew כד is attested in Rabbinic literature in the sense of 'arched or rounded' (JD 612). Cf. SG Kaf 30.

כווץ = Arab. تشنّج: 'spasm'; cf. I:6 (SP fol. 204a: SL 31, 3–4): וראוי להזהר שלא לכוות כלל הנטייה המתחדשת מן הנגוב וכווץ העצב (But cauterization [of the twisted mouth] is to be carefully avoided in that type which is due to dryness or spasm of the nerve [tendon SL]). Hebrew כווץ is derived from the root *KWṢ* 'to curl, shrink' (JD 625; SDA 556) which features in Rabbinic literature. The term features as קווץ in BM 5824 (cf. the synonym קויצה in BM 5826–7). N translates the Arab. تشنّج as כויצה, Z as כווץ or התכווץ (MA passim), and M (BMR 4:18, 27) as קיווץ; cf. KZ 65; SG Kaf 21.

כוליא = Arab. كلية: 'kidney'; cf. I:37 (SP fol. 206b; SL 107, 2–4): כשיתחדש בכליות כאב מרוח עבה או קרירות ויחסר בסבתם המשגל ראוי לכוותו במתניו על עצם הכליות כויה אחת על כל כוליא וכוליא במכוה המסמרי אשר קדם זכרו (When pain strikes the kidneys from chill or heavy vapour, and the patient's sexual vigour is impaired thereby, you should burn him right over the kidneys, once on each kidney, with the claviform cautery mentioned before). The term כוליא is Aramaic for Hebrew כליה; cf. Levy, *Chaldäisches Wörterbuch*, p. 365.[185]

---

185 J. Levy, *Chaldäisches Wörterbuch über die Targumim und einen grossen Theil des Rabbinischen Schriftthums. Unveränderter Neudruck nach der Dritten Ausgabe* (Köln 1959).

כיס: כיסים = Arab. أوعية: 'vessels (i.e. blood vessels)'; cf. II:4 (SP fol. 209b; SL 187, 22): הכיסים היורדים מן הראש אל העינים (the vessels passing from the head down toward the eyes). Hebrew כיס features in Rabbinic literature in the sense of 'receptacle, pouch, bag, purse, fund' (JD 633), and 'scrotum, crop (of a bird), cyst' (Low LVI). It also features in medieval medical literature as הכיס הקטן (i.e. gall bladder) and הכיס הגדול (i.e. urinary bladder); cf. BM 2347. N translates Arab. أوعية as כלי or כלים, while Z translates it as גידים or כיסים (MA 6:5, 91; 7:12; 10:40; 18:8; 23:1; 25:52).

-: כיס מקוה המים = Arab. مثانة: 'urinary bladder'; cf. I:38 (SP fol. 206a; SL 109, 2–4): כשיתחדש בכיס מקוה המים חולשה ורפיון מקרירות ולחויות עד שלא יוכל להחזיק השתן ראוי לכוותו כויה אחת למטה מן הטיבור על הכיס במקום שיתחיל שער הזקן התחתון (When there occurs in the urinary bladder a weakness and relaxation due to chill and humidities, so that the patient cannot retain his water, sear him once below his navel, on the bladder, where the pubic hair begins). Hebrew כיס מקוה המים is not attested in the current dictionaries. N translates Arab. مثانة as מקוה and Z as שלפוחית or הכיס של השתן (MA 1:28, 63, 65, 66, 68, 69 and passim). M (MZ fol. 93a) has מקוה just like N.

כלונס: כלונסות = Arab. رفائد: 'pads'; cf. Introduction (SP fol. 201b; SL 5, 25–7): וראיתי אחר מתעסק בזאת המלאכה בכדי חייו אצל קצת קציני ארצותינו ונתחדש לסריס שחור שנשבר שוקו קרוב מן הערקוב ונתחדשה בו חבורה ומהר הסכל בסכלותו והדק השבר על החבורה בכלונסות ובקשישים (I saw another doctor who had a regular salary from one of the high officers of our country. There had occurred to a black boy of his a fracture of the leg near the heel, together with a wound; the doctor rushed in, in his ignorance, and bound up the fracture, over the wound, very tightly, with pads and splints). The Hebrew term features in Rabbinic literature in the sense of 'poles'; cf. JD 640. Both N and Z translate the Arab. رفائد as רפידות (MA 15:65, 69, 70); cf. SG Kaf 24.

כלי: כלי ברזל = Arab. حديد: 'knife'; i.e. surgical knife; cf. II:74 (SP fol. 221a; SL 465, 5–7): וראוי לי שאזכור בזה המאמר הצמח החם אשר יקרה ברחם כשיהיה מן הצמחים המקבצים מוגלא איך תהיה דקירתו בכלי ברזל (But now in this treatise we must mention an inflamed tumour occurring in the uterus of the kind where there is a collection of pus, and the manner of its opening with the knife). Hebrew כלי ברזל, lit., an iron instrument, is not attested in the sense of 'surgical knife', a loan-translation from Arab. حديد, in the current dictionaries; cf. BM 2388–92.

-: כלי נוקב: See **מקבת**.

כף: כף הירך = I. Arab. ورك: 'hip joint'; cf. I:40 (fol. 203a; SL 113, 2–3): לפעמים תשתפכנה לחויות עבות אל כף הירך ותהיינה סבה לצאתו ממקומו (Sometimes harmful humidities reach the hip joint and result in its coming out of its place); II. Arab. حقّ الورك 'the acetabulum of the femur' (SP fol. 231b; SL 667, 109). The Hebrew term כף הירך means 'hip-socket' and features in the Bible and Rabbinic literature (BM 2480–1). The Arabic term is translated by NZ (MA 12:29; 23:14), and M (BMH 6:2) as ירך; see as well SR 34.

כרכשה = Arab. مبعر: 'rectum'; cf. II:80 (SP fol. 222b; SL 503, 5–6): ועוד יהיה ממיני הגרגתני מין מפולש אל הכרכשה ואל המעי או בלתי מפולש (These fistulae may be perforating into the rectum or bowel, or non-perforating). Hebrew כרכשה coined after the Aramaic כרכשא 'large intestines' (cf. SD 603) is not mentioned in the current dictionaries; it features, however, in BIR in an attestation from *Sefer Orḥot Ḥayyim* (הלכות אסורי מאכלות אות פד ד"ה חלב הלב).

כשיל = Arab. فأس: 'pickaxe', i.e. a phlebotome (cf. SL 624, n.1); cf. II:95 (SP fol. 229a; SL 629, 45–7): ואיכות הקזתו על מה שאגיד והוא להדק צואר החולה במצנפת עד שיראה הגיד ואחר לקחת הכלי הנקרא כשיל (Now I shall relate to you the method of cutting [of the vein in the forehead]: you bind the patient's neck until the vessel stands out; then you take the instrument called the 'pickaxe'). Hebrew כשיל features in the sense of 'a carpenter's tool for chipping, axe' in the Bible (KB 502) and Rabbinic literature (JD 675f); it is not attested in the sense of a 'phlebotome'. Cf. SG Kaf 31.

לבד: מתלבד = Arab. متلبّد: 'compact'; cf. II:82 (SP fol. 223b; SL 517, 13–14): והנמלה היא גם כן גרגתני קטן מתלבד עב הגוף הולכת בעומק מאד (A pimple is also a little compact thick prominence on the skin surface, going deep). Hebrew מתלבד, a loan translation of the Arabic متلبّد, is not attested in the current dictionaries; cf. JD 687, s.v. לבד: 'to full, to stamp' and KA 5:6: 'verbinden, befestigen, anschliessen' (to connect, attach). See התלבדות above.

לטש = Arab. جلا: 'to cleanse'; cf. III:2 (SP fol. 233b; SL 711, 105): ובכלל ראוי להרגיל מהם כל סם לוטש בלתי עוקץ (in short, in these cases use drugs whose nature is cleansing not irritating). Hebrew לטש does not feature in this sense in the current dictionaries; cf. EM 810; BM 2667. N translates Arab. جلا as מירק or צחצח, and Z as טיהר or ניקה (MA 9:30, 70, 71; 14:1; 15:24, 57; 17:38; 22:69, 70; 25:8).

לכלך = Arab. لطخ: 'to spread' (see WKAS II, 684: 'to rub, to smear, to whitewash a th., to soil, dirty, stain a th.'); cf. II:13 (SP fol. 211a; SL 223, 9–10): ורטיית הדיאכילון נתכת עם מעט מן השמנים וללכלך בה הפתילה ולרפא בה (and [employ] diachylon plaster which has been previously softened with one of the oils and spread on the packs; and treat it with this). The Hebrew term means 'to soil'; cf. BM 2678. In the sense of 'to spread' it is a non-attested semantic borrowing from the Arabic. N translates the Arab. term as טח or יצק and Z as משח or שם (MA 9:18;22:2), and M as משח (BMR 4:12).

לעוסות: לעוסה = Arab. مماضغ: 'medicaments to chew'; cf. I:10 (SP fol. 204a; SL 39, 5). The Hebrew term does not feature in the current dictionaries; however, it is possible that the term should be emended as לעיסה, לעיסות which features in Rabbinic literature in the sense of 'chewing' (cf. BM 2713–14).

מגולל is 1. Arab. مشرّب: 'soaked'; cf. I.16 (SP fol. 204b; SL 53, 25–6): ולתת תחת העין צמר גפן מגולל בחלבון ביצה וראש החולה בחיק הרופא (place also under the eye cotton wool soaked in egg-white; the patient's head being in your lap); 2. Arab. مبلول (damped); cf. I:17 (SP fol. 205a; SL 56, 5–6): ואחרי כן לשית צמר גפן מגולל בחלבון ביצה או בריר שיליות (=שיליום) על העין (Then place on his eyes cotton wool damped with egg-white or mucilage of psyllium seeds); 3. Arab. مغموس: 'soaked'; cf. I:22 (SP fol. 205b; SL 71, 8): ולתת עליו צמר גפן מגולל בחמאה (and apply cotton wool soaked in butter). The term is possibly used by Shem Tov after Biblical ושמלה מגוללה בדמים (Isa. 9:4). Both N and Z translate the Arabic مبلول and likewise مغموس as טבול (MA 9:118; 15:45 and 15:65).

מגופה = Arab. غطاء: 'lid'; cf. II:78 (SP fol. 222b; SL 497, 4): ואם לא ראוי לקחת קדרה ולהגיף אותה ולנקוב במגופה נקב ולתת בה העשבים הפותחים פי הרחם (But if not, then take a pot, close it,[186] pierce a hole in the lid, and put in it herbs that will open the womb). Hebrew מגופה is only attested in Rabbinic literature in the sense of 1. bung, stopper; 2. the clay used for sealing wine vessels (JD 726–7).

186 'close it': missing in the Arabic text.

מַגְזֵר = Arab. مقطع: 'chisel'; cf. III:2 (SP fol. 233a; SL 703, 40–1): וזה יהיה על אחד משני פנים מן המלאכה. האופן האחד הוא לכרות העצם בתחלה במגזר דק צר הפה אשר זאת צורתו. ואחר כך להרגיל מגזר אחר אחר זה המגזר יותר רחב ממנו מעט וזאת צורתו (This [i.e. the trepanning and removal of the bone] may be done in one of two ways. One way is to cut the bone with a fine-bladed chisel, this being the figure of it. Then after this one employs another chisel, a little broader). Hebrew מגזר is not attested in medical literature (cf. BM 2781, and Aram. מגזרא DA 223). It features especially in the combination מגזרי ברזל in Heykhalot literature; cf. Ma'agarim, s.v. מגזר.

מַגְזֵרָה: מגזרות = Arab. مقاطع: 'chisels'; cf. III:2 (SP fol. 233a; SL 703, 44–6): ומן הראוי להיות אצל הרופא מגזרות משתנות זאת מזאת וזה להיות קצתן יותר רחבות מקצתן וקצתן יותר קצרות מקצתן ולהיות פיותיהן בתכלית החדוד (You should have by you a number of different chisels, some broader than others and some shorter than others, their tips should be exquisitely sharp). It is possible that Shem Tov considered מגזרות as the plural of מגזר and not of מגזרה as he uses both מגזר and מגזרות but not מגזרה. See previous entry and Ma'agarim, s.v. מגזרה.

מדחה = Arab. مدفع: 'obturator' (see L 892: 'An instrument for impelling, propelling, or repelling…; an instrument used by midwifes for protruding the foetus'); cf. II:6 (SP fol. 210a; SL 199, 60–1: והרוצה להיות המדחה אשר בתוך השפופרת של נחשת עשוי בחכמה הרשות בידו (If you wish, you may make the obturator which goes in the cannula of strong bronze). The Hebrew term is a loan translation from the Arabic, and is not attested in this sense in the current dictionaries.

מזלג = Arab. نشل: 'lancet' (cf. SL p. 626, n. 3); cf. II:95 (SP fol. 229a; SL 635, 101–637, 103): זה המזלג העשוי לבקע בו יש ממנו מין רחב ומין דק כפי רוחב הגידים וצרתם ותוקח ראיה מהם על זולתם והוא אצל הרופאים מפורסם (This is the lancet for making a slit. There are broad and narrow varieties of it according to the breadth or narrowness of the vein. This one indicates what the others are like; it is well known to surgeons). Hebrew מזלג is attested as '(meat) fork (for taking meat out of the cauldron)' (KB 565; JD 755), and as an instrument for taking the child out of the womb (forceps?) (BM 2885). Another term used for 'lancet' is מסמר מזלגי; cf. s.v. מסמר. See as well SG Mem 34.

מְחַבֵּשׁ = Arab. مجبّر: ‘bone-setter’; cf. III:3 (SP fol. 233b; SL 713, 14–15): וזכרו קצת המחבשים מן הראשונים לבלול הפתילות בחמאה ולהחליפן בכל יום ואין נכון אצלי לעשות כן (Certain of the ancient bone-setters suggest that you should soak the pads in butter and change them daily, but I do not think so). Hebrew מְחַבֵּשׁ does not feature in the current dictionaries. See entry חבש.

מחבוא = Arab. مخبأ: ‘sinus’; cf. II:88 (SP fol. 226b; SL 583, 1): ומהנה נתחיב לקראו מחבוא ולא נקרא גרגתני (and hence it [i.e. the abscess] merits the name of ‘sinus’ and is not called a fistula). The Hebrew term is not attested in this sense in the current dictionaries. Arab. Plur. مخابئ is rendered by Shem Tov as מחבואות; cf. II:88 (SP fol. 226b; SL 583,1): המורסות הנקראות מחבואות (abscesses which are called ‘sinuses’ [trans. Bos]).

מחפש is 1. Arab. مدسّ: ‘explorer’; cf. II:45 (SP fol. 216a; SL343, 10–11): וראוי למתחיל ברפואת האגודה לבדוק אותה ולחפשה בתחלה במחפש (When you come to treat the cyst, you should first sound it and examine it with the instrument called the explorer); 2. Arab. مسبار ‘probe’; cf. II:46 (SP 216a; SL347, 8): וזאת צורות מחפשים (And this is the shape of the probes). The Hebrew term does not feature in these meanings in the current dictionaries.

מים: לעשות מי רגלים = Arab. بال: ‘to pass water’; cf. III:18 (SP fol. 236a; SL 771, 6–7): וכשתרצה לעשות מי רגליה ראוי להסיר הצמר גפן בנחת ולהחזירו על הענין הנזכר (and when she wants to pass water gently remove the cotton wool so she may do so). Hebrew לעשות מי רגלים is not attested in the current dictionaries. For Hebrew מי רגלים, featuring in Rabbinic literature as a euphemism for ‘urine’, cf. JD 775.

מימיות = Arab. مائية: ‘serum’; cf. II:96 (SP 231a; SL 663, 71–3): ואם יהיה בדם עובי ראוי לשרטו שתי פעמים בפעם הראשונה לפתוח דרך לדם הדק ומימיותו[187] ובשנית לחטט אחר הוצאת הדם העב (If there be a thickness of the blood he should scarify twice; the first time to make a way out for the thinner blood and serum; and the second time to complete the extraction of the thick blood). The earliest attestation of Hebrew מימיות in the sense of ‘serum’ is from Nathan ha-Me'ati's Hebrew translation of Ibn Sīnā's *K. al-Qānūn* (cf. BM 2971).

מכוה = Arab. مكواة: ‘cautery’; cf. Introduction (SP fol. 202a; SL 15, 56–8): והכויה בו יותר טובה ויותר חשובה מן הכויה בברזל כמו שאמרו אלא שהרופא כשיחמם מכוה הזהב

---

187 ומימיותו: emendation Bos ומימיותיו MS.

לא תתבאר בו חמימותו על השעור המכוון (Cauterization with it [i.e. gold] is indeed better and more successful than with iron, as they have stated; except that when you are heating the gold cautery in the fire you are uncertain when it reaches the desired temperature). The Hebrew term is not attested in the current dictionaries.

-: מכוה סכיני = Arab. مكواة سكّينيّة: 'knife-edged cautery'; cf. II:62 (SP 219b; SL 429, 50–1): ויש שעושין רפואת זה האשך גם כן בכויה חלף מן הבקוע בכלי ברזל והוא לקחת מכוה סכיני דק ולבקע בו עור הבצים (This rupture may also be treated by cautery instead of surgery. This will mean taking a knife-edged cautery and cutting with it the skin of the testicles). The Hebrew term is not attested in the current dictionaries.

מכחול: מכחל = Arab. مرود: 'probe'; cf. I:17 (SP fol. 205b; SL 77, 9–79, 1): שעושין המכוה בעל שלשה שפודין ותהיה תבנית הכויה אז שש כויות ויהיו השפודין על דקות המכחל (The cautery may be of three prongs and then the form of the cauterization will be six burns. The prongs should be of the fineness of a probe). Hebrew מכחול features in rabbinic literature in the sense of 'staff used for painting the eye' (JD 782). N uses Hebrew מכחול to render Arab. ميل which also means 'probe' (MA 9:27).

מכסה: מכסה הבטן = Arab. مراقّ البطن: 'hypogastrium'; cf. II:62 (SP 219b; SL 427, 40–429, 43): ולהכניס בפלחים צמר מן הגזה טבול בשמן זית או בשמן ורד ולתת מחוץ צמר אחר טבול ביין ושמן ולהשטיח על הבצים ומכסה הבטן (and apply to the incisions wool that has been soaked in olive-oil or oil of roses and on that again more wool that has been soaked in wine and oil, and spread that over the testicles and over the hypogastrium). Hebrew מכסה הבטן is not attested in the current dictionaries. In Rabbinic literature we find שיפולי המיעים which is translated as 'the lower part of the abdomen' (JD 1566), 'groin, lower intestines, sexual organs' (Low LXXXIV) or 'hypogastricum' (MD 370). MD (ibid.) also refers to חומש as a synonym (see above).

מלקחים = Arab. كلاليب: 'forceps' (see D 481, s.v. كلاّب); cf. II:77 (SP fol. 222a; SL 487, 12–13): תאר כלי אחר יותר נקל מזה ויותר דק עשוי מהבנים או מברוש על תבנית המלקחים (Another instrument, but smaller and lighter. It is made of ebony or boxwood in the shape of forceps). Hebrew מלקחים in the sense of forceps is attested as 'modern' in EM 956.

מסמר = Arab. مسمار: 'corn'; cf. II:82 (SP fol. 223b; SL 517, 3): המסמר אמנם הוא דבר עגול על עין הגוף דומה לראש המסמר (A corn is a round knob, the same colour as the body and resembling the head of a nail). Hebrew מסמר is only attested in this sense as featuring in Nathan ha-Me'ati's Hebrew translation of Ibn Sīnā's *K. al-Qānūn*, and in Moses ibn Tibbon's חרוזי אבן סינא, i.e. the Hebrew translation of Ibn Sīnā's *'Urğuza fī al-ṭibb* which Ibn Tibbon prepared in 1260;[188] cf. BM 3127.

-: מסמר הגרע = Arab. مبضع: 'scalpel'; cf. I:3 (SP fol. 203b; SL 23, 7): ואחר לבקע מקום הכאב מן הצדע במסמר הגרע (then cut open the side of the pain in the temple with a scalpel). The Hebrew term is attested in Rabbinic literature in the sense of 'a blood-letter's pin' (JD 809); cf. SG Mem 17.

-: מסמר מזלגי = Arab. المبضع النشل: 'lancet'; cf. II:95 (SP fol. 229b; SL 637, 113–14): ולקשור הזרוע ולבקע הגיד בקוע בנטיה במסמר המזלגי כמו שאמרתי (Then bind the arm and cut the vein obliquely with the lancet as we said). Hebrew מסמר מזלגי is not attested in secondary literature. See as well s.v. מזלג.

מסרק: מסרק היד = Arab. مشط اليد: 'metacarpus'; cf. I.44 (SP fol. 207b; SL 133, 15–16): ואם ישארו מן המכאובים באצבעות ראוי לנקוד אותם על כל פרק ופרק נקודה אחת ועל מסרק היד (If the pains remain in the fingers, pierce them once over each joint and once on the metacarpus). The Hebrew term is only attested in medieval medical literature in Nathan ha-Me'ati's Hebrew translation of Ibn Sīnā's *K. al-Qānūn fī al-ṭibb* (cf. BM 3139; MD 462; SR 26, n. 156).

-: מסרק הרגל = Arab. مشط الرجل: 'metatarsus'; cf. II:86 (SP fol. 225b; SL 563, 117–18): ואם יהיה ההפסד במסרק היד או במסרק הרגל רפואתו קשה מאד (If the disease be in the metacarpus[189] or metatarsus it is a very difficult matter treating them). Hebrew מסרק הרגל is only attested as מסרק כף הרגל in BM 3139 as featuring in *'Alilot Devarim*.

מעבר: מעבר השתן = Arab. مجرى القضيب: 'urethra'; cf. II:80 (SP fol. 220a; SL 503, 8–9): ולפעמים יהיה מהם טחורים כשיהיו בבית הפרשות מפולשים אל כיס מקוה המים ואל מעבר השתן (Sometimes also there are fistulae occurring in the perineum which penetrate to the urinary bladder and to the urethra). Hebrew מעבר השתן, lit. passage of the urine, for 'urethra' is not mentioned in the current

188 M. Steinschneider, *Die hebräischen Übersetzungen des Mittelalters und die Juden als Dolmetscher* (Berlin 1893, repr. Graz 1956), 699.

189 'metacarpus or metatarsus': 'carpus or tarsus' SL.

dictionaries, but features in BIR, a.o. in an attestation from *She'elot u-Teshuvot Sho'el we-Nish'al.* Part 1 *Yoreh De'ah. Siman* עא starting with: שאלה כיס.

מעד: לחויות ממעידות = Arab. رطوبات مزلّقة (cf. D 1:600, s.v. *zaliq*: 'glissant, visqueux, gluant'): 'synovial fluid'; cf. I:25 (SP fol. 205b; SL77, 2): כשישמט ראש פרק המרפק הנקרא בלשונם אל עצד בסבת לחויות ממעידות (When the head of the humerus is dislocated on account of the synovial fluid [note: lit. 'lubricating humidities']). For the Hebrew term ממעיד in the sense of 'synovial', possibly a semantic borrowing from the Arabic زلق, see BM 3146 with a quotation from Vidal Ben Lavi's *Sefer Gerem ha-Ma'alot*, i.e the Hebrew translation of a medico-botanical work composed by Joshua ben Joseph ibn Vives Lorki (i.e. of Lorca), a Spanish Jewish physician living around 1400. Cf. entry המעדה.

מקבת = Arab. مثقب 'drill' (see D 1:160: 'trépan, instrument de chirurgie'); cf. II:94 (SP fol. 228a; SL 617, 89–92): ואם לא יצא אחר ימים ראוי לנקוב סביב החץ בעצם עצמו מכל צד במקבת דקה כדי להרחיב לחץ ואחר למשכו (But if it [i.e. the arrow] will not come out after some days, you will have to drill away the bone from all round with a fine drill so as to make room for the arrow; then draw on it). Hebrew מקבת, i.e. 'hammer' (cf. BM 3262) is not attested in the sense of 'drill', a semantic borrowing from the Arab. مثقب, in the current dictionaries. In addition to מקבת Shem Tov uses a non-attested כלי נוקב for Arab. 'drill'; cf. III:2 (SP fol. 332b; SL 705, 57–8): אמנם איכות הנקב סביב העצם הנשבר הוא לתת הכלי הנוקב על העצם ולסובבו עד שיודע שהעצם מפולש (As to the manner of perforation round the fractured bone, you apply the drill to the bone and revolve it with your fingers until you know that the bone is pierced).

מַקּוֹר = Arab. منقاش: 'forceps'; cf. II:50 (SP fol. 217a; SL 373, 11): ואם יהיה הצמח קטון ראוי לחפשו במקור ולחתכו מן השרש (and if the tumour be small take hold of it with the forceps and cut it away by the root). Hebrew מקור means 'beak, a tool for whetting millstones' (JD 830) and features in Rabbinic literature. It is possible that the term was used by Shem Tov in the sense of 'forceps' as a loan-translation of the Arabic منقاش which designates 'an instrument with which variegated, or decorated or embellished, work is done' or 'a kind of tweezers, an instrument with which one extracts, or draws or pulls out or forth, thorns' (L 2840), but also 'an instrument used for whetting millstones' (DAS 3:252). Cf. SG Mem 51.

מְרֻבָּע: מרובע = Arab. متربّع: 'crosslegged'; cf. III:13 (SP fol. 235b; SL 753, 3–6): וכשיקרה אל המסרק שבר או ריסוק ראוי להושיב החולה מרובע ולפניו כסא ולתת היד על הכסא פתוחה (When a fracture or crushing of the metacarpus[190] occurs the patient should sit crosslegged with a chair of the right height in front of him, on which he should put his outstretched hand). Hebrew מרובע in the sense of 'crosslegged' is a non-attested semantic borrowing from the Arabic متربّع.

מַשְׁרֵט: משרטים = Arab. مشارط: 'scarifying scalpels'; cf. II:46 (SP fol. 216b; SL 355, 41): ואלה הם המשרטים אשר יבוקעו ויופשטו בהם האגודות והצמחים והם שלשה מינים גדולים ואמצעים וקטנים (these are the figures of the scarifying scalpels with which you incise and dissect away cysts and tumours. They are of three kinds: large, medium, and small). For the Hebrew term which is not attested in the current dictionaries, cf. MD 643, s.v. מַשְׁרֵט: 'scarificator'.

נחרה: נחרת הגרון = Arab. بحوحة الصوت: 'hoarseness'; cf. I:23 (SP 202a; SL 73,1): שער כג' בכויה מנחרת הגרון וצרות הנשימה (Chapter twenty-three. On cauterization for hoarseness and for constriction of the breath). Instead of the non-attested Hebrew term we find נחירות הקול in Moshe Narboni's *Oraḥ Ḥayyim* (cf. BM 3602),[191] while Arabic بحح is translated by N as צרידות הקול and by Z as חסרון הקול (MA 22:45).

נטייה: נטיית הפה = Arab. لقوة: 'twisted mouth' (see WKAS 2:1134–6: 'paralysis of the facial nerve, facial paresis, paralysis of one side of the face, crooked mouth')[192]; cf. I:6 (SP 203b; SL 31, 1): השער הששי בכוית נטיית הפה. הנטייה הראויה לרפאתה בכויה היא המתחדשת מן הלחה הלבנה על מה שזכרתי בחלוקות החליים (Chapter six. Cauterization of the twisted mouth. The twisting of the mouth which is curable with the cautery is that which arises from phlegm, as we have already noticed in the sections on sicknesses). In addition to this unattested Hebrew term Shem Tov uses the synonym עוות הפה in SG ʿAyin 31. This last term also features in Z while N merely transcribes the Arabic

190 'metacarpus': SL have 'palm of the hand' (كفّ).

191 For Moshe Narboni and his medical encyclopaedia see Gerrit Bos, 'R. Moshe Narboni, Philosopher and Physician: A critical analysis of Sefer Orah Hayyim', *Medieval Encounters* 2/1 (1995), 219–51.

192 See as well: Gerrit Bos, *Isaac Todros on facial paresis*. Edition of the Hebrew text with introduction, English translation and glossary (forthcoming: Koroth).

term as לקוה (MA 20:69), and M has ע(י)קום (BMR 4:18, 27). See as well KZ 65.

נער = Arab. صبّي: 'pupil (of the eye)' (see L 1650: 'A youth, boy, or male child'…; also signifies 'The pupil of the eye'); cf. II:23 (SP 212a; SL 253, 11): וראוי לתת שעור הכנסת המקדיח כעין שעור הרוחק אשר יהיה מן הנער אל סוף השחרות והוא עגול העין (The depth the needle goes in should measure as the distance from the pupil to the edge of the iris, which is the corona of the eye). The Hebrew נער in the sense of 'pupil of the eye' is a non-attested semantic borrowing from the Arabic. Cf. entry ראות below.

נִקְבָּס: See entry קבס.

סוף: סוף הפרשות = Arab. عجز الذنب: 'coccyx'; cf. II:80 (SP fol. 222b; SL 503, 10). Hebrew סוף הפרשות is not attested in the current dictionaries. In addition to this term, Shem Tov uses the term עצה for 'coccyx' (see below).

ספוגי: See **עצם**.

עגול: עגול העין = Arab. اكليل: 'corona'; cf. DKT 814: 'Couronne. Région ciliaire'; cf. II:23 (SP fol. 212a; SL 253, 7–8): ואחר לשית פי המקדיח קרוב מעגול העין כעובי המכחל בלובן העין עצמו מצד זנבו (Then put the tip of the needle near the corona, about the thickness of a probe away, onto the white of the eye itself, on the side of the lesser canthus); see as well previous entry. Hebrew עגול העין is not attested in the current dictionaries.

עָצָה = Arab. عصعص 'coccyx'; cf. II:96 (SP fol. 230b; SL 661, 54–5): והרבידא האחת הנתנת על העצה תועיל מטחורי פי הטבעת ומן השחין השפל ר"ל מן השחין אשר יהיה בירכים ולמטה (The application of a single cupping-vessel to the coccyx is effective for haemorrhoids of the anus and ulcers of the lower abdomen). Hebrew עצה is mentioned as featuring in the Bible in the sense of 'coccyx of the sheep' (KB 866), and in Rabbinic literature and medieval medical literature (a.o. *Sefer Asaph*) in the sense of 'backbone, spine' (JD 1102, BM 4636). However, Bar-Sela and Hoff pointed out that in *Sefer Asaph* the term apparently means 'sacrum',[193] while Singer-Rabin (SR 41–2, 320) translate the term as it features in Vesalius, *Tabulae Anatomicae Sex*, as 'coccyx'. In addition to עצה, Shem Tov uses the term סוף הפרשות for 'coccyx' (see above).

---

193 A. Bar-Sela and H.E. Hoff, 'Asaf on Anatomy and Physiology', *Journal of the History of Medicine* 20 (1965), 358–89, p. 383.

עצום: עיצום = Arab. تزحُّر: 'bearing down', i.e. contracting the abdominal muscles; cf. II:75 (SP fol. 221b; SL 473, 45–8): ואם לא יצא העובר תקח רגליה ביחד ותנענעם בחזקה ואחר כך תסחוט למעלה מן החלציים מעט מעט עד שיעלה העובר למעלה ואחר תכניס המילדת ידה ותשוה העובר מעט מעט ותצוה האשה שתרגיל העיצום עד שיצא (and if the foetus does not come out then, take both her feet and shake them violently; then press upon her costal margin until the foetus ascends; then let the midwife insert her hand and put the foetus in the right position, very gently, and bid the woman bear down, until the infant is born). Hebrew עיצום is only attested in Rabbinic literature in the sense of 1. strength, and 2. surety (cf. JD 1073–4). See as well entry בדק עצמו above.

עצם: התעצם = Arab. تزحّر: 'to bear down', i.e. to push, to contract the abdominal muscles and diaphragm during childbirth; cf. II:75 (SP fol. 221b; SL 473, 59): ואחר כך תצוה שתתעצם ותעטישנה בחנינא כי העובר יצא (then bid her bear down, and with ptarmica make her sneeze; then the foetus will come forth). Hebrew התעצם is only attested in Rabbinic literature in the sense of 1. to be closed; 2. to be headstrong towards one another; 3. to fortify each other.

עצם: העצמים הספוגיים = Arab. العظام المتخلخلة: 'ethmoid bones'; cf. II:24 (SP fol. 212b; SL 259,14–15): ואם לא יעבור הלחות על מה שראוי בידוע שבתוכו בשר מת[194] בעליון העצמים הספוגיים לא השיגו הכלי לחתכו (But if fluid does not pass through it as it should, you may know that there is a [polyp] within in the upper part of the ethmoid bones where the instrument could not reach to make an incision). Hebrew העצמים הספוגיים is not attested in the current dictionaries. For ספוגי(י) 'porous' cf. BM 4150.

עקר: עיקרי הירכים = Arab. أربيّة: 'groin'; cf II: 65 (SP fol. 220a; SL 449, 2–3): לפעמים תקרה הפיתקא בעיקרי הירכים כמו שאמרתי ויבלוט המקום (Sometimes there occurs a rupture in the groin as we have said, and the part protrudes). The Hebrew term is not mentioned in the current dictionaries, but it features in BIR, a.o. in an attestation from *Sefer Orḥot Ḥayyim* (הלכות טרפות אות ט' ד"ה ט. המעי). The same Arabic term is translated by N as אורבים (Sing. ארב, cf. BM 376) and by Z as אנגינלייא (MA 15:48). See as well ראשי הירכים.

עקץ: עוקץ החוטם = Arab. طرف الأنف: 'the end of the nose' (see FA 3218:149: 'wing of the nose'); cf. I:47 (SP 208a; SL 143,11–13): אמנם אם הגדמות כבר

194 מת: نابت SL.

נתפרסם על החולה ויראה ראייה מבוארת ראוי אז לכוותו אלו הכויות הנזכרות בראש וכויה אחת על עוקץ החוטם (If the elephantiasis be widespread over the patient and appears obvious, you should give him, as well as the cauterizations described for the head: one at the end of the nose). The Hebrew term is possibly coined by Shem Tov as a loan translation of the Arabic; cf. SG Ayin 38. In addition to עוקץ החוטם we find the same Arabic term translated as עוקץ האף; cf. II:25 (SP 212b; SL 265, 1): ביבלת הצומחת בעוקץ האף (On warts growing on the end of the nose).

ערקה = Arab. علق: 'leeches'; cf. II:97 (SP fol. 231b; SL 675, 2–3): הערקה תורגל ברוב הענינים באברים אשר לא תתכן בהם נתינת הרפידות (leeches are mostly used on those parts of the body to which application of cupping-vessels is impossible). ערקה is a non-attested Hebrew term coined after the Aramaic ערקא 'leech'; cf. SDA 883.

פדלקון = Arab. محقن 'clyster'; cf. II:83 (SP fol. 223b; SL 521, 3): ראוי לעשות הפדלקון מכסף או מנחשת נתך (A clyster may be made of silver or of cast bronze);[195] the term features often in the combination עשית הפדלקון for Arab. حقن; cf. II:59 (SP fol. 202b; SL 407,1): באיכות עשית הפדלקון לכיס מקוה המים (on the manner of irrigating the bladder). The term פדלקון which could not be identified features in SG Pe 36 as a synonym for Arab. حقنة (clyster) and Romance קלשטרי; i.e. O.Occ. or O.Cat. *clisteri* for 'clyster'. N translates Arab. حقنة as חוקן and Z as קרישטרי (= O.Occ. or O.Cat. *cristeri*, *crestiri*, *cresteri* and *cristiri*). M translates the Arab. الحقن الحادّة as קלוחים חדים (BIZ 13:5).

פדלקן: לפדלקן = Arab. حقن 'to irrigate'; cf. II:88 (SP fol. 226b; SL 583, 14–15): ואחר לקחת ממנו כפי הצורך ולטרפו במים ודבש ולפדלקן בו המחבוא (Then take as much as you need and dilute it with water and honey, and with this irrigate the sinus). פדלקן could not be identified.

פטר: הפטיר = Arab. خلّص 'to free'; cf. II:94 (SP fol. 228b; SL 619, 106–9): ואם יהיו לו אזנים ונאחז בהם ראוי להפטיר הבשר המתעכב בהם מכל צד בכל ערמה שתתכן או להשתדל אם אין יכולת להפטיר הבשר לשבור האזנים ולפתול אותם עד שיפטרו (And if it [i.e. the arrow] have two barbs by which it is held, free them from the adherent flesh all round, in any way you can; if you cannot free the tissues,

195 Cf. SL: 'A clyster may be made of silver or Chinese alloy or of cast or hammered bronze'.

try skillfully to break off the two barbs and twist them about until the arrow comes free). Hebrew הפטיר is not attested in this sense in the current dictionaries; cf. JD 1157: 1. to discard; 2. to dismiss, adjourn a meeting; 3. to read the Haftarah.

פיתקא = Arab. فتوق: 'hernia'; cf. I:45 (SP fol. fol. 202b; SL135, 1): בכוית הפיתקא (On the cauterization of hernia). פיתקא is Syriac for 'rupture; hernia' (cf. BLS 618). N (MA 9:123) and M (MZ fol. 86a) translate the Arabic term as בקיעה, and Z as בקיעה בלטין קְרֶפַּטוּרָא (MA 9:123); cf. SG Pe 48; see as well entries אשך and בֶּתֶק.

פֶּלַח = Arab. شقاق: 'cleft; fissure'; cf. I:18 (SP fol. 205a; SL 61, 1–8): שער יח' בכוית פלחי השפתים. יתחדש הרבה בשפה סדיקה תקרא השער וכל שכן בשפתי הנערים. כשירפאו אלה הפלחים בסמים במה שזכרתי במאמר החלוקה ולא תצליח הרפואה ולא תשכיל ראוי לחמם מכוה קטן סכיני על זאת הצורה ולהיות גוף המכוה על דקות הסכין ואחר כך לחממו מהרה ולכוות בו הפלח עד שתגיע הכויה אל עומקו ואחר כך לרפאו בקירוטי עד שיבריא (Chapter eighteen. On cauterization of hare lip. There often occur fissures in the lip which are given the name 'hairs'; they are particularly common in the lips of boys. When you ineffectually treated these clefts with those things that we have mentioned in their section, then heat a small edged cautery of this shape. The hollow should be as sharp as a knife. Then quickly place it, hot, right on the fissure till the burning has reached the depth of the lip. Then treat with wax plaster till healed). The plural פלחים features for Arab. شقوق in the sense of 'incisions' in, for instance, II:62 (SP fol. 219b; SL 429, 41). Hebrew פֶּלַח features in Rabbinic literature in the sense of 'segment, slice, millstone' (JD 1178), while the plural פלחים is attested in Maimonides, *Mishneh Torah, Ma'akhalot Asurot* 9:19 for 'tears' in unclean birds (cf. BM 4944). M (MZ fol. 87a) translates Arab. شقاق as בקיעה. N translates Arab. شَقٌّ (incision) as שסוע and Z as הקזה (MA 24:47).

פלח: פלחי השפתים = Arab. شقاق الشفة: 'hare lip'; cf. previous entry. The Hebrew term is not attested in secondary literature. Masie has שפה סדוקה or שפת ארנב (MD 338); the modern Hebrew term is שפה שסועה (AD 75).

פלך: פלך הארכובה = Arab. فلكة الركبة: 'the patella of the knee'; cf. III:15 (SP fol. 235b; SL 761, 2): פלך הארכובה לא יקרה בו שבר אלא על המעט (You should know that the patella is rarely fractured). פלך הארכובה is not attested in secondary literature; we do find, however פיקה (*Tosefta Ohalot* 1:6; cf. Low LXXI, s.v. פיקא) and עין הארכובה; cf. MD 551; RS 26.

פרונקא: פרונקות (Aram.: פרונקאות) = Arab. خرق: 'cloth' (see L 729, s.v. خرقة: 'a piece torn off, a rag, a ragged, patched, garment'); cf. II:10 (SP fol. 210b; SL 209, 17; 211, 1): ואם לא יראה השרנאק בתחלת הביקוע ראוי להוסיף בביקוע מעט בנחת עד שיבלוט ואחר למשכו כמו שאמרתי ולטבול אחרי כן פרונקות בחומץ ומים ולתתם על המקום ולהדקו בכלונסה (If you do not see the hydatid at the first incision, you must gently cut a little deeper, till it comes forth, then draw it out as described. Then dip some cloth in vinegar and water, apply it to the place and bind it up with pads). The Aramaic term פרונקא means 'rag' (SDA 929) and features in Rabbinic literature. cf. SG Pe 37. N translates the Arabic خرق as בגדים and Z as חתיכות בגד (MA 23:33).

פרק: פרק היד: See **פרק קנה הזרוע הסמוך ליד**.

-: פרק המרפק = Arab. عضد: 'humerus'; cf. III:11 (SP 235a; SL 741, 1–2): שער י"א בחבוש שבר המרפק. זה הפרק הוא בין המרפק אל ראש הכתף (Chapter eleven. On setting a fracture of the humerus. The humerus is what lies between the elbow and the head of the scapula). The Hebrew term, literally meaning 'the joint of the elbow', does not feature in the sense of 'humerus' in the current dictionaries. Both N and Z translate the Arab. عضد as זרוע (MA 15:62).

-: פרק קנה הזרוע הסמוך ליד = Arab. معصم: 'wrist'; cf. III:28 (SP fol. 237b; SL 809, 1): שער כ"ח ברפואת שמיטת פרק קנה הזרוע הסמוך ליד (On the treatment of a dislocation of the wrist). Another translation for the same Arab. term is פרק היד; cf. III:28 (SP fol. 237b; SL 809, 2): ישמט על הרב פרק היד והשבת שמיטתו קלה בחלוף יתר הפרקים (The carpus of the hand is often dislocated. Unlike other joints the reduction is easy). Both Hebrew terms do not feature in the current dictionaries. Masie (MD 781) mentions שורש היד or רסג היד featuring in Nathan ha-Me'ati's Hebrew translation of Ibn Sīnā's *K. al-Qānūn fī al-ṭibb*; for רסג see as well SR 25, 27.

צבות: צבות חמה (fol. 209b) = ورم حارّ: 'effusion, lit. hot swelling'; cf. II:4 (SP 209b; SL 187, 25–6): ולשית עליו כלונסה טבולה ביין ושמן או חומץ ויין כדי שלא תתחדש צבות חמה (Over all put a pad soaked in wine and oil, or vinegar and oil [= SL زيت], lest an effusion occur). The Arabic term is also translated as 'abscess' (II:6; SP fol. 209b; SL 193, 19). The Hebrew term צבות is attested in medieval literature, cf. BM 5357. In addition to צבות חמה Shem Tov translates the Arabic as צמח חם (SP fol. 210b; SL 211, 22). N translates the Arabic ورم حارّ as מורסא חמה and Z has מורסה חמה (MA passim); M has the same reading as N: מורסא חמה (MZ fol. 139a). See as well entry צמח below.

צלעות = Arab. عرج: 'to be lame'; cf. III:14 (SP fol. 235bb; SL 759, 34–5): ואם יחובש אחד מהם מבלי התחבר אליו השוק האחר על כל פנים יקרה לבעליו צלעות מתמיד (whereas if the [femur] is set alone without binding the leg to it the patient will inevitably be lame for always). Hebrew צלעות, derived from צלע 'to limp' (cf. BM 5501–2), is not attested in the current dictionaries.

צמח = Arab. خراج: 'abscess'; cf. II:45 (SP 216a; SL 3–5): ואומר כי הצמח יהיה עמו חמימות וקדחת ומכאובים מקיפים אותו מפה ומפה עד שתשקוט רתיחת המותר ויגמר העפוש ואז תשקוט הקדחת והחמימות (The abscess will be accompanied by heat and fever and fearsome pain, until the boiling-up of the superfluous matter settles down and the suppurating process is completed: then the fever and intensity will subside). Hebrew צמח means 1. 'growth, sprout, plant', and 2. 'morbid growth, swelling, ulcer, eruption' (JD 1287; Low LXXIV s.v. צמחים). In the latter sense the term features in medieval medical literature (cf. BM 5522); cf. SG Zade 1. The Arabic term خراج is translated by N as נגע, מורסה, יציאה and by Z as יציאה or צמח (MA passim), and by M as יציאה (BIZ 23:2).

-: **צמח חזירי** = Arab. ورم خنزيري: 'scrofulous tumour'; cf. Introduction SP fol. 201b; (SL 5, 19–21): וזה שראיתי רופא איש בער לא ידע וכסיל לא יבין את זאת שבקע על צמח חזירי בצואר אשה וחתך בבערותו קצת ורידי הצואר והוא לא ידע והרעיף דם האשה עד שנפלה בין ידיו ומתה (I saw an ignorant doctor incise a scrofulous tumour in a woman's neck; and he cut certain arteries in the neck so that the woman bled until she fell dead before him). For צמח see previous entry; חזירי 'scrofulous' is a non-attested adjective derived from חזירים 'scrofula', cf. BM 1485.

-: **צמח חם**: cf. the entry **צבות**.

צילחתא = Arab. شقيقة: 'migraine'; cf. I:3 (SP fol. 203b; SL 23,1): השער השלישי בכוית הצילחתא החדשה (Chapter three: On the cauterization of non-chronic migraine). Aramaic צילחתא means 'hemicrania, migraine' (SDA 960). N translates the Arab. شقيقة as פלוח הראש, Z as מגראניאה (MA 6:35); cf. SG Zade 15.

צפורן = Arab. ظفرة: 'ungula, i.e. pterygium'; cf. II:16 (SP fol. 211a; SL 231, 2–3): הצפורן תהיה על שני מינים עצביית דומה לקרום דק או בלתי עצביית דומה ללחות קפוי

לבן (Ungula occurs in two forms: either the nervous, which resembles a fine hard membrane; or the non-nervous, like a white congealed humidity). The Hebrew term is attested by Ben Yehuda (BM 5609; cf. KS 114) in medieval medical literature, e.g. in Nathan ha-Me'ati's translation of Ibn Sīnā's *K. al-Qānūn fī al-ṭibb*, and recurs in his translation of Maimonides' *Medical Aphorisms* (15.24; 23.70); similarly in Z.

קבס: נִקְבָּס = Arab. المتخوم (Mss ABM) 'someone suffering from indigestion'; cf. II:95 (SP fol. 230a; SL 641, 157–8): ואין ראוי להקיז הנקבס עד סור הקבסתו (No one suffering from indigestion should be venesected until the indigestion is over [trans. Bos]). Hebrew נקבס, i.e. Part. Nif'al from the root קבס (cf. BM 5707) is not attested in the current dictionaries. The term הקבסתו, from הקבסות, is also not attested. N translates Arab. المتخوم as בעל הקבסא and Z as הממולא (MA 9:48).

קיבה: קיבת האשה = Arab. فرج المرأة: 'female pudenda'; cf. III:18 (SP 236a; SL 771, 1): שער י"ח בשבר קיבת האשה ועצם הזקן התחתון ואמת האיש (Chapter eighteen. On fracture of the female pudenda and of the pubic bone and of the male organ). The Hebrew term is a synonym featuring in Rabbinic literature for נקבות האשה 'the female genitals' (JD 930). The Arabic term is translated by N as ערוה and by Z as ערוה/פי הרחם (MA 3:105; 16:18; 23:18, 96) and by M (MZ fol. 86a) as כלי הערוה.

קילור: קילורים = Arab. شيافات: 'eye-lotions'; cf. II:15 (SP 211a; SL 229, 9–12): ולהפריד בין העפעף והעין בפתילה של פשתן ולשית ממעלה על העין ספוג טבול בחלבוני בצים ואחר שלשה ימים ראוי להרגיל הקילורים המגלידים עד שיבריא (Then separate between the eye and the lid with a linen pad and put over the eye a piece of wool moistened with white of egg; and after the third day employ healing eye-lotions till it is better). Hebrew קילור means 'eye-salve, collyrium' and is attested in Rabbinic literature (JD 1360; Low LXXVII). See SG Qof 22. Moses Ibn Tibbon translates Arab. شياف as עִגּוּל.

קליפה: קליפות = Arab. خشكريشة: 'eschar' (see UW 270, s.v. ἐσχάρα: 'Wundschorf, Schorf'); cf. I:52 (fol. 208a; SL 155, 6–7): ואחרי כן להשהותו שלשה ימים ואחר לתת על המקומות הנכוים גפרית שחוק עם שמן זית עד שינתקו הקליפות כלן (Then let be for three days, applying to the cauterized site sulphur beaten up with oil, until the whole eschar comes away). The Hebrew term is not attested in this sense in the current dictionaries. N transcribes the Arabic as

כשכרישה; Z describes it as המקום בעצמו אשר שם כעין סובין (MA 15:9), and M translates it as סנפירות (BIZ 22:1).

קרן: קרני הראש = Arab. قرنا الرأس: 'the frontal prominences' (see DKT 825, s.v. قرن الرأس: 'Corne de la tête. Bosse frontale'); cf. I:2 (SP fol. 203a–b; SL 21,11–12): ועתיד אני לזכור עוד זאת הכויה במקומה וראוי להיות המכוה שמכ<וים> בו קרני הראש ואחוריו יותר דק מן המכוה שמכוים בה אמצע הראש (I shall describe this cauterization in its own place. The cautery for the frontal prominences and occiput must be more slender than that for the middle part.) The Hebrew term does not feature in the current dictionaries.

-: קרני הרחם or **קרנים** = Arab. بظر: 'clitoris' (see DKT 815); cf. II:71 (SP fol. 220b; SL 457, 1–2): שער ע"א בחתוך קרני הרחם הנקרא בלשונם אל בטר ובשר הבולט בקיבות הנשים. הקרנים לפעמים יוסיף שעורם על המנהג הטבעי עד שוב הרחם מכוער המראה (Chapter seventy-one. On cutting the clitoris and fleshy growths in the female genitalia. The clitoris may grow in size above the order of nature so that it gets a horrible deformed appearance). The Hebrew term does not feature in the current dictionaries.

קשיש: קשישים = Arab. جبائر: 'splints'. Cf. entry כלונס above. The Hebrew term is attested in Rabbinic literature in the sense of 'splints put about a fracture' (JD 1431). See SG Quf 28. N translates the Arab. جبائر as חבישות and Z as דבקות (MA 15:69).

קשקש = Arab. جبيرة: 'splint': cf. III:4 (SP fol. 234a; SL 717, 13–14): ואחר לתת על הלחי הנשבר הקירוטי ואחר כך לתת עליו בגד גס ולתת על הבגד קשקש גדול עשוי בחכמה (then put wax upon the fractured mandible, and upon that a double[196] dressing, and upon the dressing a large and strong splint). Hebrew קשקש is mentioned in Rabbinic literature in the sense of 'splint' (BM 6254). Cf. entry קשיש above.

ראות = Arab. ناظر: 'pupil'; cf. II:23 (SP 212a; SL 253, 10–13): וראוי לתת שעור הכנסת המקדיח כעין שעור הרוחק אשר יהיה מן הנער אל סוף השחרות והוא עגול העין כי נחשת המקדיח יראה בעצם הראות היטב לזכות הקרום הקרני (The depth the needle goes in should measure as the distance from the pupil to the edge of the iris, which is the corona of the eye; you will clearly see the metal in the pupil itself because of the transparency of the corneal tunic). The Hebrew term

196 'double dressing': translated after SL خرقة مثنيّة; Shem Tov has 'coarse cloth'.

does not feature in this sense in the current dictionaries. N translates the Arabic as רואה and Z as שומר (MA 15.30). Cf. the entry נער above.

ראש: ראש העין = Arab. ماق العين: '[inner] angle of the eye' (see MH 201); cf. I:17 (SP fol. 201b; SL 57,1): י"ז בכוית הגרגתני אשר יקרה בראש העין (Chapter seventeen. On cauterization of a fistula in the angle of the eye). The same Hebrew term features in SG Resh 23 for the Arabic الماق الأكبر, i.e. 'the inner angle of the eye'. See as well the entry זנב העין above.

-: ראשי הירכים = Arab. أربيّة: 'groin'; cf. II:40 (SP fol. 215a; SL 323, 33–4): ויש מהם מה שצריך לבקעו בקוע בעל שלש זויות <ומה שצריך> לחתוך ממנו כתבנית עלה ההדס כמו צמח ראשי הירכים (And there are some [i.e. swellings] that should be incised triangularly; and others with an incision of myrtle-leaf form; e.g. a tumour on the groin). The Hebrew term is a non-attested variant to עיקרי הירכים; see above s.v. עקר.

רבידא = Arab. محجمة: 'cupping-vessel'; cf. III:8 (SP fol. 234b; SL 731, 15): ואמרו קצתם שראוי לתת על המקום רבידא (Some of them said a cupping vessel should be applied to the place). רבידא is attested as ריבדא, meaning 'incision, scratch' (JD 1439, SDA 1072) and features e.g. in bShab 129a as: ריבדא דכוסילתא 'incision of a scalpel'. As a plural to רבידא Shem Tov uses the Hebrew term רבידות; cf. II:96 (SP fol. 230b; SL 657, 2–3): הרבידות נעשות מן הקרנות ומן העצים ומן הנחשת ומן הזכוכית (Cupping-vessels are made of horn, wood, bronze, or glass). N translates the Arab. محاجم as קרני המציצה, Z as כוסות (MA 3:85, 106; 12:37, 46; 16:11, 12), and M as כלי המציצה (MZ fol. 90a). Cf. SG Resh 20.

רגיל = Arab. حاذق: 'having skill', i.e. skilled; cf. II:86 (SP fol. 225b; SL 561, 81–2): ורפאוהו רבים מן הרופאים קרוב משתי שנים ולא היה בהם רגיל במלאכת היד (A whole host of doctors had been treating it for a matter of two years, not one of whom had any skill in the medical art). Hebrew רגיל is only attested in the current dictionaries in the sense of 'accustomed to, common, regular'; cf. BM 6409–11.

רגל: הרגיל = Arab. استعمل: 'to apply'; cf. I:3 (SP fol. 203b; SL 23, 2–4): כשיתחדש בחצי הראש כאב חזק נמשך אל העין ראוי להריק החולה בסמים המנקים הראש ולהרגיל יתר הרפואות אשר זכרתי בחלוקות החליים (When there occurs strong[197] pain in one

197 'strong pain': 'pain with headache' SL.

side of the head and the pain extends to the eye; one[198] should clear the head of the patient with purging drugs and[199] apply the other treatment that I have mentioned in the section on diseases). The Hebrew term does not feature in this sense in the current dictionaries. M translates the Arabic استعمل as עשה or לקח (BMR 3:5, 7, 8), while N translates the Arabic استعمال as עשיה, and Z as עשיה or עשות (MA 16:18, 30; 17:8).

רִסּוּק: ריסוק = I. Arab. وثء: 'contusion'; cf. I:46 (SP fol. 207b; SL 141, 1): שער מו' בכוית הריסוק (Chapter forty-six. On cauterization for contusion); II. Arab. رضّ: 'bruising'; cf. II:89 (SP fol. 227a; SL 591, 19–593, 20): ואם תקרה אל הצפורן מכה או ריסוק ונתחדש בה כאב חזק ראוי להקיז החולה בתחלה (If a laceration or bruising happen to the nail, with violent pain, you should first bleed the patient). Hebrew רִסּוּק is attested in Rabbinic literature in the sense of 'crushing, lesion' and as ריסוקי איברים in the sense of 'lesion of vital organs, internal injury' (JD 1475; BM 6626).

ריקות = Arab. فضاء: 'perineum' (see DKT 824); cf. II:70 (SP fol. 220b; SL 455, 1–4): שער ע' ברפואת האנדרוגירוס. האנדרוגינוס יהיה בזכרים על שני מינים האחד מהם שיראה במה שימשך אל הריקות או בעור הבצים במה שיש בין הבצים תבנית דומה לקיבת אשה יש בו שער (Chapter seventy. On the treatment of the hermaphrodite. There are two kinds of male hermaphrodite: one has the appearance as of female pudenda with hair in the region of the perineum; the other has the same in the skin of the scrotum between the testes). Hebrew ריקות is only attested in medieval literature in the sense of 'vacuum'; cf. BM 6581. ריקות as 'perineum' is a semantic borrowing from Arab. فضاء. In addition to ריקות Shem Tov uses בית הפרשות to render the Arabic فضاء; see above.

רְעִיפָה: רעיפת הדם = Arab. نزف: 'haemorrhage'; cf. II:55 (SP fol. 217b; SL 391, 2–3): ולהשמר בעת המלאכה מרעיפת הדם שהיא תקרה הרבה ואם תקרה ראוי להרגיל מה שיפסיקנו ולרפא החבורה עד שתבריא (And beware, in your operating, of haemorrhage, which often happens; meet it with styptics and dress the wound until it heals). The Hebrew term is attested subsequently in medieval medical literature, a.o. in Nathan ha-Me'ati's translation of Ibn Sīnā's *K. al-Qānūn fī al-ṭibb* (cf. BM 6654). The same Arabic term is translated by N a.o. as הזלת הדם and by Z as הגרת הדם (MA 15:13; 16:7, 15).

198 'one should clear the head of the patient': 'and the patient has cleared his head' SL.

199 'and to apply': 'and there has been applied' SL.

רתע: הרתיע לאחור = Arab. ردع: 'to suppress'; cf. II:87 (SP fol. 226b; SL 579, 37–8): והשתדלתי להרתיע לאחור המותר ההוא במה שנתתי על היד מן הסמים אחר הרקת הגוף ולא נרתע לאחור המותר (and I attempted to suppress the superfluity with remedies that I applied to the hand, after purging his body, but the superfluity was not to be suppressed). While Hebrew נרתע is not attested in this sense in the current dictionaries, הרתיע is attested in a medical context in BM 6771, as featuring in N (MA 3:110). Z (ibid.) translates the Arab. ردع as הזיר, and M (BIZ 14:3) translates الأدوية التي تردع (repelling remedies) as הרפואות אשר ישככו.

שבבים = Arab. شظايا: 'fragments'; cf. II:84 (SP fol. 224b; SL 535, 88–9): ואם עשתה רושם בעצם והתכה ממנו שבבים (But if there has also been injury to the bone, cutting out fragments from it…). Hebrew שבבים means 'splinters'; cf. KB 1382; BM 6820–1. It is not attested in medical literature. See as well SG Shin 30. For singular Arab. شظية Shem Tov uses the Aramaic term שיבא (see below).

שבלת: שבולת הזקן = Arab. ذقن: 'chin'; cf. II:96 (SP fol. 231a; SL 661, 43): ונתינת הרבידות מתחת שבולת הזקן מועילות מן השחין הדק אשר בפה הנקרא בלשונם אל קלאע (The application of cupping under the chin helps against ulcers in the mouth). Hebrew שבולת הזקן is attested in BM 6849 in the sense of 'a tuft of beard hair', and in the sense of 'chin' in the *Sefer ha-Ḥinnukh* which was compiled at the end of the thirteenth century.[200]

שדף: השתדף = Arab. ذبل: 'to wither'; cf. II:64 (SP fol. 220a; SL 439,15–17): ואם תקרה הזמורה לכל הכיסים ראוי להוציא אחד מן הבצים מן הכיסים פן תעדר הביצה מזון מפני חתוך הכיסים ותשתדף ולא יהיה בה תועלת (But if all the vessels are varicose then you will have to remove one testicle with its vessels lest the testicle be deprived of nourishment through cutting into the vessels; for it will wither and be of no use). Hebrew השתדף is not attested in the sense of 'to wither' in a medical context in the current dictionaries. N translates the Arabic ذبل 'to suffer from marasmus' as הצטמק and Z as ניתך ויבש (MA 25:43).

שחין: השחין הדק = Arab. بثور: 'pustules'; cf. I:55 (SP fol. 208b; SL 161, 2–3): יתחדש בגוף שחין דק מכוער מחמרים קרים עבים נפסדים (Foul pustules sometimes arise in the body, caused by heavy corrupt frigid matter). Hebrew השחין הדק (lit. a thin ulcer) is not attested in the current dictionaries. Arabic بثر is

200 See *Encyclopedia Judaica*, vol. 7, cols. 1126–7, entry 'Ha-Ḥinnukh' (Shlomo Zalman Havlin).

translated by N as צמה while Z transcribes it as בתר (MA 6:24). M translates it as שחין (BIZ 8:4) and as אבעבעות (BIZ 22:1).

שחפת = Arab. سل: 'wasting'; cf. I:24 (SP fol. 205b; SL 75, 2–3): כשיהיה השעול וחלי הריאה מלחויות קרות ולא תהיה אל החולה קדחת ולא שחפת ויהיה החלי ישן (When the cough and pulmonary disease arise from cold humidities and the patient suffers from no fever or wasting but the disease is chronic). The Hebrew term is attested in the sense of 'consumption' in the Bible (KB 1463) and medieval medical literature (Shabbetai Donnolo); cf. BM 7028. N translates the Arabic سل as שדפון or הסל הוא טישי and Z as טיציש or טישיש (phthisis) (MA 6:51; 8:58; 22:44, 70; 23:17); M has the same term as N, namely שדפון (MZ fol. 88a). Cf. SG Shin 36.

שטות = Arab. مالنخوليا 'melancholy'; cf. I:11 (SP fol. 204a; SL 41, 1–3): שער י"א בכוית השטות. כשתהיה סבתו לחויות נפסדות ולחה לבנה עבה ראוי לכוותו הכויות אשר זכרתי בבעל הפלג (Chapter eleven. On cauterization for melancholy. When the cause of the melancholy be corrupt humours and a thick phlegm, burn him with those cauterizations mentioned in the case of the paralytic). Hebrew שטות is attested in the sense of 'madness; folly' in Rabbinic literature (JD 1553). It is used by both N and Z for Arabic جنون ,madness; insanity' (MA 6:3, 32; 16:38), and by M for Arab. كلب, i.e. 'rabies'. See SG Shin 31.

שטח: השטיח = Arab. طلى 'to spread'; cf. I:49 (SP fol. 208a; SL 149, 4–6): ואחרי כן לרפאתה בקמח עדשים עם שמן ורד ועלי לשון טלה ודם יונה ודם תחמס מכל אחד חלק שוה ולערב את הכל ולהשטיחם על בגד ולתתו על המקום עד שיבריא (Then tread [i.e. the leprosy] with lentil flour, oil of roses, arnoglossa leaves, and pigeons' or swallows' blood, of each equal parts mixed all together and spread on lint; let this stick to the place till healed). The same Hebrew term is used for Arabic بسط 'to spread, h.l.: 'stretch'; cf. IV: 9 (SP fol. 238b; SL 735, 11–12): ואותות השמיטה הנשמטת לפנים שהחולה ישטיח שוקו שטיחה גמורה אלא שלא יוכל לקפלה מבלי כאב בארכובה (The sign[201] of an anterior dislocation [of the hip] is that the patient can stretch his leg fully but cannot flex it without feeling pain in the knee). Hebrew השטיח is not attested in a medical context in secondary literature; cf. BM 7053 and Ma'agarim, s.v. שטח. Arab. طلى is translated by N as רטה or שם and by Z as משח (cf. MA 8:12; 9:20; 22:21, 24, 26, 70), and by M as טח (BIZ 7:1), משח (BIZ 13:1), or חבש (BIZ 13.8).

---

201 'sign'; lit. 'signs'; cf. Arab. علامة.

שיבא = Arab. شظية 'splinter'; cf. III:6 (SP fol. 234b; SL 727, 15–16): ואם יפרד מן העצם שִׁיבָּא ותהיה עוקצת מתחת העור ראוי לבקע עליה ולהסירה (If a splinter of bone protrudes and starts to prick under the skin, cut down upon it and remove it). Aramaic שיבא is attested in Rabbinic literature in the sense of 'chip' (cf. SDA 1131). For plural Arab. شظايا Shem Tov uses שבבים; see above.

שמיטה = I. Arab. خَلْع 'dislocation'; cf. I:40 (SP fol. 206b; SL 113, 1–4): שער מ' בכוית שמיטת הירך. לפעמים תשתפכנה לחויות עבות אל כף הירך ותהיינה סבה לצאתו ממקומו. ואות השמיטה אורך השוק האחד על חברו כשיוקש אחד אל אחר (Chapter forty. On cauterization of a dislocated hip. Sometimes harmful humidities reach the hip joint and result in its coming out of place. The symptom of this is that one leg is longer than the other when one is measured against the other); II. فك (SL 787,1; 789,1; 793,1; 795,1, etc.): 'dislocation'; cf. III:23 (SP fol. 237a; SL 787, 2): השמיטה הוא צאת פרק מן הפרקים ממקומו (A dislocation is a displacement of any of the joints from its place). The Hebrew term features a.o. in Moses Ibn Tibbon's חרוזי אבן סינא (BM 7238), i.e. the Hebrew translation of Ibn Sīnā's *'Urǧūza fī al-ṭibb*. N translates the Arabic خَلْع as שמט, Z as השמטה (MA 15:46), and M as הקעה (BIZ 15:1). Arabic فك is translated by M as רסוק (BIZ 25:11).

שמיר = I. Arab. الحديد الهندي 'Indian iron'; cf. II:19 (SP fol. 211b; SL 243, 7): וכשיתגלה ויראה בו הפסד או שחרות ראוי לגרדו בכלי כזה [illustration] ויקרא העץ[202] הראש ראוי לעשותו משמיר (When bone is reached and you see necrosis or blackness, scrape it with an instrument like this [illustration]. It is called 'rough-head'[203] and is made of Indian iron). The biblical Hebrew שמיר is traditionally interpreted as a diamond, cf. KB 1562–3. However, there may have been an ancient tradition related to the Latin translation of the term as 'adamas', which can mean both diamond and steel, according to which this term does not refer to a mineral but to a metal, possibly steel; cf. Löw, *Fauna und Mineralien der Juden*, 254–6.[204] [illustration]

שקוי: השקוי הנאדי = Arab. الاستسقاء الزقّي: 'ascites'; cf I:32 (SP fol. 206a; SL 95, 2): הכויה ראויה בשקוי הנאדי בלבד (The cautery is particularly effective in ascites). N translates the Arabic استسقاء النوع الزقّي as השקוי הנואדי and השקוי הנודיי and Z as ההדרוקן הנאדי (MA 4:41; 15:36). Ben Yehuda (BM 7422) mentions השקוי הנאדי

---

202 העץ (= الخشب): الخشنة SL.

203 Translation based on the Arabic الخشنة الرأس; the Hebrew has 'wood-head'.

204 I. Löw, *Fauna und Mineralien der Juden*, Repr. with an introduction by A. Schreiber (Hildesheim 1969).

as featuring in the *Perush Ibn Rushd 'al Ḥaruzei Ibn Sina* (Ibn Rushd's commentary on Ibn Sīnā's *'Urğūza* in the Hebrew translation prepared by Solomon Ibn Ayyub in the year 1261). See as well SG Shin 32, s.v. שקוי.

שקיעה = I. Arab. عَصْر: 'squeezing'; cf II:59 (SP fol. 218b; SL 409, 27–8): ולעשות בה כמו שנעשה בכיס מקוה המים משקיעת היד עד שיגיע הלחות אל הכיס (Then tie it to the instrument and do with it as with the [camel's] bladder, squeezing until the fluid reaches the bladder of the patient); II. Arab. كَبْس 'pressing'; cf. II:63 (SP fol. 219b; SL 435, 11–12): אמנם אשר יהיה מצבות הגידים הנחים לא יתפזר ממנו מאומה בעת שקיעת האצבע עליו (The sort arising from a swelling of the vein will not disperse when you press upon it with your fingers); III. Arab. شَدّ 'to apply pressure'; cf. II:59 (SP fol. 218b; SL 409, 22–3: ולהשקיע הכיס ביד על הלחות שקיעה בחכמה עד שירגיש החולה שהלחות ההוא כבר הגיע אל הכיס (Then apply strong pressure to the bladder containing the fluid until the patient can feel the fluid has entered his own bladder); IV. Arab. غَمْز 'pressing'; cf. II:95 (SP fol. 230a; SL 667, 203–4): ויתחדש הרבה צבות ובליטה בעת הקזת הבאסליק וראוי אז לתת עליו היד ואם ימצא מתפשט בעת שקיעת היד עליו בידוע שהבליטה ההיא רעה (Often in section of the basilic vein there occurs tumour and swelling. Put your hand upon it, and if you find that it sinks when pressed then it is a harmful swelling). Hebrew שקיעה does not feature in these meanings in the current dictionaries See as well entry שקע.

שקע: השקיע = I. Arab. أمعن: 'to press'; cf II:45 (SP fol. 216a; SL 343, 14–15): ואחר להשקיע היד על הצמח כפי גדלו (then press it in proportionately to the size of the tumour); II. Arab. كبس 'to exert pressure'; cf. II:52 (SP fol. 217a; SL 377, 8): וכשיושקע עליו באצבע יתעלם (And it will disappear on digital pressure); III. Arab. شدّ 'to apply pressure'; cf. II:59 (SP fol. 218b; SL 409, 22–3: ולהשקיע הכיס ביד על הלחות שקיעה בחכמה עד שירגיש החולה שהלחות ההוא כבר הגיע אל הכיס (Then apply strong pressure to the bladder containing the fluid until the patient can feel the fluid has entered his own bladder); IV. Arab. غمز 'to press'; II:95 (SP fol. 230b; SL 649, 235–7): ואין ראוי כשיש רצון להתיר הקזת הזרוע להוציא מן הדם פעם שנית וכבר נסתם פי הגיד ותקשה יציאת הדם להשקיע עליו בחזקה ביד ולפתול אותו בכח (If you wish to loosen the arm and let blood a second time and you find that the opening of the vein is now closed up and the outflow of blood is difficult, you should not press hard upon it nor twist the arm violently). Hebrew שקע does not feature in these meanings in the current dictionaries. See as well entry שקיעה.

תונבא = Arab. خدر: 'numbness'; cf. I:48 (SP fol. 208a; SL 147, 1): שער מ"ח בכוית התונבא והיא סור חוש אבר או איברין מן הגוף (Chapter forty-eight. On the cauterization of numbness, that is the lack of feeling in a part of the body).[205] Aramaic תונבא means 'stupor, type of spirit; loss of sensation; numbness' and features in Rabbinic literature (JD 1654; SDA 1198). N translates the Arab. خدر as תרדמת האיברים or תרדמת החוש, Z as ביטול (MA 7:66; 22:38, 43; 23:22, 23), and M as תרדמה or תרדמת האיברים (BIZ 9:2; 17:2). Cf. SG Tav 15.

תלולית: תלוליות של בשר = Arab. سلع: 'cysts'; cf. II:42 (SP fol. 215b; SL 333, 4–6): ויהיה אשר יקרה מהם בצואר אחד או רבים ויתילדו קצתם מקצתם וכל חזיר מהם יהיה בתוך קרום מיוחד לו כמו שיהיה בתלוליות של בשר וצמחי הראש כמו שזכרתי (Those [i.e. tumours] occurring in the neck are sometimes single and sometimes multiple, one arising from another; and each scrofula is contained in a capsule of its own, like the cysts and tumours of the head that we have described). Hebrew תלולית is not attested in this sense in secondary literature, cf. BM 7771, and above s.v. אגודות הבשר.

תער: תער הגלבים = Arab. موسى: '(razor)'; cf. I:1 (fol. 203b; SL 6–8): וצורת הכויה להריק החולה בתחלה בסם משלשל מנקה הראש שלש לילות או ארבע כפי חיוב כחו ושניו ומנהגו ואחר להעביר שער ראשו בתער הגלבים (The manner of performing this operation [i.e. the single cauterization of the head] is first to bid the patient open the bowels with an evacuant which will also clear his head, for three or four nights, according to the strength, age, and habits of the patient. Then tell him to have his head shaved…). The Hebrew term features in Ezek. 5:1 (KB 1771). For further attestations cf. Ma'agarim (a.o.: *Sefer ha-Mitswot le-Levi, Lekeṭ Dinim* 6:2: תער הגלבים אשר שמו מוס).

תפירה: תפירות = Arab. خياطات: 'sutures'; cf. II:1 (SP fol. 209a; SL 171, 11–173, 17): ואם יהיה הלחות מתחת העצם ואותותיו הראות תפירות הראש פתוחות מכל צד והמים נשפכים לתוך הראש כשיוסחטו ביד וזה דבר בלתי נעלם מן הרופא צריך לבקע באמצע הראש שלש בקיעות על זאת הצורה (But if the humidity is beneath the bone—and the sign of that is that you will see three sutures of the skull gaping on all sides, the water manifestly yielding when you press in with your fingers — you should make three incisions in the middle of the head). The Hebrew term תפירה is only attested in this sense as modern in AD 158. Vesalius' *Tabulae* calls the sutures מחוברים, the *Fabrica* שלבים, while the Hebrew translations of Ibn Sīnā's *K. al-Qānūn* have חוליות or שלבים; cf. SR 38.

205 'that is the lack of feeling in a part of the body': addition Shem Tov.

Zeraḥyah Ben Isaac Ben She'altiel Ḥen, Hebrew translation of Maimonides' *Medical Aphorisms* (*Fuṣūl Mūsā fī l-Ṭibb*)

Introduction

Little is known about the philosopher and translator. R. Zeraḥyah ben Yiẓḥak ben She'altiel Ḥen, also known as Zeraḥyah Gracian.[206] The years of his birth and death are unknown. We know, however, that he was born in Barcelona into a prominent family which for several generations produced rabbis and sages, and at a later date emigrated to Italy. Between the years 1277–91 A.D. he was active in Rome as a teacher of philosophy, commentator of the Bible,[207] and translator. He became a recognized authority in philosophy and in philosophical Bible exegesis, and for some years taught Maimonides' *Guide of the Perplexed.* In contrast with the rabbinic leadership of the Barcelona community, which at that time was decisively influenced by the teachings of Nahmanides, the Jewish communal leadership in Rome was supportive of Zeraḥyah's rationalist-naturalist approach.[208] He corresponded with other scholars, such as Hillel b. Samuel of Verona, a talmudic scholar, philosopher, physician and translator of medical works, in a bitter controversy over Hillel's conservative interpretation of Maimonides' philosophy.[209] And when Hillel

---

206 For his life and works see M. Steinschneider, 'Ẓiyyunim le-Toledot R. Zeraḥyah ben Yiẓḥak ben She'altiel Ḥen', *Oẓar Neḥmad*, vol. 2 (Vienna 1857), 229–45; idem, *Die hebräischen Übersetzungen*, 111–14; G. Bos, *Aristotle's* De Anima. *Translated into Hebrew by Zeraḥyah ben Isaac ben She'altiel Ḥen.* A Critical Edition with an Introduction and Index, (Leiden 1994), 1–4; For a detailed account of all the relevant sources see A. Ravitsky, *Mishnato shel R. R. Zeraḥyah ben Yiẓḥak ben She'altiel Ḥen we-ha-Hagut ha-Maimunit-Tibbonit ba-Me'ah ha-Shelosh Esreh*, unpublished diss. (Jerusalem 1977). See as well the summary account by Ravitsky in *Encyclopaedia Judaica*^{2}, vol. 21, ed. by M. Berenbaum and F. Skolnik, (Detroit 2007), 514–15, s.v. Zerahiah ben Isaac ben Shealtiel.

207 In addition to his Biblical commentaries he also composed a commentary (extant only in manuscript) on parts of Maimonides' *Guide of the Perplexed* (1:1–71 and other passages, especially the 25 propositions appearing at the beginning of Book 2). See Ravitsky, *Zerahiah ben Isaac ben Shealtiel*; J. Friedman, 'R. Zerahiah ben Shealtiel Hen's Commentary on the Guide of the Perplexed', *Jacob Friedman Memorial Volume* (1974): 3–14 (Heb.).

208 Cf. Ravitsky, *Zerahiah ben Isaac ben Shealtiel.*

209 Zeraḥyah's correspondence with Hillel Ben Samuel has been published by R. Kirchheim in *Oẓar Neḥmad*, vol. 2 (Vienna 1857), 124–43. On Hillel Ben Samuel see the section on Hillel in this volume.

boasted about his theoretical medical knowledge, Zeraḥyah asked him whether he has studied the writings by Hippocrates and Galen, such as Galen's תועלת האברים (*De usu partium*), ספר החליים והמקרים (*De causis et symptomatibus*), ספר תחבולות הבריאות בחבלות ובנגעים (*De methodo medendi*): בידימיא (*Epidemics*, i.e. his commentaries to Hippocrates' *Epidemics*); ששה ספריו הגדולים (his six major works?);[210] ספר עשרה מאמרים (*De compositione medicamentorum secundum locos*), and whether it is enough for him to diagnose an illness by examining the urine of the patient and consult al-Rāzī's *K. al-Manṣūrī*,[211] or whether he also consults Ibn al-Jazzār's ספר צידת האורח (= *Sefer Ẓedat ha-Derakhim*). Little is known about his life after 1291 A.D. It is possible that around that time he returned to Barcelona in order to be buried with his ancestors.[212]

Zeraḥyah as a Translator

Zeraḥyah translated the following philosophical works from Arabic into Hebrew:[213]

1. Aristotle's *De Anima*.[214]
2. Themistius' *Paraphrase* of Aristotle's *De Caelo*.[215]

---

210 Steinschneider, *Die hebräischen Übersetzungen*, 113, n. 40, surmises that one might have to correct the number six into sixteen, and that Zeraḥyah is referring to the 16 summaries of Galenic works compiled in Alexandria around 500. These summaries, which have been lost in the original Greek and are only known through the Arabic tradition, under the name *Ǧawāmi' al-Iskandarāniyīn* (Summaria Alexandrinorum), are probably associated with those Galenic treatises, which formed a curriculum of sixteen books, that were taught with formal commentaries and read in a specific order in pre-Islamic Alexandria and in the early centuries of Islam (see G. Bos, 'Maimonides on Medicinal Measures and Weights', *Aleph*. No. 9.2 [2009], 255–76, p. 255).

211 For this work by al-Rāzī (865–932), the famous philosopher and physician, see M. Ullmann, *Die Medizin im Islam* (Leiden/Köln 1970), 132.

212 In a letter to Hillel b. Samuel Zeraḥyah states (*Oẓar Neḥmad*, vol. 2 [Vienna 1857], 124): 'Because I have the intention to return to my native country to be buried with my ancestors…'

213 For his translations cf. the bio-bibliographical literature mentioned above; see as well: M. Zonta, *La Tradizione Ebraica del* Commento Medio *di Averroè alla* Metafisica *di Aristotele. Le versioni ebraiche di Zeraḥyah ben Iṣḥāq Ḥen e di Qalonimos ben Qalonimos*. Edizione e introduzione storico-filologica, unpublished Ph.D. diss. (Turin 1995).

214 Aristotle's *De Anima* has been preserved in Greek and in Latin, but the extant Arabic version is different from that used by Zeraḥyah for his Hebrew translation, which was edited by G. Bos, *Aristotle's* De Anima.

215 Themistius' *Paraphrase* is lost in Greek and Arabic. For the Hebrew translation see ed. S. Landauer, *In libros Aristotelis* De caelo *paraphrasis hebraice et latine. Commentaria in*

3. Averroes' *Middle Commentary* on Aristotle's *Physica*.[216]
4. Averroes' *Middle Commentary* on the *Metaphysica*.[217]
5. Aristotle's *De Generatione et Corruptione*.[218]
6. Pseudo al-Fārābī's *Treatise on the Essence of the Soul*.[219]
7. Pseudo-Aristotle, *Liber de Causis*.[220]

Zeraḥyah translated Aristotle's *De Anima*, the commentaries of Averroes on Aristotle's *Physica* and *Metaphysica*, Themistius' *Paraphrase* of Aristotle's *De Caelo*, and pseudo-al-Fārābī's *Treatise on the Essence of the Soul* in the year 1284 A.D. at the request of Shabbetai b. Solomon, Rabbi of Rome and a friend and staunch defender of Zeraḥyah in his polemic with Hillel b. Samuel.

As to the question why Zeraḥyah turned to translate major works in the field of medieval philosophy during his residence in Rome, Mauro Zonta has suggested that these works were possibly part of a *Corpus Aristotelicum Hebraicum*, similar (but not identical) to the Latin *Corpus Aristotelicum*

Aristotelem Graeca, vol. 5, part 4 (Berlin 1902). This edition should now be revised on the basis of the archetype copied from the lost autograph, MS Florence, Biblioteca Nazionale Centrale, II. II. 528 (cf. M. Zonta, 'Hebraica Veritas: Temistio, Parafrasi del De Coelo. Tradizione e critica del testo', *Athenaeum* 82 [1994], 403–28).

216 Averroes' commentary is lost in Arabic, but preserved in Latin and Hebrew. Zeraḥyah's Hebrew translation of this commentary has been collated by Steven Harvey for his edition of the first two books of the Hebrew translation by Qalonimos Ben Qalonimos. Cf. S. Harvey, *Averroes on the Principles of Nature: The* Middle Commentary *on Aristotle's* Physics I–II Ph.D. diss. (Harvard University 1977).

217 This work is lost in Arabic and Latin. Mauro Zonta rediscovered the archetype copied from Zeraḥyah's lost autograph in manuscript Turin, Biblioteca Nazionale Universitaria, A. II. 13. An edition can be found in his *La Tradizione Ebraica*.

218 For the Hebrew translation of this work ,which is preserved in Greek and in Latin, but lost in Arabic, cf. A. Tessier (ed.), 'La traduzione arabo-ebraica de *De generatione et corruptione* di Aristotele', *AANLM* 184; serie VIII–vol. XXVIII, fasc. 1.

219 This treatise is lost in Arabic. The Hebrew translation, entitled *Ma'amar be-mahut ha-nefesh* was edited by Z.H. Edelman, *Ḥemdah Genuzah* (Koenigsberg 1856) and by S. Rosenthal (Warsaw, 1857). A new, revised edition was published by G. Freudenthal, 'La Quiddité de l'Âme, Traité populaire néoplatonisant faussement attribué à al-Fārābī: Traduction annotée Et commentée', *Arabic Sciences and Philosophy* 13:2 (2003), 173–237.

220 I. Schreiber (ed.), *Pseudo-Aristoteles* Liber De causis, (Budapest 1916). See as well J.P. Rothschild, *Les traductions hebraïques du Liber de Causis latin*, diss. (Paris 1985); idem, 'Les traductions du Livre des Causes et leurs copies', *Revue d'Histoire des Textes* XXIV (1994), 393–484.

diffused in Europe from 1250 onwards; they might have been intended as a sort of Jewish adaptation of the contents of that *Corpus*.[221]

In addition to these philosophical works Zeraḥyah translated the following medical works from Arabic into Hebrew:

1. Galen's *De Causis et Symptomatibus*.[222]
2. Galen's *Katagenos*, chs. 1–3.[223]
3. Ibn Sīnā, *K. al-Qānūn fi al-ṭibb*, bks. 1–2.[224]
4. Maimonides' *Medical Aphorisms*.[225]
5. Maimonides' treatise *On Poisons and the Protection against Lethal Drugs*.[226]
6. Maimonides' treatise *On Coitus*.[227]

In addition to these translations, featuring in the bio-bibliographical literature, some new hitherto unknown translations from his hand have been discovered recently. Giuliano Tamani discovered a copy of Zeraḥyah's translation of Maimonides' *Commentary on Hippocrates' Aphorisms* found in a unique manuscript in the Biblioteca Arcivescovile in Udine.[228] Mauro Zonta

221 See M. Zonta, *Zerahyah Ben Isaac Hen, Philosopher and Translator and his Role in 13th century Rome* (unpublished paper read in Jerusalem, January 1, 2007). I thank Mauro Zonta for providing me with a copy of this paper.

222 Zeraḥyah translated an Arabic paraphrase of this work consisting of four books; cf. Steinschneider, *Die hebräischen Übersetzungen*, 652.

223 The introduction to the translation was edited by Steinschneider, in: idem, *Catalog der hebräischen Handschriften in der Stadtbibliothek zu Hamburg und der sich anschliessenden in anderen Sprachen* (Hamburg 1878), 197–9; for a description of the MS, see ibidem 143–4.

224 Zeraḥyah's translation, prepared around the year 1280, was not an independent translation but was a corrected version based on the translation prepared by his colleague Nathan ha-Me'ati; cf. H. Rabin, 'Toledot Targum Sefer ha-Qanun le-'Ivrit'; *Melilah* III–IV (Manchester 1950), 133–47, esp. p. 134.

225 A critical edition of this translation by Zeraḥyah dating from the year 1277 is forthcoming.

226 Zeraḥyah's translation has been published in: Maimonides, *On Poisons* (ed. Bos-McVaugh).

227 Zerahyah's translation has been published in the past by Hermann Kroner in *Shenei Ma'amarei ha-Mishgal. Eḥad 'al 'Inyanei ha-Mishgal we-eḥad 'al Ribbuy ha-Mishgal. Ein Beitrag zur Geschichte der Medizin des XII. Jahrhunderts an der Hand zweier medizinischer Abhandlungen des Maimonides auf Grund von 6 unedierten Handschiften dargestellt und kritisch beleuchtet* (Berlin1906). Kroner's edition of the translation by Zeraḥyah is unreliable, since it suffers from editorial mistakes. A new edition is forthcoming in: Maimonides, *On Coitus*. A New Parallel Arabic-English Translation by Gerrit Bos with Critical Editions of medieval Hebrew translations by Gerrit Bos and Latin translations by Charles Burnett.

228 MS. 246. Ebraico 12, fols. 1a–29b; cf. G. Tamani, 'Codici ebraici Pico Grimani nella Biblioteca arcivescovile di Udine', *Annali di Ca' Foscari* 10 (1971), 1–25, p. 18. An edition

identified Zeraḥyah as the translator of Hippocrates' *De superfoetatione,* extant in a unique manuscript in Parma, Biblioteca Palatina.[229] I identified Zeraḥyah as the translator of Maimonides' *On Hemorrhoids*, extant in MS Parma 2642, De Rossi 354, Richler 1531;[230] *On the Regimen of Health*, extant in MS Paris BN hébr 1127 (a fragment only);[231] and *On Poisons*, extant in MSS Munich 43 and 280 (both fragmentary). I was able to identify Zeraḥyah as the author of these translations because of my edition of Zeraḥyah's translation of Aristotle's *De Anima*,[232] and because of the critical editions I prepared of Maimonides' *On Hemorrhoids*, *On the Regimen of Health*, and *On Poisons* as part of the Maimonides' project which aims at providing critical editions of his medical works in the original Arabic and medieval translations. In particular, the compilation of Arabic-Hebrew glossaries and separate alphabetical indices to the different Hebrew translations of Maimonides' medical works proved to be very useful for the purpose of identification, as it provided me with the technical terminology typical for the major translators of these works, namely Moses Ibn Tibbon, Nathan ha-Me'ati and Zeraḥyah.[233]

According to Mauro Zonta, Zeraḥyah turned to translate these medical works in order to "diffuse Greco-Arabic medicine among Italian Jewish physicians, who apparently were not yet interested in it. He may have been trying to emulate the phenomenon of Latin translations of Greek and Arabic medical works, conspicuous in Italy starting around the end of the eleventh century and continuing, especially in Southern Italy, through the first half of the thirteenth century".[234] Freudenthal remarks that Zeraḥyah translated these works in reply to the need felt by Jewish doctors to have at their disposal

---

of Zeraḥyah's translation is forthcoming in: *Maimonides, Commentary on Hippocrates' Aphorisms*. A New Parallel Arabic-English Translation with Critical Editions of medieval Hebrew translations by Gerrit Bos.

229 See M. Zonta, 'A Hebrew translation of Hippocrates' De superfoetatione: Historical Introduction and Critical Introduction', *Aleph. Historical Studies in Science and Judaism*, no. 3 (2003), 97–143.

230 See Richler, *Hebrew Manuscripts in the Biblioteca*. The translation by Zeraḥyah is forthcoming in: Maimonides, *On Hemorrhoids* (ed. Bos-Mcvaugh).

231 An edition of this fragment is forthcoming in: Maimonides, *On the Regimen of Health* (ed. Bos-McVaugh).

232 Especially the analysis of his translation technique on pp. 23–43 proved to be very useful.

233 See:www.uni-koeln.de/phil-fak/juda/forschung/forschungsprojekte/maimonides/glossare.htm

234 Zonta, *Zerahyah Ben Isaac Hen, Philosopher and Translator and his Role in 13th century Rome*.

Greco-Arabic medical works. Until the thirteenth century Jewish doctors in Italy worked within the framework of traditional medicine, transmitted from father to son. However, once non-Jewish doctors became familiar with Greco-Arabic medicine through the translations into Latin, Jewish doctors felt a growing need to gain access to this new corpus of medical literature. In the introduction to his translation of Ibn Sīnā, *K. al-Qānūn*, Zeraḥyah's colleague Nathan ha-Me'ati states that the reason for translating this work is that non-Jewish doctors ridicule their Jewish colleagues as they are not familiar with the theoretical works that form the basis for the medical art.[235]

If one studies Zeraḥyah's translations themselves, especially his translation technique, as I did in the case of my edition of his translation of Aristotle's *De Anima* mentioned above, one is perplexed by their peculiarities, inconsistencies, idiosyncrasies, and faults. In many cases his translations are so difficult and so slavishly follow the Arabic, that one cannot understand them without the original text at hand. No wonder then that his translations are only preserved in a few manuscripts, and in some cases only one.[236] One wonders whether some of these peculiarities result from his insufficient knowledge of Arabic or can also be explained as resulting from a deliberate choice to closely follow the Arabic, as is clear from his introduction to his translation of Galen's *Katagenos*: 'Before I begin to translate this work, I want the reader to know that >if< I follow the [grammatical rules of the] Arabic in many places. For instance, I use a word in the third person feminine singular [instead of the plural];...and a word in the feminine gender and vice versa.'[237] That Zeraḥyah had problems in finding the proper Hebrew terminology is clear from his own statements in two places in his translation of Maimonides' *Medical Aphorisms*. After translating Aphorism 23:25, in which Maimonides points out the failure

235 G. Freudenthal, 'Les sciences dans les communautés juives médiévales de Provence: Leur appropriation, leur role', *Revue des Études juives* CLII, facs. 1–2 (1993), 29–136, esp. p. 68. For Nathan's statement see as well, Steinschneider, *Die hebräischen Übersetzungen*, 659, n. 45; Rabin, *Toledot Targum* Sefer ha-Qanun *le-'Ivrit*, 133.

236 A notable exception is his translation of Maimonides' *Medical Aphorisms* which survives in sixteen MSS and was copied in ten Italian scripts; see B. Richler, 'Manuscripts of Moses Ben Maimon's Pirke Moshe in Hebrew Translation', *Koroth* 9, no. 3–4 (1986): 345–56, pp. 352–4 (to the fifteen MSS listed by Richler one should add MS Munich, Bayerische Staatsbibliothek 19); Bos, Maimonides, *Medical Aphorisms*. Treatises 1–5. A parallel Arabic-English edition edited, translated, and annotated. (Provo 2004), p. xxv.

237 Cf. Steinschneider, *Catalog Hamburg*, 197–9; English translation: Bos, Aristotle's *De Anima*, 23.

of Galen's commentators to distinguish between three different kinds of membranes (*aghshiyya*, *ṣifāqāt*, and *ṭabaqāt*) by using the term *ṣifāqāt* for all of them, Zeraḥyah remarks:

> Says the translator: I know that one should not translate this text from the Rabbi, of blessed memory, at all, since in our Hebrew language I cannot find [equivalents for] the terms mentioned here. For these three [kinds of] membranes as they are found in the Arabic language, namely the three mentioned in this place: *aghshiyya*, *ṣifāqāt*, and *ṭabaqāt* — although in Hebrew one [uses the terms] *qelippot* and *qerumot* for them — anyhow only the term *qerum* is applicable to them in the Hebrew language. For the term *qelippah* is not all at applicable to any of these three [membranes], because it is mostly used for the peels of edible fruits. For this reason I truely know that my translation does not at all elucidate nor clarify what the Rabbi, of blessed memory, wants to say. May the reader accept this apology of mine for the embarrassment caused to him just by this text on the explanation of the membranes.

And in Aphorism 23:107 he states:

> Says the translator: Of all these nine names [of substances] which are the result and product of milk which he mentioned in this section, I can only find two [equivalents] in the Hebrew language, namely: *he-ḥalav* and *miẓ-he-ḥalav* because the term *ḥem'ah* is not part of these nine [terms], and the terms *he-ḥalav ha-niqpa* and *he-ḥalav he-ḥamuẓ* are derivative terms: *ha-niqpa* from *ha-haqpa'ah* and *he-ḥamuẓ* from *ha-ḥimmuẓ*. For this reason I have mentioned all these nine terms in the Arabic language and they are milk, which is the highest class with seven species derived from the milk beneath it and each of the seven is different from the others; one can also call them 'individuals' when using the term 'species' for milk. The nine terms including the seven species of milk for which I do not know a Hebrew name except for *miẓ ḥalav* are respectively: *maḥīḍ* i.e. [milk] from which the butter has been removed and the rest is [called] 'maḥīḍ'; it is also called 'dūgh'. The third term mentioned by him is 'kashk', the fourth 'maṣl', the fifth 'rā'ib' and is also called 'māsit', the sixth 'ḥāriz' (= 'ḥāzir') and the seventh 'al-aqiṭ'".

Study of the Terminology Employed by Zeraḥyah in his Translation of Maimonides' Medical Aphorisms

The following study of the terminology employed by Zeraḥyah in his translation of Maimonides' Medical Aphorisms is based on my forthcoming critical edition. Next to the analysis of the terminology employed by Zeraḥyah, I shall refer to parallel terms gleaned from the following texts: 1. the Hebrew translations of Maimonides' *Medical Aphorisms* by Nathan ha-Me'ati; 2. Shem Tov Ben Isaac, *Sefer ha-Shimmush*; 3. Moses Ben Samuel Ibn Tibbon, *Sefer Ẓedat ha-Derakhim*, Bk. 7, chs. 7–30; 4. Hillel Ben Samuel, *Sefer Keritut*. The English translations are based on the Arabic text of my forthcoming edition of Maimonides' *Aphorisms* unless indicated otherwise.

List of Terms

אבה = Arab. أبه 'to pay attention'; cf. 25.64: גליאנוס לא יאבה בשום דבר מזה ולא ידענו אבל הוא מכה[238] לבד (But Galen did not pay attention to this and did not know it, since he only proceeds at random). Hebrew אבה does not feature in this sense in the current dictionaries. Nathan (a.l.) translates Arab. أبه as הבין.

אֵבֶר: **האיברים המעולים** = Arab. الأعضاء الشريفة 'the noble organs'; cf. 3.79 (see as well 10.2): מורסות האברים המעולים ממיתים (Tumours in the noble organs are fatal). Hebrew האיברים המעולים, sing. האיבר המעולה does not feature in the current dictionaries. Nathan (a.l.) has האברים המעולים or האברים הנכבדים, while in Hillel we find האיברים המיוחסים.

אֹדֶם: **אודם הביצה** = Arab. صفرة البيض 'egg yolk'; cf. 2.3: המרה האדומה צבועה הרבה או בלתי צבועה הרבה וכן כשתתרבה בה החמימות עד שתשוב כאודם הביצה תתילד בעורקים ובגידים הדופקים (The yellow bile, whether it is saturated [in colour] or not — and similarly when it is extremely heated until it becomes like egg yolk — originates from veins and arteries). Hebrew אודם הביצה does not feature in the current dictionaries. N (a.l.) has חלמון ביצה. Another term used by Zeraḥyah for 'eggyolk' is מוח הביצה (see entry מוח).

אִכּוּל: **איכול** = Arab. تأكّل: 'corrosion'; cf. 7.60: האיכול יתחדש מליחות נושכות והליחות הנושכות הם החריפות והחמוצות והמלוחות (Corrosion is caused by biting humours; biting humours are those humours that are sharp, sour and salty). Hebrew איכול is only attested in Ben Yehuda (BM 205) as occurring in medieval literature in the sense of 'itching'. Nathan (a.l.) translates Arab. تأكّل as איכול as well; cf. Shem Tov, s.v. איכול and MD 188, s.v. 'corrosion'.

---

238 מכה: يخبط a.

אכילה = Arab. تأكّل: 'corrosion'; cf. 16.7: יקרה לנשים החולי הנקרא הגרת דם בהנקות בזה הגוף כולו. וברוב יהיה זה לנשים אשר גופן יהיה לח ושמן.[239] והדבר אשר יהיה מורק בהגרת הדם בקצת העתים הוא טרי אדום ולפעמים טרי מימיי או שיהיה נוטה אל הכרכומות. אבל אם ראית אותו כדם ההקזה תרגיש אם יוכל להיות מאכילה[240] שתהיה בצואר הרחם (Sometimes women suffer from the illness called 'female flux' whereby the whole body is purged. This mostly occurs to those women whose bodies are soft and phlegmatic [in constitution]. The discharge [from the body] through this flux sometimes consists of a reddish serum, and at other times of a watery or yellowish serum. But if you observe the blood to be like the blood of venesection, investigate it carefully whether it comes from an erosion. Most often, such an erosion occurs at the neck of the uterus). Hebrew אכילה does not feature in this sense in the current dictionaries. Nathan (a.l.) translates Arab. تأكّل as התאכלות. In addition to אכילה Zeraḥyah has איכול for Arab. تأكّل. See next entry.

אוכלת: אכל = Arab. أكلة 'canker'; cf. 23.48: בגוף יתקבץ[241] הפסד גדול עם[242] החבלה ליחה רעה או מרות מלינקוניקי או זינגארי שורץ וילבש מה שסביבו מן האברים עד שיאכל האבר הבריא אשר סמוך לאבר החולה. וזה החולי נקרא האוכלת (Sometimes because of the severe corruption of an ulcer a malignant humour or black bile or verdigris green bile accumulates in the body, and spreads and affects the parts around [the diseased part] until the healthy part adjacent to this diseased part becomes corroded. This illness is called 'ukla' [canker]). Hebrew אוכלת does not feature in the current dictionaries. In Low XXXVI we find Aram. אוכלא in the sense of: 'A sickness (perhaps consumption or spreading cancer)'; but cf. SDA 88: 'dimness of the eye'. Nathan (a.l.) translates Arab. أكلة as איכול.

אספוגות = Arab. تخلخل 'looseness; porousness; rarefaction'; cf. 3.99 (see as well 7.14; 23.99): בהתקבץ דקות הליחה והאספוגות האבר וחמימות האויר הסובב וכח הרפואה הנעשית והוזק כח החולה אז תתיר המורסה במהרה ואפשר שתתיר פתאם (If fineness of the humour, looseness [of the substance] of the organ, heat of the surrounding air, strength of the medicine applied, and abundant strength in the patient combine, the tumour is quickly and sometimes suddenly

---

239 ושמן: البلغميات a.

240 מאכילה שתהיה: من تأكّل وأكثر ما يعرض التأكّل a.

241 יתקבץ הפסד: يجتمع... عن فساد a.

242 עם: في a.

dissolved). Hebrew אספוגות is a non-attested variant to ספוגיות which features in medieval literature, for instance in Samuel Ibn Tibbon's Hebrew translation of Maimonides' 'Guide of the Perplexed' 2. 21 (cf. BM 4150). Nathan translates تخلخل as חלחול or רפיון.

אֹפֶל: אופל = Arab. كسوف 'eclipse'; cf. 24.1: ספר כאבי הנשים לאבקראט הוציאו חונין וביארו גליאנוס ונמצא תוספת באותו הספר הוציאו זולתי חונין וביארו זולתי גליאנוס ונמצא באותו התוספת עניינים זרים מהם שאמר שפוריפיריוס אמר שהיה לשמש בסקליאה אופל גדול ובאותה השנה קרה שהנשים ילדו בנים משונים בצורתם בעלי שני ראשים ושקצת הנשים קרה להם שרואות דם ווסתן מפיהן בקיא (In the *Book on Women's Diseases* composed by Hippocrates, translated by Ḥunayn and commented upon by Galen I found an addition which is not part of Ḥunayn's translation nor of Galen's commentary. In that additional commentary there are strange things. Among them that he says: Porphyry has related that there was a great eclipse of the sun in Sicily [and that] in that year women gave birth to abnormally shaped babies that had two heads. And that some women menstruated from their mouth through vomiting). Hebrew אופל only features in the current dictionaries in the general sense of 'darkness'; cf. KB 79. Nathan (a.l.) translates Arab. كسوف as the standard לקות. See as well entry יצא.

בֵּאוּר: **ביאור** = Arab. تبيين 'distinction'; cf. 6.8: אמר משה הסתכל איך שם הפרש בין החיכוך והפלצות והריגור מדרגות חידוד הליחה לבד. ובזה תוספת ביאור ממה שאמרו במאמרו ברעדה וברפפות ובריגור ובכיווץ (Says Moses: Consider how only the [different] degrees of sharpness of the humour are turned by him [Galen] into that which forms the difference between itch, shivering and rigour. There is another distinction between these diseases that he makes in his treatise *De tremore, palpitatione et convulsione*). Hebrew ביאור in the sense of 'distinction' is a non-attested semantic borrowing from the Arabic تبيين.

בִּטּוּל = Arab. خدر 'numbness'; cf. 22.38: אכילת ראשי הארנבת כל מה שאפשר יועיל מן הרעש ונמצא בנסיון שיועיל כמו כן מבטול והפלג ואכילת בשר הארנבת ישבר החול (The consumption of the heads of hares, as much as one is able to eat from it, is beneficial for trembling. I found by experience that it is also beneficial for numbness and hemiplegia. The consumption of hare meat crumbles [kidney] stones). Hebrew בִּטּוּל does not feature in this sense in the current dictionaries. Nathan (a.l.) translates Arab. خدر as תרדמת האברים. Cf. entry בטל, and ZA 27.

בטח: הבטיח = Arab. رجا 'to hope'; cf. 8.22: ובאלהים כי כל מי ששתה המים הקרים מאותם שאני הבטחתי שיהיו ניצלים ניצלו ונתרפאו (And I swear by God, all those who drank cold water and whom I had hoped would recover [actually] recovered and regained their health). Hebrew הבטיח does not feature in this sense in the current dictionaries. N translates Arab. رجا with the standard Hebrew synonym קיוה.

(בטל) ביטל = Arab. خدّر 'to benumb'; cf. 8.39: זאת הרפואה המחוברת לשכך הכאב אשר יכנסו בה הדברים המבטלים החוש ראוי לאדם שיכוין בחיבורה אל ג' סגולות: האחת שיבטל החוש (When one compounds remedies with narcotics to alleviate pain, one should consider three things: first that [by means of which] one should benumb the sensation [of pain]…). Hebrew ביטל does not feature in this sense in the current dictionaries. N (a.l.) translates Arab. خدّر as הרדים; cf. entry בִּטּוּל.

(בטל) התבטל = Arab. خدر 'to turn numb'; cf. 23.23: הביטול הנקרא בערבי כדר בכף רפה הוא דבר מורכב מעוצר[243] החוש ועוצר[244] התנועה ויהיה מקרירות האויר ומלחיצת הגופות העצביות וממישוש הבעל חיים הימיי. והאברים יקרה להם תחלה שיתבטלו ואחרי כן ישובו אין להם חוש ולא תנועה ויאמר לזה המין מההזק רפיון בערבי איסתירכא ברפה הכף (Numbness is something composed of difficulty of sensation and difficulty of movement. It arises from coldness of the air, from compression of the nervous parts of the body, or from [the shock caused by] contact with a sea creature. The bodily parts first turn numb, then loose their sensation and movement. This kind of harm is called 'paralysis'). Hebrew התבטל does not feature in this sense in the current dictionaries. Nathan (a.l.) translates Arab. خدر as נרדם.

בֶּטֶן = Arab. بطن 'hollowness'; cf. 15.3: אין ראוי שיהיה[245] אבר שיהיה לו עומק או בטן ואין בגוף אבר אלא ולו בטן עם עומק מלבד הידים והרגלים והחלצים (One should not cauterize a part of the body that has depth or hollowness, and all bodily parts have depth or hollowness except the hands, feet and loins). Hebrew בטן does not feature in this sense in the current dictionaries. According to EM 154 it can have the meaning of פנים/תוך/מעמקים (inside; interior; depth) in Biblical literature. Nathan (a.l.) translates Arab. بطن as חלל.

---

243 מעוצר: من عسر a.

244 ועוצר: وعسر a.

245 שיהיה: أن يكوى a.

מובטן (בטן) (Part. Hofʿal) = Arab. مبطون 'abdominal patient'; cf. 23.93: בהתחדש במעים הדקים מורסא קשה או סתימה גדולה ממותר עד שיקיא האדם צואתו אותו החולי נקרא איליאוס ומעט הם שיהיו נצלים ממנו. ובהתבטל המעים כולם והאסטומכא ולא יוכל להחזיק מה שבהם ואפילו שעה מועטת ולא תהיה החולי עוקץ אותו החולי נקרא המעדת המיעים וחוליי הבטן. ונקרא בעל זה החולי כמו כן מובטן (If the small intestines are affected by a hard tumor or by a severe obstruction of faeces so that the patient vomits his faeces, that illness is called 'ileus' and hardly anyone can be saved from it. If all [parts of] the intestines and the stomach fall ill and one cannot retain their contents even for a short time, or if the illness does not come with biting [pain], that illness is called 'lientery'. It is also called 'abdominal affections'. The patient suffering therefrom is called 'abdominal patient'): Hebrew מובטן does not feature in the current dictionaries. Nathan (a.l.) translates Arab. مبطون just like Zeraḥyah as מובטן.

בלבול הדעת :בלבול = Arab. اختلاط العقل 'delirium'; cf. 6.37: סימני קראניטס י"ו עלאמה והם התעורה או השינה המצטערת ובלבול הדעת (The signs of phrenitis are sixteen: sleeplessness or disturbed sleep and delirium…). Hebrew בלבול הדעת does not feature in the current dictionaries. Masie (MD 211) mentions בלבול השכל as featuring in Tobias Kohen's (1652–1729) *Maʿaseh Tuviyyah* which was printed in Venice 1709. Nathan (a.l.) translates Arab. اختلاط العقل as ערבוב השכל (cf. BM 4707), while Moses Ibn Tibbon has ערבוב שכל for Arabic تخليط 'delirium' (cf. Moses Ibn Tibbon, s.v. ערבוב). See as well ZA 135: 'mental confusion'.

בקיעה = Arab. فتق 'hernia'; cf. 9. 123: זכר התמימי בספר הנקרא אלמרשד זה העניין מרפואת הבקיעה קודם שיאריך (In his book entitled *al-Murshid* al-Tamīmī mentions the following way of treating a hernia before it becomes chronic). Hebrew בקיעה only features in the current dictionaries in the sense of 'cleaving, cleft, that which is cloven' (JD 186). Nathan (a.l.) translates Arab. فتق as בקיעה as well. A synonym for Arab. فتق, namely قيلة is translated by Zeraḥyah as כיס (see entry כיס below).

בַּשָׂמוּת = Arab. عطرية 'fragrance'; cf. 20.75: הפירה יחזק האסטומכא ויש להם סגולה שהם מכבים הצמא כשהם נאכלים אחר המזון ומיצם כשיונח ישוב חומץ שיחזק האסטומכא חיזוק מופלא ולא יזיק בעצבים מפני שיש בו מן הקיבוץ והבשמות (Pears strengthen the stomach and have the special property to quench the thirst when eaten after a meal. If one lets their juice stand, it turns into vinegar which strengthens the stomach in a wonderful way and does not harm the nerves because of the astringency and fragrance which it contains). Hebrew בשמות only features in the current dictionaries in the sense of 'the manufacturing of perfumes, spices' (cf. EM 206; BM 643). Nathan (a.l.) translates Arab. عطرية as בשמיות.

גחלת = Arab. جمر 'carbuncle'; cf. 23.38: הגחלת הוא מן המורסות החמות אלא שתולדת הגחלת תהיה בקרות לדם כמו הרתיחה עד שהעור יהיה נשרף ויחדש עם זה קרושטא (38) (A carbuncle is an inflammation, but it is formed if the blood is affected by something similar to boiling to such a degree that the skin is burned and that an eschar is formed with it). In the sense of 'carbuncle' Hebrew גחלת is a semantic borrowing from the Arabic جمر and is mentioned in BM 749 in the sense of 'Pestblatter, charbon, furoncle' in an attestation from Nathan ha-Me'ati's Hebrew translation of Ibn Sīnā's *K. al-Qānūn* prepared in Rome in 1279. גחלת is also used by Nathan in his translation of this particular aphorism.

גיד, Plur. **גידים** = I. Arab. عروق 'vessels'; cf. 6.6: הגידים הנראים יהיו מליאים מתמשכים ולא יהיו הפנימיים כן (Sometimes the outer vessels are full and stretched while the inner ones are not); II. Arab. قضيب 'penis'; cf. 16.10: כל הגידים הדופקים ושאינם דופקים בכל הגוף מהזכרים והנקיבות הם על דמיון אחד לא במספר לבדו אלא ביצירתם ותכונתם ומקומם אבל ישתנו בכלי ההריון ויתבאר בניתוח כי כלי ההריון בזכרים ובנקבות זה נוכח זה בדמיון כי בזכרים יוצאים ובנקבות הם בפנים עד שהרחם אילו נתהפך שטחו הפנימי לחוץ היה דומה לכיס הביצים והביצים אשר בצדי הרחם יהיו בתוך כיס ויהיה צואר הרחם דומה לגיד (All the pulsatile and non-pulsatile vessels in the entire body of both male and female are the same, not only in number but also in structure, form and location. However, [male and female] are different in their reproductive organs. [Yet] it is clear from anatomy that the reproductive parts of the male and female correspond to each other and resemble each other, but in the male they protrude whereas in the female they are internal. [This is true] to such a degree that if the female [reproductive] organs were reversed so that their internal side would be external, the uterus would as it were become the scrotum, and the testicles[246] which are on the sides of the uterus would be located inside this pouch and the neck of the uterus would correspond to the penis). For a summary account of the different meanings of this term in medieval medical literature,

246 I.e. the ovaries.

see Shem Tov, entry גיד; see as well Lieber, *Asaf's Book of Medicines*, p. 238, n. 42.[247]

גיד: גיד הדופק = Arab. العرق 'artery'; cf. 4.21: בהיות בגיד הדופק רוע המזג משתנה כי החלק ממנו שהוא יותר לחות וחמימות יהיה דפקו יותר גדול ויותר מהיר (If a [varying] bad temperature occurs in an artery, that part of it containing more moisture and heat has a pulse that is greater and more rapid). Next to גיד הדופק Zeraḥyah (4.22) has גיד שלדופק . Cf. Shem Tov, s.v. גיד.

גפן: **גפנים** = Arab. دوال 'varicose veins'; cf. 23.47: כל המורסות הסרטניות אמנם תהיה תולדתם ממותר מלינקוניקו. ואם יטה אותו המותר אל שפל הגוף וידחהו הכח הדוחה אשר בגידים מפיותיהם אשר בפי הטבעת או ברחם[248] נקרא זו ההרקה טחורים שיצא מהם הדם. ולפעמים תדחה אל הרגלים ותעשה חולי הנקרא גפנים (All cancerous tumours especially develop from a melancholic superfluity. If that superfluity tends to the lower part of the body and the expulsive faculty in the vessels expels it from the openings [of the vessels] in the anus or vagina, then [the parts from which] this evacuation [takes place] are called 'haemorrhoids', and blood flows from them. Sometimes those superfluities are forced to the legs and cause varicose veins). Hebrew גפנים is a non-attested semantic borrowing from the Arab. دوال. The Arabic term is not translated by Nathan (a.l.).

גרד = Arab. حكّ 'to rub'; cf. 22.53: ואבן עקיק כשתשחקנו ותגרד בו השנים ילבנם וימנע איכולם (If a carnelian is pulverized and the teeth are rubbed with it, it makes them white and prevents their corrosion). Hebrew גרד only features in the current dictionaries in the sense of 'to scratch, to scrape, to comb' (JD 265) or 'to scratch, to shave' (BM 834). Nathan (a.l.) translates Arab. حكّ as חכך.

גרידה: גרידת המעים = Arab. خراطة الأمعاء 'shreds of intestinal tissue'; cf. 6.82: שלשול הדם הבא מחולי הכבד יתחדש פתאום. אבל אותו שיבוא מהמעים לא יתחדש פתאום אבל יתחדש שלשול מרות ינשוך בתכלית הנשיכה ואחר כן יהיה נמשך אחר זה גרידת המעים (Bloody diarrhoea due to a liver disease may occur suddenly. But if it comes because of [a disease of] the intestines, it does not happen suddenly, but rather begins as a bilious diarrhoea which is extremely acrid; this is followed

247 E. Lieber, 'Asaf's Book of Medicines: A Hebrew Encyclopaedia of Greek and Jewish Medicine, Possibly Compiled in Byzantium on an Indian Model', in J. Scarborough (ed.), *Symposium on Byzantine Medicine* (Dumbarton Oaks Papers. No. 38, 1984 [Washington 1985]), 233–49.

248 ברחם: في القبل a.

by shreds of intestinal tissue). Hebrew גרידת המעים does not feature in the current dictionaries. גרידה features in BM 841 (= EM 266) in an attestation from Nathan's Hebrew translation of Ibn Sīnā's *K. al-Qānūn* prepared in Rome in 1279. גרידת המעים also features in Nathan's translation of Arab. خراطة الأمعاء in our aphorism.

גרעין, Plur. **גרעינים** = Arab. حبّ 'pills'; cf. 13.13: כשתרצה להריק הגוף ממה שיש בו מן הליחות ותנקה הראש עמו עד שלא ירד ממנו קטרא ראוי לך שתהיה הרפואה מחוברת מרפואה משונה בכחותיה כמו הגרעינים אשר חברנו אנחנו (If you want to cleanse the body from the [bad] humours in it and at the same time want to cleanse the head so that no defluction descends from it, the remedy must be compounded from ingredients of varying strength, such the pills which I compounded…). Hebrew גרעין, Plur. גרעינים only features in the current dictionaries in the sense of 'kernel' (BM 848). Nathan (a.l.) translates the Arab. حبّ as גרגרים.

נדבק (דבק) = Arab. انجبر 'to heal (of broken bones)'; cf. 15.63: העצמות במי שהוא בחור יהיו נדבקים קודם מהיותם נדבקים בילדים כי הילדים צריכים אל חומר יגדלו בו ויחליפו במקום מה שהותך מהם. זכר זה אסקליביוס במאמר הראשון מפירושו לספר הדבקות ([Broken] bones of young people heal sooner than those of children, because children need material for their growth and to replace the matter which has been dissolved. This was mentioned by Asklepios in the first treatise of his commentary on [Hippocrates'] book on [fractures] and their setting). Hebrew נדבק does not feature in a medical sense in the current dictionaries. Nathan (a.l.) translates the Arab. انجبر as נחבש.

דִּבֵּק (דבק) = Arab. جبر 'to set (broken bones)'; cf. 15.64: כל עצם שישבר שילך עליו ד' ימים ויותר לא תחשוב לדבקו כי היה[249] גובר על החולה הזק גדול (Do not attempt to set any broken bone if only four days have passed, lest you cause the patient severe harm). Hebrew דִּבֵּק does not feature in this sense in the current dictionaries. Nathan (a.l.) translates Arab. جبر as חבש.

דבקה: דבקות = Arab. جبائر 'trusses'; cf. 15.69: ראוי שתקשור תחלה תחת הרפידות ותתחיל ממקום החולי ותכלה אל המקום העליון למען מנוע הרקת הלחויות ויהיה מונע המורסא. ואחרי כן תשים הרפידות ואחר כן תרפד[250] ממעלה לרפידות כדי שלא יסתער ותתחיל ממקום המחלה ותכלה למטה לדחוק הדם המעופש מן האבר החולה עד הקצה. ואחר

249 היה גובר: تجلب a.

250 תרפד: تربط a.

זאת הקשירה השנייה תשים[251] והיא תקיים ותחזק כל מה שהוא מאחריה ויסמוך אותו. ויהיה כל אשר יקיף באבר ארבעה דברים. הקשירה הנעשית על האבר והרפידות והקשירה שעליהם והדבקות ([In cases of fracture] first put a bandage below the pads. Begin from the spot of the injury and end higher up to prevent moistures from streaming [to that part] so that it does not become inflamed. Then apply the pads, and then put a bandage above the pads, so that they do not become disordered, and begin with the spot of the injury and end downwards in order to force the putrid blood from the injured limb to its extremity. After this second bandage, apply the trusses which secure and support all that is behind it. Thus, there are four things which surround the limb: The bandage which has contact with the limb, the pads, the bandage on these, and the trusses). Hebrew דבקה: דבקות does not feature in the current dictionaries. Nathan (a.l.) translates Arab. جبائر as חבישות and Shem Tov (s.v. קשיש) as קשישים. See as well SG Quf 28.

דְּבֵקוּת = Arab. جَبْر 'setting (of broken bones)'; cf. entry נדבק (דבק). Hebrew דבקות does not feature in this sense in the current dictionaries. Nathan (a.l.) translates Arab. جَبْر as חבישה and Shem Tov (s.v. השבה) as השבת השברים.

דבקות הזהב = Arab. لصاق الذهب 'chrysocolla'; cf. 23.101: הרפואה אשר תחמם ותלחלח עד שתפסיד מה שתמצא היא באמת הרפואה המעפשת. וכן נקראות כמו כן כל הרפואות החמות היבשות העבות בעצמותם בהיותם נושכים מעט או שורפות מעט מבלתי חדש כאב נקראות מעפשות כי הם יתיכו ויאכלו הבשר ויעשו בו מה שיעשה המעפשת באמת והם כמו הארסניץ ודבקות הזהב והפיניי[252] וממית הזאב (Remedies which warm and moisten until they corrupt what they encounter are truly called 'putrefying remedies'. Similarly, all remedies which are hot and dry and whose substance is thick, if they bite or burn somewhat without causing pain, are called 'putrefying' because they dissolve and corrode the flesh. They have the same effect on it as the truly putrefying remedies. These include the two types of arsenic, chrysocolla, stinging or urticating caterpillar of the pinewoods, and aconite). Hebrew דבקות הזהב, a loan translation of the Arab. لصاق الذهب does not feature in the current dictionaries. Nathan (a.l.) translates the Arab. as מדביק הזהב, just like Shem Tov (SG Mem 63). :-

251 תשים: الجبائر add a.

252 והפיניי: ودود الصنوبر a.

דקירה = Arab. انبثاق 'bursting'; cf. 15.39: החבלות אשר יתרבה יציאת הדם מהם מפני דקירת העורקים יפסיק אותו הדם בכויה או ברפואה שיהיה כחה כח הכויה או בדבר שיקבץ וימעט[253] או כשיעתיק החומר אל מקום אחר קרוב או במשכו אל הפך הצד או בקררו לכל הגוף וכל שכן לקרר האבר שבו החבלה (When an excessive amount of blood is streaming from wounds because of a bursting of the vessels, the flow of the blood can be stopped either by cauterization or by drugs whose strength is equal to cautery or by something that closes and agglutinates, or by transferring it to a nearby site, or by attracting it to the opposite side, or by cooling the whole body, and especially the part of the body where the wound is). Hebrew דקירה does not feature in this sense in the current dictionaries. Nathan (a.l.) translates انبثاق as החנק (is: اختناق).

דקר = I. Arab. بتر 'to cut'; cf. 12.38: וכשידוקר הגיד הדופק על רחבו בשני חצאיו אין בו פחד כי הוא יתקווץ כל אחד משני קצותיו אל הצד אשר הוא בו (When a pulsatile vessel is cut in its width, it is not dangerous because every part contracts to its own side); II. Arab. بطّ 'to lance'; cf. 15.8: כשתדקור שום מקום והריקות מה שיש בו מן הטרי תהיה נזהר באותה שעה ובמה שאחריה מעשותך השמן עם[254] המים (If you lance a site and evacuate the pus from it, be careful at that moment and thereafter not to use oil or water [to wash the wound]). Hebrew דקר only features in the current dictionaries in the sense of 1) 'to dig, bore, pierce'; 2) 'to spread, branch off' (JD 320) or 'to pierce' (BM 988). Nathan (a.l.) translates Arab. بتر with the Hebrew parallel בתר and Arab. بطّ as כרת.

הבטחה = Arab. ثقة 'confidence'; cf. 8.22: הייתי מקדים על הרבה בני אדם וקצתם השקיתים המים הקרים בהבטחה ונאמנות בכל זמן שהם חולים ומהם בזמן בלתי זמן עם שזולתי מן הרופאים היו מניחים מהשקותם אילו (In the case of many people I behaved daringly [in my treatment]. With confidence and certainty, I gave some of them cold water all the time they were ill, and I gave it to others from time to time, although other physicians refrained from letting their patients drink cold water). Hebrew הבטחה is only attested in the sense of 'confidence' in the current dictionaries for Rabbinic literature (BM 1026; EM 339). In addition to הבטחה for Arab. ثقة Z uses בֶּטַח; cf. ibid.: אבל מי שהיתה קדחתו שורפת גמורה ולא היה בשום אחד ממיעיו מורסא הייתי משקהו המים הקרים בתכלית הבטח והאמונה (With utmost confidence and trust, I let someone who suffered

253 וימעט: يسدّ a.

254 עם: أو a.

from pure ardent fever but had no tumour in any part of his viscera drink cold water). See as well entry (בטח) הבטיח.

הגרה: הגרת הדם = I. Arab. اختلاف الدم 'bloody diarrhoea, dysentery'; cf. 6.90: בתחלת הגרת הדם יקרה בטול תאות המזון (Sometimes a lack of appetite occurs in the beginning of bloody diarrhoea [dysentery]). Hebrew הגרת הדם only features in BM 1041 in the literal sense of 'the streaming of blood'. Nathan (a.l.) translates Arab. اختلاف الدم as שלשול הדם (lit. diarrhoea of blood). According to Masie (MD 238) Nathan has Hebrew הפשט הדם in his translation of Ibn Sīnā's *K. al-Qānūn* prepared in Rome in 1279; II. Arab. نفث الدم 'hemophtysis'; cf. 9.61: בעל האיקטריזיאה יועילנו המראים הירוקים שהם יתירו הקולורא. והרחיקו בעלי הגרת הדם מראות המראה[255] האדום כי הם ישלחו הדם (Sometimes a jaundice patient benefits from [looking at] yellow colours because this dissolves the yellow bile). A patient with hemoptysis should be forbidden to look at colours that are primarily red, because this will make the blood stream forth). Nathan (a.l.) translates Arab. نفث الدم as רקיקת הדם.

-: הגרת הדם מהאף = Arab. رعاف 'nosebleed'; cf. 9.2: לא תמתין בהגרת הדם מהאף עד שיפול כח החולה (In the case of a nosebleed you should not wait for the strength [of the body] to collapse). Hebrew הגרת הדם מהאף does not feature in the current dictionaries. Nathan (a.l.) translates Arab. رعاف as רעיפה. Masie (MD 509) refers to 'nosebleed' as דמם האף. Another term used by Zeraḥyah for Arab. رعاف is הטפת דם מהנחירים (see s.v. הטפה).

הזרה = Arab. رَدْع 'restraint, repulsion'; cf. 3.85: ולא ארמוז בהזרתו לעולם אלא לעתים רחוקות שנזיר במעט הזרה כשלא יהיה שם כאב ויהיה הגוף נקי (I never advise application of a restraining treatment, except for a light one when there is no pain and when the body is clean). Hebrew הזרה does not feature in the current dictionaries. Nathan (a.l.) translates the Arabic رَدْع as ארתעה. Cf. entry (זור) הזיר.

הטפה: הטפת דם מהנחירים = Arab. رعاف 'nosebleed'; cf. 12.42: הנשים אשר יתחיל להם ההדרוקן בסבת העצר הווסת וכן מי שקרה לו זה מהעצר דם שהיה נגר מפיות העורקים או בהטפת דם מהנחירים ראוי שתתחיל בהקזתם קודם שהכח יחלש ויפול (In the case of women in whom dropsy begins because of the retention of their menstruation as well as in the case of those in whom dropsy occurs because of a retention of the blood which was streaming from the mouths of the veins or through a

255 המראה: الأَوْلي add a.

nosebleed, one should hurry to bleed them before their strength dissolves and collapses). Hebrew הטפת דם מהנחירים does not feature in the current dictionaries. Nathan (a.l.) translates Arab. رعاف as רעיפת דם נחירים. Another term used by Zeraḥyah for Arab. رعاف is הגרת הדם מהאף; see entry הגרה.

הידרוקן = Arab. استسقاء 'dropsy'; cf. 6.45: מי שהוא בטבעו דומה לבעל ההידרוקן ההידרוקן ימהר אליו (If someone resembles a person suffering from dropsy in his nature, he is quickly affected by this disease). Hebrew הידרוקן is only attested for Rabbinic literature, cf. JD 335; 557. Nathan (a.l.) translates Arab. استسقاء as שקוי. See as well Shem Tov, glossary 1 (SG He 10).

המעדת המעים: המעדה = Arab. زلق الأمعاء 'lientery'; cf. 23.80: אנמם שינוי המזונות באסטומכא אל איכות אחרת לא אל אותם אשר בטבע ויאמר לו רוע העיכול והוא האמפונימינטו בערבי תכמה. וביטול הכח העוצר מן האסטומכא הוא שלא תתקבץ האסטומכא כלל ולא[256] תרחף על המזון ולא תאסוף עליו בדבקות ואסיפה. וזה יקרה לה בחולי הנקרא חלקות או המעדת המיעים (If the foods change in the stomach into a quality different from the natural one, it is called 'dyspepsia', i.e. bad digestion. If the retentive faculty of the stomach becomes inactive, it means that the stomach does not contract at all and does not wrap itself around the foods in a tight and firm manner. This happens to the stomach in the illness called 'lientery'). Hebrew המעדת המעים, a loan translation of Arabic زلق الأمعاء, does not feature in the current dictionaries. In addition to המעדת המעים Zeraḥyah has מעידת המעים (see s.v. מעידה) and חלקות המיעים (see s.v. חלקות). Nathan (a.l.) translates زلق الأمعاء, just like Zeraḥyah as המעדת המעים. The same term features in Shem Tov (cf. SG He 11), while Moses Ibn Tibbon has הגרת המעים in his translation of Maimonides' *On the Regimen on Health*; cf. BMR IV, 22.

הנחה = Arab. موضوع 'subject'; cf. Introduction: המאמר הראשון ישלם על פרקים יהיו נתלים בהנחת המלאכה (The first treatise contains aphorisms which concern the subject of the [medical] art). הנחה does not feature in this sense in the current dictionaries. Nathan (a.l.) has נושא, which also features in Samuel Ibn Tibbon's Hebrew translation of Maimonides, *Guide of the Perplexed* 1.60,90; cf. EP 88.

הפך ל-: הפך = Arab. ضادّ 'to have a contrary effect on'; cf. 21.42: הקנמון הוא רפואה דקה מאד פותחת שבילי האסטומכא ויטהר הליחות וידקדקם ויהפך לטרי המוסרח כולו

256 ולא תרחף על המזון ולא תאסוף עליו בדבקות ואסיפה: ولا تلتحف على الأغذية التحاف ضمّ ولزوم a.

כשישנהו ויתירהו (Chinese cinnamon [Cinnamomum ceylanicum] is a very fine drug; it opens the passages of the stomach, cleanses and attenuates the humours and has a contrary effect on all the putrefactive serous discharges by changing and dissolving them). Hebrew הפך does not feature in this sense in the current dictionaries. Nathan (a.l.) translates the Arab. ضادّ as ניגד.

הפרדה: הפרדת הדבקות = Arab. تفرّق اتّصال 'a dissolution of continuity'; cf. 7.6: סבות הכאבים הוא או הפרדת הדבקות או שינוי מה שיהיה פתאום (The causes of pain are a dissolution of continuity or a sudden change). Hebrew הפרדת הדבקות does not feature in the current dictionaries. Nathan (a.l.) translates Arab. تفرّق اتّصال as פרוק חבור, while Hillel (s.v. התרה) translates the Latin parallel 'solutio continuitatis' as התרת הדבקות.

הקדמה: הקדמת ההכרה = Arab. تقدمة المعرفة 'prognosis'; cf. 6.94: ותנהיג זה הפרק בהשגחה גדולה כי הוא יספיק על חלקים הרבה מהקדמת ההכרה (Consider this aphorism carefully, for it contains many things relevant to prognosis). Hebrew הקדמת ההכרה does not feature in the current dictionaries. Nathan (a.l.) translates the same Arabic term as הקדמת הידיעה.

הקפאה = Arab. جمود 'catalepsy'; cf. 23.59: בהתחזק הקרירות על המוח ויתערב בו לחות יתחדש ממנו השרסאם הקר והוא ליתרגיאה. וכשיתערב עם הקרירות יובש יתחדש ההקפאה (If cold dominates the brain and moisture becomes added thereto, lethargy develops therefrom. If dryness is added to the cold, catalepsy develops from it). Hebrew הקפאה features in the sense of 'congelation' in BM 1174 in an attestation from Nathan's Hebrew translation in his translation of Ibn Sīnā's *K. al-Qānūn* prepared in Rome in 1279. Nathan (a.l.) translates Arab. جمود as קפאון.

הרגל: הרגלים = Arab. رياضيات 'mathematics'; cf. 25.59: והוא בלא ספק כלומר גליאנוס הרגיל בהרגלים (He, I mean Galen, has undoubtedly trained himself in mathematics). In the sense of 'mathematics' Hebrew הרגלים is an unattested loan translation from the Arabic رياضيات. Nathan (a.l.) translates the Arabic رياضيات as למודיות.

הרגשה = Arab. حدس 'conjecture'; cf. 11.1: זמני החולי הכוללים הם ארבעה: התחלה ותוספת ועמידה וירידה. ולפי[257] עמוד על ידיעת הזמן ההווה מזמני החולי בהרגשה אמתית אי זה מזמניו הוא עתה (The periods of a disease are four altogether: beginning,

257 ולפי עמוד על: وبكذ ما يوقف على a.

increase, culmination and decline. It is only with great toil that one can come to know the actual period of a disease at a certain moment through an exact conjecture). Hebrew הרגשה only features in the current dictionaries in the sense of 'sensation, sentiment' (BM 1184; cf. KT 1:212) Nathan (a.l.) translates Arab. حدس as אומד.

הריון = Arab. تناسل 'reproduction'; cf. entry גיד. Hebrew הריון only features in the current dictionaries in the sense of 'conception, coition' (JD 367) or 'conception' (BM 1193). Nathan (a.l.) translates Arab. تناسل as הולדה.

הִשְׁוָיוּת = Arab. مساواة 'equality'; cf. 8.45: רוע המזג המתחדש בכל אחד מן האברים הוא חולי אשר באברים המתדמים החלקים וימנע וייצר בכח בלתי כח מכחות אותו האבר ויהיו הליחות מורקות בעבור זה בזמנים משתנים אל אברים משתנים על בלתי השויות ועל בלתי הסדר (A bad temperament occurring in any part of the body is an illness of that[258] part. It forms an obstruction and obstacle now for one and then another of that part's powers. Because of this, humours stream towards various parts at various times unequally and irregularly). Hebrew הִשְׁוָיוּת, a parallel to הַשְׁוָיָה (cf. BM 1206), does not feature in the current dictionaries. Nathan (a.l.) translates Arab. مساواة as שווי.

השמטה = Arab. خَلْع 'dislocation'; cf. 15.46: ועל זה המשל כשיקרה בפרק מן הפרקים הגדולים השמטה עם חבלה נרפא החבלה עד שתתרפא ואע"פ שאי אפשר דבקות ההשמטה אחר מכן כי אנו אם נחשוב להשיב ההשמטה עם החבלה ימצאהו כיווץ ברוב העניין (Similarly, when a major joint suffers from a dislocation in combination with an ulcer, we treat the ulcer [first] until it is healed, even if it is not possible to treat the dislocation afterwards. For if we try to combine the reduction of the dislocation with the treatment of the ulcer, the [patient] is mostly affected by spasms). Hebrew השמטה features in the sense of 'dislocation' in EM 415 in an attestation of Rashi on tb*Ḥulin* 28. Nathan (a.l.) translates Arab. خَلْع as שמט, Shem Tov as שמיטה, and Moses Ibn Tibbon as הקעה. Hillel uses the same term as Zeraḥyah, i.e. השמטה for translating Latin 'dislocatio'.

השקעה = Arab. استغراق 'torpor'; cf. 23.64: ביטול הדמיון נקרא ההשקעה וההקפאה והגרת[259] האף נקרא ערבוב (The loss of imagination is called 'torpor' and

258 Lit. of the homogeneous parts; cf. Gerrit Bos, *Maimonides, Medical Aphorisms. Treatises 6–9*. A parallel Arabic-English edition edited, translated, and annotated (Provo 2007), 51 and 119, n. 85.

259 והגרת האף: وجريانه المنكر a.

'catalepsy'. Its bad functioning is called 'delirium'). Hebrew השקעה in the sense of 'torpor' is a semantic borrowing from the Arab. استغراق which does not feature in the current dictionaries. Nathan (a.l.) translates the Arab. استغراق as שקיעה.

השתדלות הרפואה: השתדלות = Arab. حيلة البرء 'De methodo medendi' (*On the Method of Healing*); cf. 25.55: מקום הקושיא היותו מבאר בהשתדלות הרפואה כי מזון הטחול יותר עב ממזון הכבד[260] (The point of doubt is that in *De methodo medendi* he explains that the nourishment of the spleen is thicker than that of the liver whereas in *De usu partium* he explains that the nourishment of the spleen is thinner than that of the liver). Hebrew השתדלות הרפואה does not feature in the current dictionaries. Nathan (a.l.) translates Arab. حيلة البرء as תחבולת הרפואה.

התיתרות = Arab. توتّر 'stretching'; cf. 1.70: ואמנם המושקולי שלחזה ולבטן הוא הפך למושקולי של הידים והרגלים כי כשיתיתר יתרחב כי ימצא תחתיו גופות חלקים יכפפו לו בזמן התיתרותו (But something happens to the muscles of the chest and abdomen which is opposite to [that which happens to] the muscles of the arms and legs—namely, when they stretch they flatten because below them are soft organs that sink when these muscles stretch). Hebrew התיתרות in the sense of 'stretching' is a non-attested loan translation of Arab. توتّر. Nathan (a.l.) translates Arab. توتّر as המתח. See as well entries יתר and מְיֻתָּר.

התכה = Arab. ذبول 'marasmus'; cf. 8.58: ואני מכיר אדם אחד הלך[261] למרחץ אחד[262] מאילו המימות המעורבות מלח או ניטרי או גפרית כדי שיריק גופו. והיה עם זה הנהיג לצד הרקת המרות ולא היה יודע שהיה ראוי שיכניס על כל איכות גובר ויצא מהעניין הטבעי הפכו ושזה יותר טוב מן ההרקה ולא קיבל מי שהודיעו בזה והביאו זה אל יובש גדול באיבריו השרשיים עד שמצאו ההתכה והטיסיס ואחר כך מת (I know a man who relied upon bathing in waters mixed with salt or borax or sulphur in order to evacuate his body [of yellow bile]. In the rest of his regimen he [equally] pursued the evacuation of the bile, but he did not know that every dominating unnatural [humoural] quality should be opposed by the opposite quality and that this is much better than evacuation. Nor did he listen to those who told him so. As a result the main organs [of his body] dried so much that he was afflicted by phthisis and marasmus and then died). Hebrew התכה only features in the

---

260 הכבד: وبيّن في منافع الأعضاء أنّ غذاء الطحال ألطف من غذاء الكبد add a.

261 הלך: ركن a.

262 אחד מאילו המימות: بهذه المياه a.

current dictionaries in the sense of 'melting, dissolution' (cf. BM 1229–30) or of 'Verminderung, Abnahme, Diminutio, Auflösung, Zersetzung u.a.; Zergliederung, Analyse' (cf. KT 1:236). Nathan (a.l.) translates Arab. ذبول as צִמּוּק.

התכי = Arab. ذوباني 'wasting'; cf. 7.11: ועצם האברים יהיה ניתך או באורך חליים ארוכים או בחידוד חליים חדים או בקדחות התכיות (The substance of the organs is dissolved either because of prolonged chronic diseases or because of acute diseases or because of wasting fevers). Hebrew התכי, an adjective coined from התכה (cf. entry התכה) does not feature in the current dictionaries. Nathan translates Arab. حمّيات ذوبانية as קדחות שהם מהמס האברים.

התרה: התרת הבטן = I. Arab. الاستطلاق 'diarrhoea'; cf. 7.42: חולשת הכח שהוא סבת הרעש אינו סבה אחת אבל סבותיו מרובות. יוכל להיות בסבת המזון כמו שיהיה בשלשול הנק' איניישטיאון והתרת הבטן הגדולה (A weakness of the force that is the cause of a tremor does not have one cause but many causes. Sometimes it is caused by malnutrition, as happens in the case of cholera, severe diarrhoea…). Hebrew התרת הבטן does not feature in the current dictionaries. N (a.l.) translates Arab. الاستطلاق with the standard Hebrew term for 'diarrhoea ', i.e. שלשול.

-: התרת השתן = Arab. استطلاق البول 'polyuria'; cf. 24.39: התרת השתן והוא הנקרא דיאביטיס והצמא החזקה הוא החולי שאינו נמצא כי אם בזמן מועט ולא לעתים רחוקים כי אני עד היום הזה לא ראיתיהו אלא שני פעמים לבד (Polyuria, also [called] 'diabetes' or 'severe thirst' is an illness that is only rarely found, and which I until now have only observed twice). In the sense of 'polyuria' Hebrew התרת השתן is a semantic borrowing from the Arab. استطلاق البول which does not feature in the current dictionaries. Nathan (a.l.) translates Arab. استطلاق البول just like Zeraḥyah as התרת השתן. Masie (MD 590) has רבוי שתן for 'polyuria'.

הזיר (זור) = Arab. ردع 'to restrain'; cf. 3.85: ולא ארמוז בהזרתו לעולם אלא לעתים רחוקות שנזיר במעט הזרה כשלא יהיה שם כאב ויהיה הגוף נקי (I never advise application of a restraining treatment, except for a light one when there is no pain and when the body is clean). Hebrew הזיר does not feature in this sense in the current dictionaries. Nathan (a.l.) has הרתיע. Hillel (s.v. זור) uses המזירים in the sense of restraining ingredients or repercussive remedies.

זיו: זיו האדם = Arab. سحنة 'external condition'; cf. 12.3: לא יקיז הנער קודם י"ד שנה ולא אחר השבעים שנה ולא ישמור אל מספר השנים לבד אבל ישמור עם זה בזיו האדם (Do not bleed children below fourteen years nor [anyone] older than seventy. Do not consider the number of years only but also the external condition [of the body]. Hebrew זיו features in the current dictionaries in the sense of 'splendour' (cf. BM 1319–20). In addition to 'splendour, glory' Jastrow (JD 392) refers to the fact that זיו also features in Rabbinic literature in a sense similar to that of 'external condition', namely 'countenance'. Nathan (a.l.) translates the Arab. سحنة as תואר הפנים.

זַכּוּת = Arab. 'acumen'; cf. 25.59: ובטוב שכלו וזכותו אשר שימש ברפואות והיותו מצא מה שידעו הוא בקצת מיני[263] הדפק והניתוח והתועלות והפעולות יותר אמת מאשר שזכרו אריסטו' בספריו בלא ספק לפי דעת מי שיודה על האמת והביאו אותו המאמר[264] לדבר בעניינים שהוא בהם קצר מאד וישמש[265] זריזותו בהן (His excellent intellect and acumen which he directed towards medicine, and his discoveries of some of the conditions of the pulse, anatomy and the usefulness and functions [of organs] — which are undoubtedly more correct than what Aristotle mentions in his books if one looks at them impartially — have induced him to speak about things in which he is very deficient and about which the experts have contradictory opinions). Hebrew זַכּוּת only features in the current dictionaries in the sense of 'clarity, purity'; cf. KT 1.260: 'Reinheit, Lauterkeit'.

זרוע = Arab. مأبض 'the inner side [of the arm]'; cf. 25.53: במאמר החמישי מהתחבולה אמר בהתחילו לספר איך ירופא רקיקת הדם מן הריאה אמר מאמר זה לשונו: וצוה לחולה שלא יתנפש ניפוש חזק ושיעשה המנוחה והשלווה תמיד ויקיז מיד גיד הזרוע (In the fifth book of *De methodo medendi*, when he begins to describe how someone suffering from hemoptysis from the lungs should be treated, he says the following and these are his words: Tell the patient not to take deep breaths and to adhere to [a regimen] of constant rest and repose and immediately phlebotomize him from the vein at the inner side [of the arm]. Hebrew זרוע does not feature in this sense in the current dictionaries. Nathan (a.l.) transcribes Arab. مأبض as מאבץ.

חיבוש: חִבּוּשׁ = Arab. تضميد 'the application [of a poultice]'; cf. 15.51: המורסא הנקראת חמרה תקררנה בתחלת העניין. וככלות חומו ונתבטלה רתיחתו אז תועילנו השריטה והחיבוש בתחבושת יהיה נעשה בקמח השעורים מחומם ([In the case of] the inflammation which is called 'ḥumra',[266] one should, first of all, apply

263 מיני: أحوال a.

264 המאמר: om a.

265 וישמש זריזותו בהן: وتضارب المهرة فيها a.

266 'ḥumra'; i.e. erysipelas.

cooling. When its seething heat subsides, scarification and the application of a poultice made from barley (*Hordeum vulgare* and var.) meal and then heated is beneficial). Hebrew חיבוש only features in EM 495 as a modern term in the sense of 'binding'. Nathan (a.l.) translates Arab. تضميد as עשה.

(חבל) (1): התחבל = Arab. قرح 'to develop an ulcer'; cf. 6.72: כשיתחבל מעי מן המיעים מן המרה השחורה לא יהיה לו רפואה (When one of the intestines develops an ulcer caused by black bile, it cannot be cured). Hebrew התחבל does not feature in this sense in the current dictionaries; cf. JD 419–20 s.v. חָבֵל: 'to injure, to wound'; s.v. התחבל: 'to be spoiled, ruined'. Nathan (a.l.) translates the Arabic قرح as התנגע.

(חבל) חיבל = Arab. قرّح 'to ulcerate'; cf. 23.46: הסרטן שני מינים והוא מורסא נולדת מהמרה השחורה ובהשתפך המרה השחורה אל הבשר ותהיה נושכת תאכל כל העור אשר סמוך לה ותחבלנו והוא הסרטן המתחבל ובהיותה ממוצעת תחדש סרטן בלתי מתחבל (Cancer consists of two types, namely a tumour that arises from black bile, and when the black bile streams into the flesh and is biting, it corrodes the entire adjacent skin and ulcerates it, and this is the ulcerous cancer. But when [the black bile] is moderate, it produces a cancer that is not ulcerous). Hebrew חיבל does not feature in this sense in the current dictionaries. Nathan (a.l.) translates the Arabic قرّح as השחין.

(חבל) (2): התחבל = Arab. احتال 'to exercise one's skill'; cf. 15.17: כשתקרה עקיצה בעצב מן העצבים על כל פנים יכאב כאב מרובה מפני[267] חוש העצב. על כן תתחבל לשכך הכאב ולמנוע ככל יכולתך שלא תתחדש שם מורסא (If someone is pricked [directly] into a nerve and he suffers unavoidably because of the great sensitivity of the nerve from severe pain, exercise your skill to alleviate the pain and to prevent an inflammation [of the site]). Hebrew התחבל does not feature in this sense in the current dictionaries; cf. BM 1425: 'to act wickedly, to hurt'. Nathan (a.l.) translates the Arabic احتال as הערים. Cf. ZA 137: 'to do recourse (to devices)' (sic).

חָבָל/חֵבֶל Plur. **חבלים** = Arab. جراحات 'wounds'; cf. 15.33: אמנם רפואת חבלי העצבים אני עושה בה הגפרית אשר לא נגעהו אש עם השמן עד שובו עבה כטיט[268] כתלי המרחץ (As medications for nerve wounds I use sulphur that has not been affected by fire, [mixed] with olive oil until it assumes the consistency of bath-sordes).

---

267 מפני חוש: لفضل حسّ a.

268 כטיט כתלי המרחץ: وسخ الحمّام a.

Hebrew חָבָל is attested for Rabbinic literature in the sense of 'injury' (BM 1426, EM 497), and חֵבֶל as '1) writhing, throes of birth, agony; 2) damage, injury' (JD 420); cf. BM 1426: 'labour-pains'.

חֲבָלָה, Plur. **חבלות** = I. Arab. قروح 'ulcers'; cf. 3.76: החליים הארוכים כמו צרות הניפוש והחול והטחורים באף וההבלות הרעות ודומיהם כי רוב אילו הכאבים אשר יתילדו לנערים ולילדים יתרפאו עד מ' יום או לז' חדשים או ז' שנים (Concerning chronic illnesses such as orthopnea, stones, tumors in the nose, bad ulcers, and the like, most of these afflictions occurring to youngsters and children are cured in forty days or seven months or seven years); II. Arab. جراحات 'wounds'; cf. 12.32: הרפואה היותר מועילה לחבלות העצבים והיותר מתקנת להם הוא מה שהוא מייבש והוא במעט חמימות ותהיה חמימותו מספיק[269] ומייבש עם כל זה (The most beneficial and appropriate medication for nerve wounds is that which dries while it is slightly warming, or one in which the heat is not noticeable but which dries just the same). Hebrew חבלה features in Even Shoshan (497) as Rabbinic in the sense of 'wound' or 'fine' (cf. JD 420: 'injury, mayhem; damages for mayhem'), and as modern in the sense of 'trauma'. Nathan (a.l.) translates Arab. قروح as שחינים, and Arab. جراحة as חבורה. Hillel (s.v. חבלה) uses Hebrew חבלות for Latin ulcera 'ulcers'.

חוט = I. Arab. ليف 'fibre'; cf. 1.12: אלו השלשה כלים והם העצב והיתר והקישור כלם הם לבנים ומעשה מקשה נעדרים מהדם וכשתתירם יותרו אל חוט הולך אל האורך מלבד מה שיהיה מן הקישורים קשה מאד כי אי אפשר שיתיר וישוב חוט (These three structures — namely, nerve, tendon, and ligament — are all white, solid and bloodless. If you dissect them, they separate into lengthwise fibres, except for the very hard ligaments, for [these] cannot be taken apart into fibres); II. (Plur.) חוטים = Arab. شظايا 'fibres'; cf. 1.74: החוטים בכל אחד מן המעים הם עגולים יכרכו ברוחב בשתי כרומות כלם כי המעים אמנם יקיפו על מה שבהם לבד ויאספהו ולא ימשכו שום דבר מן הדברים (The fibres within each of the intestines are circular and are altogether intertwined in its two layers widthwise, for the intestines merely surround and hold their contents and do not attract anything). Hebrew חוט is only attested in Rabbinical literature in a medical sense as 'sinew' (cf. JD 431; BM 1462). N (a.l.) translates Arab. ليف as פתילים וליפים and شظايا as פתילים; for ליף cf. MD 288.

---

269 מספיק (= كافية) : خافية a.

חול = Arab. حصاة 'stone(s)'; cf. 3.76: החליים הארוכים כמו צרות הניפוש והחול והטחורים באף והחבלות הרעות ודומיהם כי רוב אילו הכאבים אשר יתילדו לנערים ולילדים יתרפאו עד מ' יום (Concerning chronic diseases such as orthopnea, stones, tumors in the nose, bad ulcers and the like, most of these afflictions occurring to youngsters and children are cured in forty days…). Hebrew חול does not feature in this sense in the current dictionaries. Nathan (a.l.) translates the Arabic term as חצץ.

חיזק (חזק) = Arab. وقى 'to protect'; cf. 1.44: חוט של שדרה כלומר הגוף החלק אשר יצא מן המוח בחליות השדרה כלה יקיף בו אותן הקרומות בעצמן המקיפין במוח ואחד משתי הקרומות דבק באחר ויקיף בהם קרום כרוך עליהם מנראיהם כמו קרום שלישי חזק קשה מסוג העצבים לחזקו מפני חוזק תנועתו וכחו וקשייו (The spinal cord — in effect, the soft substance which emerges from the brain and runs down the entire spinal vertebrae — is surrounded by exactly the same two membranes as those surrounding the brain. One membrane adheres to the other, and both are surrounded by a third tunic that is coiled around them from the outside just like a third membrane — strong, hard and sinewy — to protect the spinal cord because of its intense, vigorous and strenuous movement). Hebrew חיזק does not feature in this sense in the current dictionaries. Nathan (a.l.) translates Arab. وقى as שמר. See as well entry מְחֻזָּק.

חֵלֶב = Arab. ثرب 'omentum'; cf. 9.102: אבל תראה ותדע כי הכיס אשר ירד בו הקרום אשר על האסטומכא והמיעים והוא החלב הוא חולי גדול וחזק אע"פ שמקומו אינו גדול (Rather, consider and know that a hernia in which the membrane that covers the intestines and stomach, namely the omentum, descends, is a serious and grave illness, although the size of the hernia may not be large). Hebrew חֵלֶב is not attested in the sense of 'omentum' in the current dictionaries; cf. JD 464; 'fatty concretion, esp. that abdominal fat of cattle which it is forbidden to eat'; Low LI: 'fat (abdominal)'; BM 1553–4: 'suet'. Nathan (a.l.) translates the Arab. ثرب just like Zeraḥyah as חלב. Masie (MD 522) has פדר for 'omentum'.

-: החלב המכסה הקרב = Arab. ثرب 'omentum'; cf. 1.60: החלב המכסה הקרב הוא אחד מן האברים שאינם מוכרחים במציאות הבעל חיים ותועלתו בגוף מעוטה (The omentum is an organ that is not necessary for life to exist; its usefulness for the body is slight). The Hebrew term is not attested in the current dictionaries. Nathan (a.l.) translates the Arab. ثرب as החלב המכסה, and Shem Tov (s.v. חלב) as החלב המכסה את הקרב or החלב אשר על הקרב.

חלול: חלולים = Arab. تجاويف (MSS EL) 'the ventricles' (of the heart); cf. 4.18: וכן הלב בעצמו יזדמן כמה פעמים שיהיה הלב בעצמו יותר קר ממזגו הטבעי ויהיה העצם אשר יקיף עליו חלוליו יותר חד או בהפך (Similarly, the body of the heart itself is sometimes cooler than its natural temperament, while the substance contained in the two ventricles of the heart is warmer; or the reverse [may occur]). Hebrew חלול only features in the current dictionaries in the sense of 'hollowed' (BM 1560–1; JD 465) or of 'pipe, channel' (JD 465). Nathan (a.l.) translates the Arab. تجاويف as חללים.

חֳלִי = Arab. آفة 'harm'; cf. 25.72: והפלאו קהל בעלי העיון איך נוכל להאמין בזה הספור עם האמיננו לו במה שזכר בפרק חמישי מההכרות והוא האמת והוא אומרו שם כי על כל פנים יבוא ללב חולי בבוא המות (Be amazed you who belong to the community of those who engage in speculation. How can we believe him in [what he says in] this statement and at the same time believe him in what he says in the fifth [treatise] of *De locis affectis,* and [this last] statement is correct? For there he remarks that it is in any case unavoidable that the heart suffers harm when death occurs). Hebrew חֳלִי does not feature in this sense in the current dictionaries. Nathan (a.l.) translates Arab. آفة as פגע. See as well BA 154: 'egritudo; occasio; infirmitas'.

-: **חֳלִי: חולי הצד** = Arab. ذات الجنب 'pleurisy'; cf. 4.42: איני יודע ששום אדם ימלט מחולי הצד בהיות דפק בעליו קשה בתכלית הקושי קטון ומתואתר מאד (I do not know anyone who was saved from pleurisy when his pulse was extremely hard, small, and very dense). Hebrew חולי הצד does not feature in the standard dictionaries. Nathan (a.l.) translates the Arab. ذات الجنب as בעלת הצד, while in his translation of Ibn Sīnā's *K. al-Qānūn* prepared in Rome in 1279 we find חולי הצד (MD 578). The term בעלת הצד is also used by Shem Tov (SG, Beit 17).

חָלָל = Arab. مقعّر 'concave [part]'; cf. 7.57: הצמא הגדולה שתהיה נעדרת מהתרת הבטן סבתו הראשונה רוע מזג חם או יבש או שניהם יחד יתחדש באסטומכא ובייחוד פיה. וסבתו השנית אחר האסטומכא כשיתחדש בה רוע מזג בכבד וכל שכן בחללו (The first cause of a severe thirst without diabetes is a hot or dry bad temperament, or both, occurring in the stomach and especially in the cardia of the stomach; and after the stomach, the second cause is that this bad temperament affects the liver and especially its concave part). Hebrew חָלָל only features in the current dictionaries in the sense of 'cavity, empty space, hollow' (JD 470). The term also features in the sense of 'concavity' in R. Samuel Ibn Tibbon's translation of Maimonides' *Guide of the Perplexed* (cf. Sarfatti, *Munaḥei ha-Matematikah*, p. 178 (no. 231).[270] Nathan (a.l.) translates the Arabic مقعّر as מקוער, a loan translation from the Arabic (cf. BM 3284: earliest reference is the *Moreh ha-Moreh* by Shem Tov Ibn Falaquera), while Shem Tov Ben Isaac has חללות for Arab. تقعير: 'concavity' (cf. Shem Tov, s.v. חללות).

חלצים: מתחת החלצים = Arab. ما دون الشراسيف 'hypochondria'; cf. 6.52: סימני המראקיא שיהיה לו אחר אכלו רוטו חמוץ ורקיקה לחה בשיעור ושריפה מתחת החלצים (The indications of hypochondriac melancholia are that the ingestion of food is followed by sour eructations, watery sputum in a large quantity, a burning sensation in the hypochondria…). Hebrew מתחת החלצים is not attested in the current dictionaries. Nathan (a.l.) translates the Arab. as מה שלמטה מצדי הכסלים while Shem Tov (s.v. חלצים) translates Arab. تحت الشراسيف as תחת החלצים. Another term used by Zeraḥyah for Arab. ما دون الشراسيف is מה שתחת הצלעות (see entry צלעות).

חָלָק = Arab. ليّن 'soft'; cf. 1.9: היתרים יותר הם חלקים מן הקשרים ויותר הם קשים מן העצבים (Tendons are softer than ligaments but harder than nerves). Hebrew חלק only features in the current dictionaries in the sense of 'bald; smooth, slippery' (BM 1596–7; but cf. BM 1600 s.v. חָלַק: 'to be soft'). Nathan (a.l.) translates Arab. ليّن as רך. See as well BA 154, s.v. חלק: 'lenis, durus, mollis'. Zonta's (ZA 137) translation of the term as 'smooth' should be corrected as 'soft'.

(חלק) החליק: להחליק הבטן = Arab. إلانة البطن 'prescribing laxatives'; cf. 12.8: אבל באדם[271] אחר נקצר ויספיק לנו למנוע ממנו המאכל. ובאדם אחר יספיק לנו למעט לו המאכל ובאדם אחר יספיק לך שתחליק בטנו או שתשלשלהו או שתרבה לו להכניסו במרחץ או שיספיק לו הטורח לבדו או שתעשה החפיפה המרובה (Rather for such a person one should limit oneself and be content with withholding food <from him>.[272] In the case of someone else one should limit oneself to diminish his food

270 Gad B. Sarfatti, *Munaḥei ha-Matematikah ba-Sifrut ha-Madda'it ha-'Ivrit shel Yemei ha-Benayyim. Mathematical Terminology in Hebrew Scientific Literature of the Middle Ages* (Jerusalem 1968).

271 באדם אחר: في ذلك الشخص a.

272 I.e. putting him on a diet.

<intake> and in yet another one should limit oneself to prescribe laxatives or purgatives or frequent bathing in the bathhouse or exercise only or much massage). Hebrew החליק הבטן does not feature in the current dictionaries. Nathan (a.l.) translates Arab. إلانة البطن as רכוך הבטן.

החליק הטבע: החליק (חלק) = Arab. ليّن الطبيعة 'to soften the stools'; cf. 17.33: ראוי להקדים תחילה מכל מה שהאדם אוכל ושותה מה שיהיה מחליק לטבע כמו היינות המתוקים והירקות המחליקות הנעשות עם השמן והכותח (From any food or drink one should first of all take that which softens the stools like sweet wines and softening vegetables prepared with olive oil and garum). Hebrew החליק הטבע does not feature in the current dictionaries. Nathan (a.l.) translates Arab. ليّن الطبيعة as ריכך הבטן.

חֲלָקוּת (BM 1602) or **חַלְקוּת** (EM 548) = I. Arab. لين 'softness'; cf. 1.11: הקרומות כלם הם בתכלית הדקות והחלקות (All membranes are extremely thin and soft); II. Arab. تليين 'softening effect'; cf. 9.72: קושי הכבד ראוי שתהיה הרפואה המחליקה ברפואותיה חלושה מאד ויגבר בהם הדברים אשר יחממו וידקדקו יותר ממה שיגבר ברפואת קושי שאר האברים כי גוף הכבד אמנם הוא כמו לחות נקפא ואם החליקנו חלקות חזק יתכו כחותיו (Of the remedies for hardness of the liver, the softening ones should be very weak, and those remedies that heat and refine should be more predominant than in the case of the treatment of hardness of the other organs. For the substance of the liver is indeed like congealed moisture, and if those remedies soften it greatly, its powers dissolve). Hebrew חֲלָקוּת or חַלְקוּת only features in the current dictionaries in the sense of 'smoothness'; cf. BM 1602: סגולת דבר חלק. Nathan (a.l.) translates Arab. لين as רכות and Arab. تليين as רכוך.

חלקות המיעים :- = Arab. زلق الأمعاء 'lientery'; cf. entry המעדת המיעים. Hebrew חלקות המיעים does not feature in the current dictionaries. See entries המעדת המיעים and מעידת המיעים.

חימוץ האתרוגים: חִמּוּץ = Arab. حمّاض الأترج 'The acidic inner part of the lemon'; cf. 22.52: חימוץ האתרוגים יסיר הצמא והוא חזק בהסרת הקולורא מחזק לנפש (The acidic inner part of the lemon eliminates thirst, vigorously subdues yellow bile, and strengthens the soul). Hebrew חימוץ האתרוגים features in BM 1616 in an attestation from Meir Aldabi, *Shevilei Emunah* which was completed in 1360. Nathan (a.l.) translates the Arabic حمّاض الأترج just like Zeraḥyah as חימוץ האתרוגים.

חֶנֶק = Arab. خوانيق 'angina'; cf. 25.11: ומפני זה העיקר הגדול בתועלת יצוינו גליאנוס שנקיז גיד הראש הנקרא קיפאל בחוליי העין החזקים ובחנק ודומה (And because of this very beneficial fundamental rule Galen instructs us to bleed the cephalic vein in the case of severe illnesses of the eye, and angina, and the like). Hebrew חֶנֶק only features as a medical term in BM 1661 in the sense of 'hysterical suffocation'. Nathan (a.l.) translates Arab. خوانيق as מחנקים.

חפז = Arab. حفز 'to become urgent'; cf. 8.41: המקרים המזיקים בכח אשר ראוי לכוין להם כשהם חופזים מאד (Some symptoms are harmful to the strength and should be attended to [immediately] when they become urgent). Hebrew חפז is attested in the current dictionaries in the sense of 'to act with haste a. fright' (BM 1684). In the sense of 'to become urgent' it is a non-attested semantic borrowing from the Arabic حفز. Nathan translates Arab. حفز just like Zeraḥyah as חפז.

חפיפה = Arab. دلك 'massage'; cf. 8.12: הרקת הגוף כולו יהיה בהוצאת הדם או ברפואה המתירה לבטן או ברפואה המקיאה או בחפיפה המרובה (A complete evacuation of the body is [effected] through bloodletting or laxatives or emetics or frequent massage…). Hebrew חפיפה features in Rabbinical literature in the sense of 'cleansing the head' (JD 491). As 'massage' it features in BM 1686 in an attestation from Nathan ha-Me'ati's translation of Ibn Sīnā's *K. al-Qānūn* prepared in Rome in 1279. In the same sense it occurs in Moses Ibn Tibbon (see Moses Ibn Tibbon, s.v. חפיפה).

חשב = I. Arab. اتّهم 'to have doubts'; cf. Introduction: ובהיותו חושב שום אדם לשון אותו הפרק או ענינו ישוב לאותו המאמר בנקלה (So, if someone has doubts about the wording of that aphorism, he can easily look up that section); II. Arab رام 'to call for, to strive, to seek'; cf. 8.43: הדרך אשר תלך בו תמיד הוא שתחשוב להריק ולהתיר מה שהוא חוץ מהטבע ואם לא יהיה יכול להשלים זה בעבור טבע האבר או בסבת שהחולי לא יקח בו רפואה תשים ידך לעפש אותו הדבר שהוא חוץ מהטבע ולהביאו לידי מוגלא (The method one should always apply is to seek the evacuation and dissolution of the unnatural [substance in the body]. If this is impossible because of the nature of the [affected] organ or because the illness is incurable, one should let the unnatural substance suppurate and putrefy); III. Arab. أوهمه أنّ 'to imagine'; cf. 9.57: מי שיהיה מן הממולאים וזולתם ימצא באסטומכתו שרפה חזקה עד שתחשוב שיהיה שם מורסא חמה הצרותו העשוי בשמן[273] ורדים או בשמן

273 בשמן ורדים או: om a.

חבושים יועיל לו (If someone suffers from indigestion and the like and from a burning in the stomach that is so severe that one imagines that there is an inflamed tumour there, he will benefit from a salve prepared with quince oil). IV. ادّعى 'to pretend'; cf. 25.61: ולא עמד[274] על כל[275] זה הגדר אלא מחוזק הנאתו במה שנראה לו מקצת תועלת האברים חשב להתנבאות ואמר כי מלאך בא אליו מאת השם ולמדהו כך וצווהו כך (He did not stop at this limit, but because of the excessive pleasure he took in what became evident to him about some of the uses of organs, he pretended to be a prophet and said that an angel came to him from God and taught him such and such and ordered him such and such). Hebrew חשב does not occur in these senses in the current dictionaries. Nathan (a.l.) translates Arab. اتّهم as פקפק; Arab. رام as השתדל; Arab. أوهمه أنّ as דמה בלבבו; and Arab. ادّعى as התבאר.

נחתך (חתך) = Arab. تقطّع 'to stop'; cf. 24.24: אשה הרה אחר ההריון בקצת חדשים ראתה תחלה דם ואחר כן טרי רקיק מוסרח ואחר האריך בה הזמן הפילה ואחר מכן הוציאה מן השילייא בכל יום מעט כי השילייא נתעפשה בפנים. ואחר שנחתכה מה שנשאר מן השלייא חשבו המילדות וכל[276] הרופאים זולתי שהאשה נקתה לגמרי (A woman who was pregnant for some months at first saw blood, then thin, fetid blood serum. With the passing of time she miscarried. After this, every day part of the placenta was extruded because it had putrefied internally. When the remains of the placenta stopped [coming out], the midwives and all the attending physicians except me thought that she was completely cleansed). In the sense of 'to stop' Hebrew נחתך is a non-attested semantic borrowing from Arab. تقطّع. Nathan (a.l.) also translates Arab. تقطّع as נחתך.

חתם = Arab. ختم 'to cicatrize'; cf. 9.95: כשתגיע מורסא בכליות ותתבשל וישתין החולה טרי יגיע ריחו[277] מהרעי[278] אבל על כאב[279] מחבלת הכליות. ותשמור[280] עצמך שלא תאחר מחתום אותה החבלה (If an abscess forms in a kidney and ripens and the patient micturates pus, he will find relief from his pain, but he should be wary of an ulcer in that kidney. Therefore, one should attempt its cicatrization by all means). In the sense of 'to cicatrize' Hebrew חתם is a semantic borrowing

274 עמד על: وقف عند a.
275 כל: om a.
276 וכל הרופאים: وجميع من حضر من الأطبّاء a.
277 ריחו: راحة a.
278 מהרעי: من الوجع a.
279 כאב (= وجع): وجل a.
280 ותשמור עצמך שלא תאחר: فاحرص بكل حيلة a.

from Arab. ختم that does not feature in the current dictionaries. Nathan (a.l.) translates the Arab. ختم just like Zeraḥyah as חתם. Masie (MD 163) has the entry צלק or הצטלק for 'to cicatrize'.

טיבולים: טִבּוּל = I. Arab. نطولات 'fomentations'; cf. 8.2: הדברים אשר יעזרו על בשול הליחות הם כל הדברים אשר יחממו במיצוע קצתם הם מזון וקצתם הם משקים וקצתם טיבולים וקצתם תחבושות (The things that help to coct the humours are all those that heat moderately; some of these are foods, some are beverages, some are fomentations and some are poultices); II. Arab. تكميد = 'the application of a hot compress'; cf. 9.81: רפואת חולי הצד בהקזה ובטיבול וחלקות הבטן (Pleurisy should be treated through bleeding, the application of a hot compress, and softening of the stool). Hebrew טִבּוּל is only mentioned in the current dictionaries as featuring in Rabbinic literature in the sense of '1) dipping, luncheon, antepast; 2) the act which makes foods subject to priestly gifts' (JD 529) (see as well ibid. Aram. טִבּוּלָא: 'dipping, immersion, bathing'). Nathan (a.l.) translates Arab. نطولات as יציקות and Arab. تكميد as הנחות חמות. In addition to טִבּוּל, Zeraḥyah uses Hebrew משיחה to render Arab. تكميد; cf. 10.5: המוקדח שהביאך ההכרח שתקיזנו או תשלשלנו או תשכך בו כאב בתחבושת או במשיחה הנק' תכמיד בער' אין ראוי שתאכילנו גרישי שעורים הנק' כשך בער' ולא מימיו עד שתעשה לו זה (If you find it necessary to bleed a fever patient or to purge him or to alleviate a pain he is suffering from with a poultice or a hot compress, you should not give him barley groats or barley gruel before doing the aforementioned).

טבל = I. Arab. نطل 'to foment'; cf. 9.6: בהיות המותרות הניגרים מן האף מימיות בלתי מבושלים היותינו מתקנים אותם יהיה בדברים אשר תטבול הראש כדי שיחמם המוח ועם הדברים אשר תשאף ואשר יריק באוזן (If a mucus discharge from the nose is watery and uncocted, we stop it with things with which we foment the head in order to heat the brain, and with those things that are inhaled through the nose, and with those things that are dripped into the ears); II. Arab. كمّد 'to apply a compress'; cf. 9.22: ראוי שתרחץ העין באספוג במים שנתבשל בו האזמרינו ופינוגרקו ואם היה הכאב נקל תמשחנו פעם או פעמים ביום אחד. ואם היה הכאב חזק תטבלנו פעמים רבות וכל שכן בימים הארוכים ([For eye pain] one should apply to the eye a warm compress with a sponge [dipped] in water in which melilot and fenugreek have been cooked. When the pain is mild, apply the compress once or twice a day, and when the pain is severe apply it many times, especially during the long [summer] days). Hebrew טבל only features in the current dictionaries in the sense of 'to dip; to immerse, to bathe for purification' (JD 517; BM 1838: 'to immerse'). Nathan (a.l.) translates Arab. نطل as טבל and Arab. كمّد as הניח. See as well entry משמש.

טָחוּל = Arab. مطحول 'spleen patient'; cf. 23.89: הרופאים באמרם טחולים ירצו לומר במי שיקרה בטחולו קושי ואבנינות מבלתי מורסא (When speaking of 'spleen patients' physicians mean those patients whose spleen is affected by induration and calcification without an inflammation). Hebrew טָחוּל does not feature in the current dictionaries. Nathan (a.l.) translates the Arab. مطحول as מוטחל.

טֹרַח: טורח = Arab. رياضة 'exercise'; cf. 3.11: ובתנאי שישגיחו בהגרת המותרות מגופותם בטורח (This is [only] on condition that they take care to expel the superfluities from their bodies through exercise...). Hebrew טורח only features in the current dictionaries in the sense of 'toil, labour, trouble, painstaking preparations' (JD 526), or: 'charge, burden' (BM 1922). Another term used by Zeraḥyah for 'exercise' is תנועה; cf. 7.45: עשה התנועה for Arab. استعمل الرياضة. Yet another term used by him for رياضة is the Romance סירסיציאו (cf. 8.28). Nathan (a.l.) translates Arab رياضة as התעמלות and استعمل الرياضة as עשה ההתעמלות.

טרח = Arab. ارتاض 'to exercise'; cf. 12.7: הגוף אשר יהיה הדם הטוב בו מעט והליחות הנאות הרבה מאד אין ראוי שיתנועע בשום דבר כלל ולא יכנס למרחץ מפני שההקזה תוציא הדם הטוב ותמשוך הדם הרע המקובץ בעורקים הראשונים אשר בכבד וישלחהו בגוף כולו. אבל הרפואה המשלשלת יחדש לבעלי זה העניין נשיכה[281] ועקיצה והתעלפות ולא ישלשלנו דבר בעל שיעור. והליחות בעבור עבים יתקדמו ויסתמו המעברות ומפני זה אין ראוי שיטרח ולא יכנס למרחץ (If someone's body contains a small amount of good blood and a very large quantity of raw humours, [venesection should not be applied] and he should not carry out any activity at all and not enter the bathhouse. For venesection removes the good blood from it and attracts the bad blood collected in the primary [non pulsatile] vessels of the liver and disperses it throughout the body. When one gives a purgative to such a patient, it causes colic, biting pain and fainting but does not evacuate anything in a [significant] quantity. For the humours precede [the matter to be evacuated] and obstruct the passages because of their thickness. For this reason he should not exercise, nor enter the bathhouse). Hebrew טרח only features in the current dictionaries in the sense of 'to run about, be busy, to take pains,

281 נשיכה: مغسا a.

prepare' (JD 551) or 'to load' (BM 1923). Nathan (a.l.) translates the Arab. ارتاض as התעמל.

יוצא = Arab. خارج 'exterior'; cf. 1.56: על האסטומכא קרום יקיף בבשר היוצא וזה הקרום יקשרנו עם הגב (There is a membrane over the stomach surrounding its exterior, fleshy layer, and this membrane attaches to the spinal column). Hebrew יוצא in the sense of 'external' is a non-attested semantic borrowing of Arab. خارج; cf. BA 157; ZA 138. Nathan (a.l.) translates Arab. خارج as חיצון.

יערה: יערת הדבש = Arab. شهدة 'honeycomb'; cf. 23.54: בעור הראש תתחדש חולי מסוג המורסא יהיה בה חורים קטנים מליאים לחות רקיק ויסקוסו יאמר לו האלצעפא. ויתחדש בעור הראש חולי דומה לאילו בראייה ונקביו יותר גדולים ויותר רחבים מנקבי האלצעפא והם מליאים מלחות דומה ביערת הדבורים וזה נקרא יערת הדבש (54. The skin of the head is affected by a type of swelling which has fine, small openings filled with a thin, viscous liquid. [This disease] is called 'saʿfa' [cradle cap]. [Another] illness occurs on the skin of the head which resembles the former in its appearance but the openings are larger and wider than the openings of cradle cap and they are filled with a honey-like moisture, and this [illness] is called 'honeycomb'). Hebrew יערת הדבש does not feature in a medical sense in the current dictionaries. Nathan (a.l.) translates Arab. شهدة as יערית.

הוציא (יצא) = Arab. أخرج 'to translate'; cf. entry 24.1: ספר כאבי הנשים לאבקראט הוציאו חונין וביארו גליאנוס ונמצא תוספת באותו הספר הוציאו זולתי חונין וביארו זולתי גליאנוס (In the *Book on Women's Diseases* composed by Hippocrates, translated by Ḥunayn and commented upon by Galen I found an addition which is not part of Ḥunayn's translation nor of Galen's commentary). Hebrew הוציא in the sense of 'to translate' is a semantic borrowing from the Arabic أخرج which does not feature in the current dictionaries. Nathan translates Arab. أخرج as העתיק. See as well entry אִפֵּל.

ירידה: ירידת המים בעין = Arab. نزول الماء 'cataract'; cf. 7.69: הלחות הלבנית אם היא יותר או פחות מן הראוי תזיק בראות העין. ואם יתעבה תחסר הראות עד שלא יראה הדברים הרחוקים ולא יתבאר הדברים הקרובים. ואם יתעבה בתכלית כמו שיקרה בירידת המים בעין ימנע הראות (If the albuminoid humour is larger or smaller [in quantity] than necessary, it harms vision. When this humour becomes thick, clarity of vision is diminished so that distant objects cannot be seen [at all] and close objects cannot be seen clearly. When it becomes extremely thick, as happens in the case of a cataract, it makes vision impossible). Hebrew ירידת המים (בעין) in the sense of 'cataract' is a semantic borrowing from the Arab. نزول الماء which does not feature in the current dictionaries. Nathan (a.l.) translates the Arab نزول الماء as ירידת המים.

ירקנות = Arab. خضرة 'greenness'; cf. 15.50: המורסות הבאות מסבת דם המתחדשות מבלתי סבה מבחוץ כשתשרטנו תביא על בעליהם רעה רבה וכל שכן אם תרצה לעשותה בתחילת החולי. אבל כשהחולי יאריך אינו רע שתשרטנו. וכן המורסא הנקראת ריזיפילא בערבי חמרה כשתגיע עניינה לשחרות או למראה העופרת או לירקנות טוב לשרט (If you scarify bloody inflammations which occur without an external cause, the one affected by it suffers from a grave affliction, especially if you do so at the outset. But if the illness lasts for a long time, there is no objection to scarification. Similarly, when the inflammation known as 'ḥumra', has reached the condition of lividness, greenness or blackness, it should be scarified). Hebrew ירקנות, formed from יָרֹק 'green' does not feature in the current dictionaries. Nathan (a.l.) translates Arab. خضرة as ירוקות.

יָשָׁר = Arab. معتدل 'moderate'; cf. 8.2: הדברים אשר יעזרו על בשול הליחות הם כל הדברים אשר יחממו במיצוע קצתם הם מזון וקצתם הם משקים וקצתם טיבולים וקצתם תחבושות והחפיפה הישרה והמרחץ הממוצע הוא מזה הסוג (The things that help to coct the humours are all those that heat moderately; some of these are foods, some are beverages, some are poultices, and some are fomentations. Moderate massage and moderate bathing equally belong to this category). Hebrew יָשָׁר in the sense of 'moderate' is a non-attested semantic borrowing from Arab. معتدل which is not mentioned in the current dictionaries. Nathan (a.l.) translates Arab. معتدل as שָׁוֶה.

התיתר (יתר) = Arab. توتّر 'to become tense'; cf. 1.25: אמר משה זה שגמר[282] דעתו במאמרו באלו הארבעה תנועות הוא שהרצון כשישלח הכח הנפשיי בעצבים נוכח מושקולו מן המושקולי כשירצה להכפיל בהם אותו האיבר לצד התחלתו יכפול האבר ההוא. וכן כשירצה להשאיר האבר נמשך[283] תפשוט הרצון אותו המושקולי עם המושקולי שהוא נכחו ויתיתרו יחד (Says Moses: A summary of his words about these four movements is [thus]: When one's will sends the psychical faculty through a nerve to the muscle with which it wants to flex a specific limb, that muscle contracts toward its origin, so that the limb is flexed. Similarly, when one wants that limb to

---

282 שגמר דעתו: الذي تلخّص a.

283 נמשך: مشالا add a.

remain stretched and raised, the will stretches that muscle, together with its antagonistic muscle, so that they both become tense). Hebrew התיתר in the sense of 'to become tense' is a non-attested loan translation of the Arabic توتّر. Nathan (a.l.) translates Arab. توتّر as נמתח. See as well entries מיותר and התיתרות.

יֶתֶר, Plur. **יתרים** = Arab أوتار 'tendons'; cf. 1.7: הקשרים העגולים והיתרים יחשוב מי שאין לו עיון בניתוח שהן עצבים ולא היינו כמו כן מכירים אחד מהם לולי רפואת הניתוח (Someone who is not knowledgeable in anatomy supposes the round ligaments and tendons to be nerves. I would also have been unable to distinguish between them if I had not occupied myself with anatomical dissection). Nathan (a.l.) translates the Arab. أوتار as מיתרים (cf. MD 708). In the sense of 'tendon' Hebrew יֶתֶר is only attested for biblical Hebrew; cf. KB 452: 'still wet tendon of a slaughtered animal'; Ben Yehuda (BM 2202) quotes Maimonides, *Iggeret Teiman* for יתרים in the sense of 'nerves'.

כִּוּוּץ = I. Arab. تقلّص contraction'; cf. 1.71: לתנועות כל המושקולי צד אחד והוא הכווץ והקבוץ אל התחלתו (The movements of all muscles have one aspect [in common] — namely, contraction and gathering to their origin); II. Arab. تشنّج 'spasm'; cf. 3.10: הגופות שהם מקבלים מהר הקיווץ ומוכנים לו הם גופות הנערים מפני חולשת עצם העצבים בהם (Most susceptable to spasms are the bodies of children because of the weakness of the body of the nerves in them). Nathan (a.l.) translates both Arab. تقلّص and Arab. تشنّج as קויצה. Hebrew כווּץ features in BM 2279 as synonymous with כויצה which is translated as 'spasm'. Cf. Shem Tov, s.v. כווּץ and Hillel s.v. קִווּץ.

כותח = Arab. مرّي 'garum';[284] cf. entry חלק: החליק הטבע. Cf. Krauss, *Talmudische Archäologie*, vol. 1, p. 472, n. 430: 'כותח bestand sonst aus Molke, Salz und (verschimmeltem) Brot';[285] *Arukh ha-Shalem*, vol. 4, p. 357, s.v. כתא: 'Sauermilchspeise, Zuthat zu den Speisen'.[286] Nathan (a.l.) renders Arab. مرّي as מוריים. Cf. SG Zade 12.

284 I.e. a fish sauce common in the classical Mediterranean world of Greco-Roman times. But actually two varieties of *murrī* were known in the Arabic/Islamic tradition, one made from fish, and the other from cereals. The cereal-based preparation was called *murrī al-ḥinṭa* while the fish-based condiment, 'fish-brine, garum' was called *murrī al-ḥūt*.

285 S. Krauss, *Talmudische Archäologie*, 3 vols (Leipzig 1910–12).

286 A. Kohut, *Arukh shalem. Aruch Completum*, and Krauss, *Tosefet he-Arukh*. Additamenta. Repr. in 9 vols (Tel Aviv 1970).

כיס = I. Arab. قيلة 'hernia'; cf. 9.102: ויש[287] חולי קטון ומקומו גדול והכיס אשר ירדו בו מעט מן המעים יותר גדול ויותר חזק וכן בשאר החליים (A hernia that encloses water is a minor illness, although it may reach a large size. And a hernia into which a portion of the intestines has descended is very grave and serious. The same applies to the other illnesses); II. (Plur. כיסים) = Arab. أوعية 'vessels'; cf. 18.8: מי שהרבה במנוחה יוליד בגופו מזה שני מיני המילוי כולם כלומר המילוי אשר לפי הכיסים והמילוי אשר יהיה לפי הכח (If someone indulges excessively in idleness, two kinds of overfilling develop in his body as a result of that, namely that which pertains to the vessels and that which pertains to the strength [of the body]). Hebrew כיס features in Rabbinic literature in the sense of 'receptacle, pouch, bag, purse, fund' (JD 633), and 'scrotum, crop (of a bird), cyst' (Low LVI). It also features in medieval medical literature as הכיס הקטן (i.e. gall bladder) and הכיס הגדול (i.e. urinary bladder); cf. BM 2347. Nathan (a.l.) translates Arab. قيلة as הגרה and Arab. أوعية as כלים; likewise Shem Tov (s.v. כיס). In addition to כיס Zeraḥyah uses בקיעה (see entry בקיעה) for Arab. فتق in the sense of 'hernia'.

כיס הבשר :- = Arab. قيلة اللحم 'sarcocele'; cf. 23.57: קושי הבצים נקרא כיס הבשר כמו שנקרא הלחות המימיי המתקבץ בקרומות אשר סביבות הבצים כיס המים. אבל כיס החלב וכיס המעים והחולי המורכב מהם כלומר כיס החלב והמעים הם שמות בדויים מן הרופאים החדשים אשר קורין כל המורסות המתחדשות במה שסמוך הביצים כיס בערבי קילה (A hardening of the testicles is called 'sarcocele',[288] just as the watery fluid accumulated in the tunics around the testicles is called 'hydrocele'.[289] Epiplocele[290] and enterocele[291] and the illness consisting of both of these, i.e. epiploenterocele, are names invented by more recent physicians, who call all the swellings which occur in the area of the testicles 'hernia'). Hebrew כיס הבשר does not feature in the current dictionaries. Nathan (a.l.) translates Arab. قيلة اللحم as קילה אללחם כלומר הגרת הבשר. Masie (MD 641) translates 'sarcocele' as שבר הבשר.

287 ויש חולי קטון ומקומו גדול: والقيلة التي هي ماء مرض يسير وإن كانت عظيمة الحجم a.

288 'sarcocele'; i.e. a fleshy excrescence on the testicles.

289 'hydrocele', i.e. water in the scrotum.

290 'Epiplocele'; i.e. hernia of the omentum.

291 'enterocele'; i.e. intestinal hernia.

-: **כיס החלב** = Arab. قيلة الثرب 'epiplocele'; cf. entry כיס הבשר. Hebrew כיס החלב does not feature in the current dictionaries. Nathan (a.l.) translates Arab. قيلة الثرب as קילה החלב. Masie (MD 263) translates 'sarcocele' as שבר הפדר.

-: **כיס המים** = Arab. قيلة الماء 'hydrocele'; cf. entry כיס הבשר. Hebrew כיס המים does not feature in the current dictionaries. Nathan (a.l.) translates Arab. قيلة الأمعاء as קילה אלמא כלומר הגרת המים. Masie (MD 361) translates 'enterocele' as הדרקון/הדרקון האשכים/ מים באשכים.

-: **כיס המעים** = Arab. قيلة الأمعاء 'enterocele'; cf. entry כיס הבשר. Hebrew כיס המעים does not feature in the current dictionaries. Nathan (a.l.) translates Arab. قيلة الثرب as קילה המעי. Masie (MD 258) translates 'enterocele' as שבר המעים.

נכנס (כנס) = Arab. تمكّن 'to be firmly established'; cf. 9.65: בכל מיני ההדרוקן הכבד בעצמו הוא אשר לא ישנה מה שיבואנו מן המזון אל הדם בסבת רוע מזג קר שולט[292] על אחד מכלי המזון או אחד מכלי הניפוש וישוב ממנו אל מה שקרוב ממנו מן האברים עד שיגיע הקור בעצם הכבד בשיתוף הגידים והמחלה תכנס בכבד בעצמו ויתחדש ההדרוקן (In all [the various] types of dropsy, the liver itself fails to transform the food that reaches it into blood because of a cold bad temperament that dominates it. Sometimes this cold bad temperament dominates one of the digestive organs or one of the respiratory organs and passes from there on to the neighbouring organs until it reaches the substance of the liver through the common vessels. As a result the illness settles in the substance of the liver and produces dropsy). Hebrew נכנס does not feature in this sense in the current dictionaries. Nathan translates Arab. تمكّن as נקבע.

כָּפוּל = Arab. مثني 'flexed'; cf. 1.25: ואמנם תנועת הפישוט היא רצונית והיא תנועת המושקולי במקרה[293] כי הרצון כשירצה לפשוט האבר הכפול תבטל הכח הנפשיי מן המושקולי אשר נכפל מקווץ ושולח אותו הכח למושקולי הנכחי (The movement of extension is a voluntary and deliberate movement of the muscle; for when one's will wants to stretch a flexed limb, it stops the psychical faculty in the flexed, contracted muscle and sends it to the antagonistic muscle. Hebrew כפול in the sense of 'flexed' is a non-attested semantic borrowing from the Arabic مثني. Nathan (a.l.) translates Arab. مثني as כפוף.

---

292 שולט: عليها. وقد يكون ذلك السوء مزاج البارد استولى a add.

293 במקרה: = بالعرض a بالغرض Bos conj.

כפל = Arab. انثنى 'to be flexed'; cf. entry (יתר) התיתר. Hebrew כפל in the sense of 'to be flexed' is a non-attested semantic borrowing from the Arabic انثنى. Nathan (a.l.) translates Arab. انثنى as נכפף.

נכפל (כפל) = Arab. انثنى 'to be flexed'; cf. entry כָּפוּל. Hebrew נכפל in the sense of 'to be flexed' is a non-attested semantic borrowing from the Arabic انثنى. Nathan (a.l.) translates Arab. انثنى as נכפף.

הכפיל (כפל) = Arab. ثنى 'to flex'; cf. entry (יתר) התיתר. Hebrew הכפיל in the sense of 'to flex' is a non-attested semantic borrowing from the Arabic ثنى. Nathan (a.l.) translates Arab. ثنى as כפף.

כת: הכת הקרניי = الطبقة القرنية 'the hornlike tunic'; cf. 3.52: הלחות הכפורי והביציי הזכוכיי וכן הכת הקרניי אין בו גידים בשום פנים (The crystalline, vitreous, and albuminoid humours, and likewise the hornlike tunic, do not contain any vessels at all). Hebrew כת does not feature in this sense in the current dictionaries. It is possibly an abbreviation of כתנת; cf. Kaufmann, *Die Sinne*, p. 97:[294] quoting this passage he corrects the Hebrew term כת as: [']כת. Nathan (a.l.) translates Arab. الطبقة القرنية as העור הקרניי.

כתות = Arab. طبقات 'layers': cf. 1.43: וזאת השכבה היא כתות הרבה (This network consist of many layers). See previous entry. Nathan translates Arab. طبقات as עורות.

לקח = Arab. أخذ ; cf. entry (נשג) השיג. Hebrew לקח in the sense of 'to begin' is a non-attested semantic borrowing from Arab. أخذ which does not feature in the current dictionaries. Nathan (a.l.) translates Arab. أخذ just like Zeraḥyah as לקח.

מבואר: מְבֹאָר = Arab. مباين 'different'; cf. 3.40: וישובו אילו הגידים המשותפים התחלתם מבוארת להתחלת שאר העורקים (The origin of these joined vessels are different from those of the other vessels). Hebrew מבואר only features in the current dictionaries in the sense of 'explained'; cf. BM 455. Nathan (a.l.) translates Arab. مباين as נבדל.

מוגלי: מֻגְלִי = Arab. صديدي 'serous'; cf. 6.78: ואם יהיה הדם אשר יצא דקיק מוגלי מורה על שהכבד יחלש ממנו מעשה הדם (If the blood is thin and serous, it indicates that the liver is too weak to make blood). Hebrew מֻגְלִי, derived from מֻגְלָה 'serum'

294 David Kaufmann, *Die Sinne: Beiträge zur Geschichte der Physiologie und Psychologie im Mittelalter aus hebräischen und arabischen Quellen* (Budapest 1884), 97.

(cf. BM 2783–4; JD 738, s.v. Aram. מוגלא: 'pus, tenacious matter' [cf. SDA 645]) does not feature in the current dictionaries. MD 653 mentions Hebrew נסיוב for 'serum'. Nathan (a.l.) translates Arab. صديدي as חלודיי.

מֹחַ: מוח הביצים = Arab. مخ البيض 'eggyolk'; cf. 2.4: המרות העבות האדומות אשר[295] אינם אדומות מאד הוא אשר יקראו קצת בני[296] אדם במוח הביצה (The thick and pure red bile is the one some physicians call 'eggyolk-like'. Hebrew מוח הביצים, possibly a loan translation of Arab. مخ البيض features in BM 2891 in an attestation from the *Halakhot Pesuqot*, an early medieval legal code from the geonic period and in an attestation from Meir Aldabi, *Shevilei Emunah,* which was completed in 1360. Another term used by Zeraḥyah for 'eggyolk' is אודם הביצה (see above). Nathan (a.l.) translates Arab. مخ البيض as חלמון ביצה.

מְחֻבָּר: מחובר = Arab. مؤلّف 'compounded'; cf. entry גרעין. Hebrew מחובר does not feature in the current dictionaries in the medical sense of 'compounded' in relation to medicines. Nathan (a.l.) translates Arab. مؤلّف just like Zeraḥyah as מחובר.

מְחֻדָּד: מחודד = Arab. مخروط 'conic'; cf. 4.44: לא תדמה תנועת הדפק בשלשה קצוותיו כתנועתו בגוף המרובע או המחודד וזולתם אלא תחשוב שהיא תנועה אחת והקפה אחת כתנועת הכדור כי תנועת הגיד תתבאר לחוש עגולה מאד (Do not imagine the movement of the artery in three dimensions as a movement in a cubic body or a cone or a similar body, but think of it as a singular movement and a singular rotation, as the movement of a sphere; for the movement of the artery as it appears to the senses is that of a perfect rotation). Hebrew מחודד does not feature in the sense of 'conic' in the current dictionaries. Samuel Ibn Tibbon uses the variant חדודית in his translation of the *Guide of the Perplexed* 1.60, 90 (EP 46). Another term for 'conic' found in medieval Hebrew mathematical literature is חרוט; cf. Sarfatti, *Munaḥei ha-Matematikah*, no. 134: גולם חרוט (cone). Nathan (a.l.) translates Arab. مخروط as המחודד הנקרא החרוט.

מְחֻזָּק: מוחזק = Arab. موقاة 'protected'; cf. 1.18: וכל העצבים והיתרים והגידים המוגבלים מן העצם מוחזק מכוסה בקרומות חזקים (All the nerves, tendons, and veins which lie in bony grooves are covered and protected by strong membranes). Hebrew מוחזק does not feature in this sense in the current dictionaries. Nathan (a.l.) translates Arab. موقاة as מוסתר. Cf. entry חזק.

---

295 אשר אינם אדומות מאד: الناصع a.

296 בני אדם: = الناس BELPS الأطبّاء a.

מחשבה = I. Arab. تهمة ‘suspicion’; cf. 6.95: כשתקרה לבריאים תורה על החולי וכשתקרה לחולים תורה על בריאות. ותאות המזון החזקה כשתקרה לבריאים תהיה מקום מחשבה וראיה על חולי וכשתקרה לחולים תהיה ראיה טובה (When it (i.e. sleep which is longer and deeper than usual) occurs to healthy people, it indicates illness, and when it occurs to sick people, it indicates health. And when a strong appetite occurs to healthy people, there is reason for suspicion, as it indicates a disease, and when it occurs to sick people, it is a laudable sign); II. غمّ ‘anxiety’; cf. 7.2: הדברים המחלישים הכח ויפסידו עליו הם שבע[297] סבות: הראשונה הצום. השנית התעורה. השלישית המחשבה (The things which weaken and diminish one’s strength are eight: (1) fasting, (2) sleeplessness, (3) anxiety…). Hebrew מחשבה does not feature in these senses in the current dictionaries. Nathan (a.l.) translates Arab. تهمة as חשש, and Arab. غمّ as דאגה.

מיץ: מיץ המזון = Arab. صفو الطعام ‘the purified food’: cf. 3.34: מיץ המזון אשר יגיע מן האסטומכה אל הכבד ירתח ויתבשל בכבד וישתנה לדם (The purified food which arrives from the stomach into the liver is boiled and cocted in the body of the liver and turned into blood). Hebrew מיץ only features in the current dictionaries in the sense of ‘[that which is won by squeezing,] juice’ (JD 778). Nathan a.l. translates Arab. صفو الطعام as סנון המאכל.

מְיֻתָּר: מיותר = Arab. موتّر ‘tense’; cf. 1.24: כל מיני תנועות המושקולי ארבעה וזה או שיתקבץ או שיתפשט או שיתעקם או שישאר נמשך מיותר (There are altogether four [different] kinds of movements of a muscle, namely [these]: it is either contracted, or it is extended, or it is twisted, or it remains stretched and tense). Hebrew מיותר in the sense of ‘tense’ is a non-attested calque of the Arab. موتّر. Nathan (a.l.) translates Arab. موتّر as נמשך כמתר. Cf. entries יתר, התיתרות.

התמלא (מלא) = Arab. تخم ‘to suffer from an indigestion’; cf. 9.44: המחלה הנופחת ישים בעליה כואב ודואג רעת התוחלת מתיאש מהטובה ובכלל עניינה כעניין בעל השעמום המלינקוניקו בעבור שיתוף פי האסטומכא למוח. ותתחזק חליים כשיתמלאו ורובם הם בעלי טחול (A gassy disease makes the patient suffering from it depressed, sad, hopeless, and despairing of good. In short, their condition is like that of those suffering from melancholic delusion because of the connection between the cardia of the stomach and the brain. Their affliction becomes [even] more severe when they suffer from indigestion. Most of these patients suffer from

297 שבע: ثمانية a.

an affection of the spleen). Hebrew התמלא does not feature in this sense in the current dictionaries. N (a.l.) translates Arab. تخم as קרהו קבסא.

מִלּוּי: מילוי = Arab. تخمة 'indigestion, dyspepsia'; cf. entry מרקחת. Hebrew מילוי only features in the current dictionaries in the sense of 'filling' (JD 774; EM 946). Nathan translates Arab. تخمة as קבסא. 'Indigestion' features as הפרעת העכול or as אי עכול in Masie, MD 382.

ממית הזאב = Arab. قاتل الذئب 'aconite'; cf. entry דבקות הזהב. Hebrew ממית הזאב, a loan translation of the Arabic قاتل الذئب does not feature in the current dictionaries or secondary literature. Nathan (a.l.) translates the Arab. قاتل الذئب as הורג הזאב.

מְמֻלָּא: ממולא = Arab. متخوم 'someone suffering from indigestion'; cf. 9.56: כשתרצה לחזק אסטומכת הממולאים ודומיהם ואפילו יהיה עמהם קדחת יום תשים הדברים המחזקים על האסטומכה (If you want to strengthen the stomach of those suffering from indigestion and the like even if they have ephemeral fever, put strengthening substances upon the stomach). Hebrew ממולא does not feature in this sense in the current dictionaries. Nathan (a.l.) translates Arab. متخوم as בעל הקבסא.

מְמֻרְסָם: ממורסם = Arab. وارم 'tumorous'; cf. 3.109: ברופאים כת שחושבים כי כל אשר יהיה יותר קובץ בחוזק יהיה יותר טוב במה שירצו בו לעשות דברים מקבצים וכן מה שהיה מן הרפואות יותר מתיר שהוא יותר טוב ומועיל יותר במה שירצו להתירו. ולא יבינו כי כל אחד משתי אילו הכחות כל אשר הוא יותר חזק יהיה מה שיתחדש באבר הממורסם מן הכאב יותר חזק (There are physicians who think that the stronger a medicine is in astringency, the more effective it is, when astringency is required. They also think that the more dispersing a medicine is, the more effective and beneficial it is, when dispersion is required. They do not understand that the stronger either of these powers is, the stronger the pain in the tumorous part of the body). Hebrew ממורסם does not feature in the current dictionaries. Nathan (a.l.) translates Arab. وارم as בעל המורסא. Cf. entry מרסם.

מנע = Arab. نهى 'to forbid'; cf. 25.48: אמר משה: בני אדם מקשים לגליאנוס באומרו כי ההקזה היא טובה בכל הקדחות המעופשות והנה מנע ההקזה במאמרו שעשה בהקזות ובמקומות אחרים בקדחת הפליאומטיקה הפשוטה כיון שהליחות פגות. וכן ימנע ההקזה בקדחת הרביעית הפשוטה אלא אם היה נראה בו סימני הדם[298] (Says Moses: One may doubt [Galen's]

298 סימני: كثرة add a.

approval of venesection in [the case of] all putrid fevers. In his treatise *De venae sectione* and other places he [himself] forbids venesection in pure phlegmatic fever because the humours are raw and crude. He also forbids bloodletting in pure quartan fever, unless there is a clear indication for excess of blood). Hebrew מנע does not feature in this sense in the current dictionaries. Nathan (a.l.) translates Arab. نهى as הזהיר מן. See as well BA 166: 'prohibere; impedire'.

מָסָךְ = Arab. حجاب 'husk'; cf. 13.51: מדבריו: הקולוקינטידא תיקונה[299] יהיה בליבות[300] הפסתק ואחריו לבות השקדים נתאמת זה בניסיון ארוך. ומסך התורפיד[301] פרח הנילופר ואם יחבר לו שמן השקדים היה זה טוב (He further said: <In the case of> the rind <enclosing> the pulp of colocynth and kernels of pistachio, followed by almond kernels this[302] has been confirmed by long experience. [The same applies to] husks of hellebore (Helleborus) [and] nenuphar (Nymphae) blossoms. And if one adds almond oil thereto, it is a good decision). Hebrew מָסָךְ only features in a medical sense in the current dictionaries as 'diaphragm' or 'Velamenti cerebri, Meninges'; cf. BM 3119 and SG Pe 37. In the sense of 'husk' it is a non-attested semantic borrowing from Arab. حجاب. Nathan (a.l.) translates Arab. حجاب as קליפה.

מעידה: מעידת המעים = Arab. زلق الأمعاء 'lientery'; cf. 22.36: לשתות משקל תשעה גרעיני חיטה מהזמרד שחוק ומנופה יבלענו במים על הריקנות יפסיק שלשול הסמום ואם יתלנו על מי שיש בו שלשול או מעידת המעים ירפאנו (The ingestion of nine granules of emerald, pulverized and filtered, in a mouthful of water on an empty stomach stops the diarrhoea caused by poisons. If it is hung [around the neck] of someone suffering from diarrhoea or lientery, it cures him). Hebrew מעידת המעים, a loan translation of Arabic زلق الأمعاء, does not feature in the current dictionaries. In addition to מעידת המעים Zeraḥyah has המעדת המעים (see s.v. המעדה) and חלקות המיעים (see s.v. חלקות).

הכח המפרנס: מפרנס = Arab. القوة الغاذية 'the nutritive faculty'; cf. 1.72: והכח אשר יפרנס האבר עד שיצמח ויגדל או שיחליף עליו מה שהותך ממנו הוא הכח המפרנס (And the faculty that feeds the organs so that they grow or replaces what has been

299 תיקונה יהיה: om a.

300 בליבות: لبّ a.

301 התורפיד: الخربق a.

302 I.e., what he stated above (13.49) that these purgatives should not be mixed with musk, nor with wine.

used up by them, is the nutritive faculty). Hebrew מפרנס only features in the current dictionaries in the sense of 'sustaining'; cf. EM 1019. Nathan (a.l.) translates Arab. القوة الغاذية as הכח הזן. See as well entry פרנס.

מצב = Arab. انتصاب 'orthopnea'; cf. 24.38: פגשתי יום אחד רופא אחד מפורסם במלאכת הרפואות ומששתי לו הדפק ומצאתי בו כל מין ממיני השינוי בלא קדחת ולא היה מרגיש בניפושו שום דבר כלל. ואמרתי לו אני רואה שזה השינוי יהיה מדוחק וצרות שיהיה בגידים אשר בריאה או בעבור סתימה מליחות עבות דבקות או מתולדת צמח שלא נתבשל. ואמר לי אם כן היה ראוי שהיה לי בניפוש מצב מרימפלי. ואמרתי לו כי המצב יהיה בהתקבץ הליחה הדבקה בחלקי קנה הריאה לא בהתקבצו בגידים הדופקים (One day a person famous for his medical practice met with me. I felt his pulse and noticed therein all kinds of irregularities but without fever and without feeling anything at all during respiration. I told him that in my opinion this irregularity arose from a pressure and stenosis of the pulsatile vessels in his lungs, [and that this was caused] either through an obstruction of thick, sticky humours or through the development of an abscess that was not ripe. He said to me: Then I should be suffering from an asthmatic orthopnea. I then said to him that orthopnea arises from the accumulation of a thick, viscous humour in the subdivisions of the trachea (i.e. bronchial tubes) but not from their accumulation in the pulsatile vessels). In the sense of 'orthopnea' Hebrew מצב is a semantic borrowing from Arab. انتصاب which does not feature in the current dictionaries. Nathan (a.l.) translates Arab. انتصاب as התיצבות (cf. Masie (MD 529): התיצבות הנשימה (Nathan's translation of Ibn Sīnā's *K. al-Qānūn* prepared in Rome in 1279)).

מצעת = Arab. مصفاة 'sieve'; cf. 1.42: אבל העצם אשר יגן בעד המוח סמוך לפנים ולחיך הוא חלול ובעלי הנתוח יקראוהו המצעת (The bone which protects the brain and is close to the face and palate is hollow; the anatomists call it the 'sieve'). Hebrew מצעת, coined from מצע 'to press, squeeze' (JD 827) does not feature in the current dictionaries. Nathan (a.l.) translates Arab. مصفاة as מסננת.

מקום = Arab. حجم 'size'; cf. 9.102: אל יפחדך במלאכת היד גודל החליים אבל תעיין בסכנתה וכוחה וחולשתה. מזה שאין ראוי שיפחדך גודל החולי[303] ותחשבנו חולי חזק אבל תראה ותדע כי הכיס[304] אשר ירד בו הקרום אשר על האסטומכא והמיעים והוא החלב הוא חולי גדול וחזק אע"פ שמקומו אינו גדול (Do not be frightened of the severity of

303 החולי: القيلة a.

304 הכיס: القيلة a.

illnesses when performing surgery; rather, consider whether these illnesses are dangerous and serious or minor. For instance, you should not be frightened of a large hernia and think that it is a serious illness. Rather, consider and know that a hernia in which the membrane that covers the intestines and stomach, namely, the omentum, descends, is a serious and grave illness although the size of the hernia may not be large. Hebrew מקום does not feature in this sense in the current dictionaries; cf. KT 2:265–6. Nathan (a.l.) translates Arab. حجم as שעור.

מקומי = Arab. وضعي 'conventional'; cf. 25.59: מבעלי זה החולי הכולל נמצא מינים[305] מבני אדם בעלי זריזות והבנה שידעו אחת מהחכמות הפילוסופיות או[306] העיוניות[307] או שידעו אחת מהחכמות המקומיות (Because of this common illness we find that individuals who possess cleverness and alertness and have learned one of the philosophical, theoretical or speculative sciences, or one of the conventional sciences). Hebrew מקומי does not feature in this sense in the current dictionaries. Nathan (a.l.) translates Arab. وضعي as מונח.

מקור: מקורים = Arab. معادن 'minerals'; cf. 7.72: אמר משה זה אמת כי השחוק מסגולות האדם. וידוע כי כל סגולה היא נמשכת אחר הצורות המיניות בין שיהיו אותם הסגולות לאי זו מין ממיני בעל חיים או הצמחים או המקורים (Says Moses: This statement is correct because laughter is a specific characteristic of human beings. It is well-known that each specific property belongs to the generic form, regardless of whether it belongs to the species of animals or plants or minerals). Hebrew מקור is mentioned in BM 3275 as a synonym of מחצב (see BM 2924: 'quarry, mineral' a.o. in an attestation from Samuel Ibn Tibbon's Hebrew translation of Maimonides' *Guide of the Perplexed*). Nathan (a.l.) translates the Arabic معادن as the standard Hebrew מחצב.

מקורי = Arab. معدني 'mineral'; cf. 9.97: והרפואה המקררת המייבשת ברוב היא עוצרת והעוצר יהיה נושך והוא לא יסבול הנשיכה ועל כן הטוב שברפואותיה הוא המקוריות שאינם חמות כשיגיעו[308] (However, cooling and drying remedies are mostly astringent, and astringent [drugs] are biting, and the anus cannot tolerate biting. Therefore, the best medications consist of mineral substances that are not hot when they are washed). Hebrew מקורי features in the sense of 'mineral' in

---

305 מינים: أشخاصا a.

306 או: om a.

307 העיוניות: أو العلمة add a.

308 כשיגיעו (= وصولت): صوّلت a.

BM 3276, a.o. in an attestation from Efodi's commentary on Maimonides' *Guide of the Perplexed* 1.58.

מַרְאֶה = Arab. لون 'colour'; cf. 9.8: הכתמים אשר יראה האדם לפני עיניו הם מן הליחות עצמותם ומראיהם מנגד ללחות הביציי ויתקבצו בין הכפורית והקרנית (The sparks that a person sees before his eyes result from humours whose consistency and colour are contrary to the albuminoid humour that gathers between the crystalline humour and the hornlike [tunic]). Hebrew מראה is attested in the sense of colour in Rabbinic literature only; cf. JD 834. Nathan also translates Arab. لون as מראה. The same term features in Moses Ibn Tibbon (See Moses ibn Tibbon, s.v. מַרְאֶה).

מרוצה = Arab. مجرى 'channel'; cf. 1.67: וזה העצב החלול...כלומר ראש האמה מרוצתו[309] רחוק מהגיד[310] ומרוצת הזרע בו ממה שסמוך הצד השפל משוך בארך באמצעיתו (This hollow nerve…I mean, the penis — is embedded far from the anus, and the channel for the semen extends longitudinally in its lower parts and is centrally located). Hebrew מרוצה does not feature in this sense in the current dictionaries. Ben Yehuda (BM 3320) states that מרוצה has the same meaning as מרוץ and one of its meanings given by him is 'corridor'. Nathan (a.l.) translates Arab. مجرى as מעבר.

מֹרֶךְ: מורך = Arab. سخافة 'emaciation'; cf. 9.116: אשר יקרה להם העילוף בעבור מורך גופם ורוב התרת הרוח תפרנס במזון שאינה ממהרת ההתרה (Those who are stricken by syncope because of the emaciation of their bodies and the severe weakening of the pneuma should be nourished with foods that do not decay rapidly…). Hebrew מורך only features in the current dictionaries in the sense of 'weakness' (BDB 940), 'faintness, cowardice' (JD 750), esp. as מורך הלב (cowardice) (BM 3333). Nathan (a.l.) translates Arab. سخافة as רפיון.

מרכב: מירכב = Arab. عقيد 'thickened juice'; cf. 21.61: רפואה שתטהר ותנקה מבלתי נשיכה כמו השורבו העשוי מן הפולים ומים שלפארי מהשעורים וזרע הפשתן הקלוי והמירכב העשוי מן התאנים היבישים. אבל מירכב הענבים כחו שיטהר[311] וידבק[312] והוא רחוק מהנשיכה יותר מכל דבר (Drugs which cleanse without biting are similar to soup prepared from beans (*Vicia faba*), barley gruel, roasted linseed (*Linum usitatissimum*)

309 מרוצתו: = مجراه L مجراها E مغرّزة a.
310 מהגיד: من الدبر a.
311 שיטהר: تطلق a.
312 וידבק: وتغذّي a.

and thickened juice prepared from dried figs. Concentrated grape juice has relieving power and is nourishing. It is one of the least biting substances). Hebrew מירכב does not feature in the current dictionaries. Nathan (a.l.) translates Arab. عقيد as דבש and תירוש respectively.

התמרסם (מרסם) = Arab. تورّم 'to have a tumour'; cf. 3.61: בהאריך לעמוד הלחויות המורקות אל המקום הפנוי באברים אשר נתמרסמו יתחדש בהם שינויים משונים מאד (If fluids stream into the cavities of organs that have tumours and remain there for a long time, they undergo a great variety of transformations). Hebrew מרסם does not feature in the current dictionaries. Nathan (a.l.) translates Arab. تورّم as עלה בנפיחה כמורסא; cf. entry ממורסם.

מרקחת = Arab. جوارش 'stomachic'; cf. 9.47: המילוי אשר ישתלשל עמו הטבע עד שיתרבה ויחטוף הכח תפרנסנו בדברים עוצרים בסדר והרבה פעמים תפול תאות המזון עם אחד ממיני השלשול הנק' דרב וצריך שיקח החולה מרקחת החבושים ודומיהו. ([In the case of] indigestion associated with diarrhoea so severe that it harms one's strength, one should feed oneself with things that are astringent more and more. Often diarrhoea goes with loss of appetite. In this case the patient should take a stomachic of quinces and the like). Hebrew מרקחת only features in the current dictionaries in the sense of 'drug, poison' (JD 847) or 'aromatic oil; ointment; confiture' (BM 3347–8). Nathan (a.l.) translates Arab. جوارش as מרקחת as well.

נמשך זו אחר זו: משך = Arab. مترادف 'synonymous'; cf. 23.21: אמר משה בהיותך משתכל מה שזכר גליאנוס בספרו הנקרא הרעד והרפפות והריגור והכיווץ ובאר זה כי שם הרעד והרעש שתי שמות נמשכות זו אחר זו (Says Moses: If you consider what Galen mentions in his treatise *De tremore, palpitatione, rigore et convulsione*, it will be clear to you that the terms 'riʿda' (tremor) and 'riʿsha' are synonyms). Hebrew נמשך זו אחר זו does not feature in the sense of 'synonymous' in the current dictionaries. Nathan (a.l.) translates Arab. مترادف as נרדף.

המישמוש בידים: משמוש = Arab. التكميد 'a warm compress'; cf. 23.33: המישמוש בידים או בדבר אחר ונקרא בערבי תכמיד והוא נופל על מה שיחמם הגוף מחוצה ומיניו חמשה ([The term] hot compress applies to everything that warms the body externally. There are five kinds of it). Hebrew המישמוש בידים does not feature in the current dictionaries. Nathan (al.) translates Arab. التكميد as ההנחה החמה.

משמש = كمّد 'to apply a hot compress'; cf. 23.33: והממוצע הוא שיוקח שעורים וכרסנה תשחקם ותבשלם בחומץ חזק ומזוג יותר חזק יהיה מאותו ששותים בני אדם ותשימנו בכיס ותמשמש בו האברים וכן תעשה בסובין. (The intermediate [hot compress] one is that prepared with barley and bitter vetch; they should be pulverized and boiled with acid vinegar mixed with it to a degree that is stronger than could be drunk. Put this in a bag and apply it as a hot compress to the parts of the body [you want to treat]. The same [should be done] with bran). Hebrew משמש does not feature in this sense in the current dictionaries. Nathan (a.l.) translates Arab. كمّد as חימם. See as well entry טבל.

מְשֻׁעֲמָם = Arab. موسوس 'someone suffering from delusions'; cf. 20.74: התפוחים להריח אותם יחזקו הלב והמוח וריחו יועיל לבעלי הרישפיצי והמשועממים (The smell of an apple strengthens the heart and the brain and is beneficial for those suffering from marasmus and delusions). Hebrew מְשֻׁעֲמָם is mentioned in EM 1087 as featuring in Rabbinic literature in the sense of 'melancholic'. Nathan (a.l.) translates Arab. موسوس as נחשל. See as well entry שעמום.

המתין על (מתן) = Arab. صبر على 'to bear'; cf. 20.65: הדברים אשר להם שמנונית ודבקות כמו החלבים מיד שיגיעו אל האסטומכא בתחלת אכלם הם שובעים וימלאו גוף האוכל אותם. ואחרי כן ישובו וימעטו התאוה למזון והאדם לא ימתין על התמדתם (Things which are greasy and sticky such as the [different kinds of] fat satiate and fill someone who eats them from the outset, as soon as they reach the stomach. And then they diminish and lessen his appetite. A human being cannot bear to eat such food constantly). Hebrew המתין only features in the current dictionaries in the sense of 'to wait' (BM 3450) or '1. to last, remain fresh, keep; 2. to keep, to let (fruits) lie over; 3. to wait, tarry, postpone; 4. to be slow, patient' (JD 863). Nathan (a.l.) translates Arab. صبر على as יכול.

הֵנִּיחַ מן (נוח) = Arab. اجتنب عن 'to refrain from'; cf. entry הבטחה. Hebrew הֵנִּיחַ מן does not feature in this sense in the current dictionaries. However, in the Bible (cf. KB 680: 'let go one's hand from') and modern Hebrew literature (cf. EM 1130) we find the term as הֵנִּיחַ ידו מן in a similar meaning. N (a.l.) translates Arab. اجتنب عن as להרחיק עצמו מן.

נֶחְבָּא = Arab. محتقن 'congested'; cf. 9.54: תתחדש כמו כן תאות המשקים הרעים כמו שיתחדש זה למזונות הרעים כי בהיות ליחה רעה נחבאת בתוך קרומותיה או שתהיה הליחה מלוחה או מרירייה (A craving for bad and detestable beverages can also occur in the same way as it occurs for bad foods. This is the case when a bad humour, either salty or biliary, is congested in the coats of the stomach). Hebrew נֶחְבָּא does not feature in this sense in the current dictionaries. Nathan (a.l.) translates Arab. محتقن as נעצר.

נֵיּוּת = Arab. خام 'crude' (matter); cf. 5.19: והשתן הדשן יורה על התכת השומן והדומה לשתן הבהמות יורה על ריבוי הניות (Oily urine indicates dissolution of the fat. Urine similar to that of animals indicates a large amount of crude matter. Hebrew נֵיּוּת (is נאות), an abstract noun derived from נא (cf. BM 3460–1) is not attested in secondary literature. Nathan (a.l.) translates Arab. خام as הליחה הנקראת כאם.

נְכָאוּת = Arab. كآبة 'sadness'; cf. 6.52: סימני המראקיא שיהיה לו אחר אכלו רוטו חמוץ ורקיקה לחה בשיעור[313] ושריפה מתחת החלצים וקולות לא תתחדש אלא אחר האכילה בשעה אחת ויתחדש ריעות נפש ונכאות ויקרה לשכלו כמו מקרה השעמום המלינקוניקו (The indications of hypochondriac melancholia are that the ingestion of food is followed by sour eructations, watery sputum in large quantity, a burning [sensation] in the hypochondria and a gurgling sound not occurring until one hour after the ingestion of food. Despondency and sadness also occur while the mind is affected by something similar to melancholic delusion). Hebrew נְכָאוּת in the sense of 'sadness' is only mentioned as modern in EM 1153. Nathan (a.l.) translates Arab. كآبة as עצבון. The same Arab. term features in 9.110 where it is translated by Zeraḥyah as כאב לב and by Nathan as עצבון.

הכה (נכה) = Arab. خبط 'to proceed randomly'; cf. entry אבה. In the sense of 'to proceed randomly', Hebrew הכה is a non-attested semantic borrowing from the Arabic خبط. Nathan (a.l.) translates Arab. خبط as נבוך.

הכיר על (נכר) = Arab. استدلّ على 'to conclude from'; cf. 11.30: משׁשה דברים תכיר על הבחראן השלם (From six things one can conclude that a crisis is complete and perfect). Hebrew הכיר על does not feature in this sense in the current dictionaries. Nathan translates Arab. استدلّ على as קיבל מופת.

נמלה = Arab. نملة 'shingles'; cf. 9.105: מה שתהיה מן הנמלה עמה איכול תהיה רפואתה רפואה מקררת לא מלחלחת כשאר מיני הנמלה (The kind of shingles that is associated with corrosion should be treated with remedies that are cooling but not moistening, just like the other kinds of shingles). The Hebrew term features a.o. in *Sefer ha-Refu'ot* by Asaph (BM 3678) and is defined by Ben Yehuda

313 בשיעור: كثير المقدار a.

(ibid.) as שיחוש האדם בחלי כמו נמלים הלכים על בשרו (in this disease it feels as if ants creep over one's flesh). The same Hebrew term is used by both Nathan (a.l.) and Hillel (s.v. נמלה).

נִמְשָׁךְ: See **משך**.

נִפּוּשׁ = Arab. تنفّس 'respiration'; cf. entry מצב. In the sense of 'respiration' Hebrew נִפּוּשׁ is quoted in BM 3717 in an attestation from Shem Tov Ibn Falaquera, following Kaufmann, *Die Sinne*, p. 70. Even Shoshan (EM 1171) only mentions נִפּוּשׁ as occurring in medieval literature in the sense of 'animation'. Nathan (a.l.) translates Arab. تنفّس as נשימה. See as well entry צרות הניפוש, and BA 173: 'anelitus, inspiratio'.

נִפְסָק: See פסק.

נקירה = Arab. نخر 'caries'; cf. 7.25: הליחות החדות או הרפואה המחודדת אשר יעבה האברים כשיהיה עמם מותר כח מרובה שיחום(?)[314] באברים הבשריים חבלות ובעצמות נקירה (When sharp humours or sharp drugs that make the organs rough are excessively strong, they produce ulcers in the fleshy parts of the body and caries in the bones. Hebrew נקירה is attested in Rabbinic literature in the sense of 'picking, bite' (JD 933). Nathan translates Arab. نخر as נגע.

השיג (נשג) = Arab. استدرك 'to correct'; cf. 25.43: ואמר בזה המאמר בדברו על עניין זה האיש בעצמו זה המאמר אמר: אין ראוי שיהיה היובש נשאר כמו שהוא לבדו ויהיה החמימות והקרירות משתוים לא[315] יחסר דבר כי האברים כשאינם מתפרנסים יתקררו בזמן קצר. זה לשונו כמו כן שם וזהו האמת. ובזוכרו מה שקדם לו ממאמרו בזה האיש שהוא היה בין החמימות והקרירות בריא לקח להשיג זה בזה הלשון (In his discussion of this very same man in this treatise he says the following and these are his words: It is impossible that dryness remain on its own and by itself while heat and cold are counterbalanced without any blemish, for organs, if not nourished, become cold very rapidly. These too are his words there and this is correct. But when he remarked in his earlier statement about this man that he was healthy in terms of heat and cold in his body he started to correct this with the following words). In the sense of 'to correct' Hebrew השיג is a semantic borrowing from the Arab. استدرك that does not feature in the current dictionaries. Nathan (a.l.) translates Arab. استدرك just like Zeraḥyah as השיג.

---

314 שיחום(?): أحدثت a.

315 לא יחסר דבר: لا يذمّ من أمرهما شيء a.

נשך = Arab. نخس 'to prick'; cf. 15.10: האבר כשהוא מת ולא ירגיש כשאתה תנשכנו או תחתכנו או תשרפנו באש בלא ספק כי זה האבר ישתחר ועל כן ראוי שתמהר לחתכו כדי[316] שלא יפסיד המקום הבריא אשר[317] לצדו (When a limb dies to the point that one does not feel it when it is pricked, cut off or burned with fire and inevitably turns black, hasten to cut it off at the point where it touches the connected healthy site). Hebrew נשך only features in the current dictionaries in the sense of 'to bite' and 'to take interest' (BM 3828–9). Nathan (a.l.) translates Arab. نخس as the standard עקץ.

התיר (נתר) = I. Arab. حلّل 'to dissolve'; cf. 15.25: החולי שבעין הנקרא ברדה צריכה לחיתוך. וכן הטרי המקובץ בעין בחולי הנקרא אלכמנא ברוב תרופא ברפואה מתירה לא בדבר שמייבש יובש חזק כי הוא יריק הרוב ויקפיא הנשאר (Hailstone in the eyelid requires excision. The same applies to the pus collected in the eye in the illness called 'kumna'. However, in most cases it can be treated with dissolving medications that do not have a strong drying effect because these evacuate most of the pus and congeal the rest). Hebrew התיר only features in the current dictionaries in the sense of 1) 'to loosen, untie, unscrew'; 2) to permit, declare permitted'; 3) to free, surrender, outlaw, proscribe' (JD 946; cf. BM 3887: 'to loose'). Nathan (a.l.) translates Arab. حلّل as התיך; II. Arab. أطلق in the expression أطلق القضية 'to state definitely'; cf. 25.36: ומקום הספק מבואר מאד והוא היותו מתיר הגזרה בתועלת האברים בעצבי העור אמנם הוא מן המושקלי[318] אשר יבוא למושקולי הפנימי. ובשלישי מהההכרות יאמר כי עצב יבוא לעור מן היד זולתי העצבים אשר יבואו למושקלי המניע היד. וזה פלא אם יהיה מיוחד ליד מבין שאר האברים איך לא זכר זה (The point of doubt is very clear in that in *De usu partium* he definitely states that the nerves of the skin are only [subdivisions] of the nerves that reach the muscles beneath the skin. And here in book three of *De locis affectis* he says that the nerves which reach the skin of the hand are different from the nerves which reach the muscles that move the hand. I wish I knew whether this only applies to the hand amongst all the organs and [if this is the case] why he did not mention it). The expression התיר הגזרה is a semantic borrowing from the Arab. أطلق القضية which does not feature in the current dictionaries. Nathan (a.l.) translates Arab. أطلق القضية as אמר במוחלט.

---

316 כדי שלא יפסיד: من حيث يلقى a.

317 אשר לצדו: الذي يتّصل به a.

318 המושקלי: العصب a.

נִתַּר (נתר) = Arab. تحلّل 'to dissolve'; cf. 15.20: הצמחים אשר ברוב יתחדשו בשטח הגוף הכוונות הכוללות ברפואתם הם שלושה: ההתרה או העיפוש או לחתוך בברזל. והדבשית מהם תצטרך אל אחת מאילו לבד. אבל אשר תהיה בתוכה כדמות קמח מבושל במים ראוי[319] לך שתחתכנה והוא עובר שתעפשנה והדומה לחלב או לשומן תרפאנה בברזל לבדו אחר שאי אפשר בה שתתעפש ולא שתהיה ניתרת (The therapy of abscesses which mostly occur on the surface of the body has three common goals: dissolution, putrefaction, or surgery. For honey-like [abscesses] one only needs either one of these [forms of therapy]. Those [abscesses] whose contents resemble meal boiled in water may be either excised or allowed to putrefy. Fat-like [abscesses] can only be treated through surgery since they cannot putrefy nor dissolve). Hebrew נִתַּר only features in the current dictionaries in the sense of 'to be torn loose, be released; to be untied, released from an obligation; to become permitted' (JD 945).

סַמּוּת = Arab. سمّية 'poisonous effect'; cf. 13.50: אמר משה זה אמת כל זמן שיהיה השלשול ברפואה בעלת סם או חזקה כמו הקולוקוינטידא והתורפד מפני סמותם או הקטפוץ מרוב כחו (Says Moses: This is correct if the purgation is done by poisonous drugs, such as pulp of colocynth or turbith (Ipomoea turpethum) because of their poisonous effect, or [by strong drugs, such as] laurel (Laurus nobilis) because of its strength). Hebrew סַמּוּת does not feature in the current dictionaries. It was possibly coined by Zeraḥyah for Arab. سمّية. Nathan (a.l.) translates Arab. سمّية as ארסיות.

סמרות = Arab. اقشعرار 'shivering'; cf. 19.37: התרחץ במרחץ בקדחות כולם ראוי שתכווין בו שלשה כוונות: האחד שלא יחדש פלצות ולא סמרות בהכנסתו. והשני שלא יהיה אבר שפריטואלי חלוש. והשלישי שלא יהיה בגידים הראשונים מהליחות הניות שיעור מרובה מקובץ וכלוא (In the case of all fevers one should pay attention to three things concerning bathing in the bathhouse: one is that the patient is not affected by a shivering fit when he takes a bath; secondly that none of the vital organs is weak, and thirdly that the primary vessels are not congested by a large quantity of crude humours). Hebrew סמרות, derived from סמר 'to shiver' (cf. BM 4118: 'to shudder, to bristle') does not feature in the current dictionaries. Nathan (a.l.) translates Arab. اقشعرار as סמור.

סַעַר = Arab. كرب 'distress'; cf. 13.47: ותעלה בדעתך כי מי ששוקה רפואה משלשלת וליחותיו גסות והאויר קר כי יחדש לו סער והמיה וכאב באסטומכא ובמיעים ולא ישלשלנו

319 ראוי לך: فيجوز a.

(Imagine someone with coarse humours who is given a purgative while the weather is cold, for he suffers from distress and disturbance and pains in the stomach and intestines, but does not respond to the medicine). Hebrew סַעַר features in the sense of רעש/מהומה/צרה (tumult; disturbance, confusion; trouble, misfortune) in EM 1260. Nathan (a.l.) translates Arab. كرب as צער. See as well BA 176: 'tristitia'.

סערה = I. Arab. اضطراب 'disturbance'; cf. 6.86: הרעי אשר יהיה בו קצף יורה על אחד משני עניינים: או על חמימות מרובה תתיך הגוף ויתחדש הקצף בעבור הדבר אשר ירתיח לחויות הגוף אשר התיכם החמימות המרובה או על סערה מרובה מפני התנגד רוח עב ללחות (A foamy stool indicates one of two things: either extreme heat melting the body, whereby foam results from the boiling of the body moistures which were boiled[320] by the extreme heat, or from an anomalous disturbance resulting from the struggle between thick flatulence and moisture). In addition to סערה Zeraḥyah (13.47) has המיה for Arab. اضطراب (see entry סַעַר). Nathan (a.l.) translates Arab. اضطراب as התגעשות; II. كرب 'discomfort': cf. 7.55: כשתאכל מזון ולא יקרה לך ממנו נפיחה ולא רעם ולא רפפות ולא שנגלוצו אבל יהיה מוצא אותך באסטומכתך סערה אין לך בו תועלת ויכבד באסטומכא (If you take food without suffering from intestinal rumblings or inflation or palpitation or hiccups, but you do have an unusual feeling of discomfort in your stomach — the food weighs heavily on it —…). Nathan (a.l.) translates Arab. كرب as מצוק. In addition to סערה Zerahyah uses סַעַר to translate Arab. كرب (see entry סַעַר). Hebrew סערה in a medical sense features in BM 4141 as סערת החולי in an attestation from *Sefer ha-Refu'ot* by Asaph and from Meir Aldabi, *Shevilei Emunah*. However, Ben Yehuda does not explain its meaning. See as well entry סַעַר.

הספיג (ספג) = Arab. سخّف 'to rarefy'; cf. 21.62: הרפואה המשככת לכאבים באמת יהיה סבת הכאב ליחה או רוח קרים או חמים באי זו עצם שתהיה הליחה הם הרפואה אשר חומה כחמימות הגוף או חמימות שיהיה בראשונה ויהיה עמו דקות עצם עד שתספיג ותדקדק ותבשל ותריק מה שנתבשל ויוציא מן הנקבים ועל כן ראוי שלא יהיה בו קיבוץ כלל (Drugs which really alleviate pains, whether the cause is a cold or hot humour or a cold or hot wind and whatever the consistency of the humour, are those drugs whose heat is like the heat of the body or which are hot in the first degree. In addition, their substance is so fine that it rarefies, refines, concocts and

320 boiled, lit. 'melted'.

evacuates the concocted material and expels it through the pores. Therefore, these drugs should not have any astringency at all). Hebrew הספיג features in JD 1011 in the sense of 'to wipe, dry; to receive drippings, collect' and in BM 4143 in the sense of 'to clean off, dry'. Nathan (a.l.) translates Arab. سخّف as הרפה החלקים.

עיבה (עבה) = Arab. خشّن 'to make rough'; cf. entry נקירה. Hebrew עיבה only features in the current dictionaries in the sense of 'to make thick, fat' (cf. BM 4263). Nathan (a.l.) translates Arab. خشّن as הנחיר (to make rough); cf. Ben Yehuda (BM 3599, s.v. נִחוּר).

עוֹדֵף = Arab. وافد 'epidemic'; cf. 23.16: החליים הנקראים העודפים הם חליים כוללים מתחדשים ביושבי אחד מן המקומות ובקצת שנים והם נמשכים אחר שינוי מתחדש באויר או במים או במזונות המורגלים או בשלשתם (The diseases which are called 'epidemic' are general diseases which occur to the inhabitants of a certain city in certain years. These [diseases] are consequential upon a change occurring in the air or in the water or in the usual nutrition, or in all three of these). Hebrew עודף in the sense of 'epidemic' is a semantic borrowing from the Arabic وافد that does not feature in the current dictionaries. Nathan (a.l.) translates Arab. وافد as מתרגש.

עונה = Arab. نوبة 'attack, paroxysm' (of a disease); cf. 3.103: אותם שימותו בלא בחראן ימותו ביום העונה ויש מהם שימותו בתחלת עונות הקדחות ויוכל למות בעמידת העונה ויוכל למות בירידת העונה בהתיך הכח (The death of those who die without a crisis occurs on the day of the paroxysm [of the disease]. Some of them die in the beginning of fever attacks, others die when the attack reaches its peak, and yet others [die] when the attack is receding and their strength is eroded). Hebrew עונה in the sense of 'attack, paroxysm' is a semantic borrowing from the Arabic نوبة and is mentioned without any further explanation by Ben Yehuda (BM 4381) in, a.o. an attestation from Nathan's Hebrew translation of Ibn Sīnā's *K. al-Qānūn* prepared in Rome in 1279. Nathan (a.l.) translates Arab. نوبة as עונה as well.

עוֹתֵק = Arab. مقلع 'intermittent'; cf. 19.37: הזמנים המשובחים בהכנסת המרחץ בכל הקדחות שהם עותקות כשיהיה עובר היותו נכנס במרחץ הוא זמן שתתחיל הקדחת להתיר כי המרחץ אז יכין הגוף מיד ויתקנהו להתפרנס. (For all intermittent fevers the best time to take a bath, if one is allowed to do so, is when the heat of the fever begins to dissolve, for then the bath immediately prepares the body and makes it fit to be nourished). Hebrew עתק does not feature in this sense in the current dictionaries. This section is missing in Nathan.

עָיַן: עין בעין = Arab. لحظ 'to regard'; cf. 25.59: וכל שכן אם היה אותו האיש נזדמן לו מזל מן המזלות הנחשבים ובני אדם עוינים אותו בעין הגדולה[321] והמעלה וההקדם (This is especially the case if that person happens to achieve one of the alleged felicities of being regarded as someone with authority and preeminence). Hebrew עין בעין does not feature in the current dictionaries. Ben Yehuda (BM 4447) refers to עָיַן only in the sense of 'to look askance'. Nathan (a.l.) translates Arab. لحظ as ראה.

עֲלִיָּה = Arab. تزيّد 'getting worse; increase' (of a disease); cf. 9.20: ליתרגס ככלות עלייתו לך למשוח הגרון ברפואות חזקות וחריפות (When the lethargy stops getting worse, smear strong and sharp medications on the palate…). In the sense of 'getting worse; increase' (of a disease) Hebrew עֲלִיָּה features in Ben Yehuda (BM 4514) in an attestation from Nathan's Hebrew translation of Ibn Sīnā's *K. al-Qānūn* prepared in Rome in 1279. Nathan (a.l.) translates Arab. تزيّد as תוספת.

עמידה is I. Arab. منتهى 'culmination'; cf. 9.18: בעמידת מורסת המוח מי שתהיה חוליו עם תעורה וערבוב תשפוך על ראשו מישרת הפאפויר ותשים בקצה נחיריו ופניו מה שיקרר המוח (When a brain tumour reaches its culmination, one should rub the head of the person whose illness is accompanied by sleeplessness and delirium with a salve prepared from poppy, while the corner of the nostrils and face should be rubbed with substances that cool the brain); II. Arab. انتهاء 'culmination; climax'; cf. entry הרגשה; III. Arab. مكث = 'staying'; cf. 9.97: חוליי פי הטבעת קשים להתרפא מפני ד' סבות והם ריבוי הרגש האבר והיותו מקום שיריקו בו המותרות נושכות ומיעוט עמידת הרפואה בו ומפני היות מזגו חם ולח (The diseases of the anus are difficult to heal because of four reasons: this part of the body is hypersensitive; it is the outlet for biting humours; drugs hardly stay there; and its temperament is warm and moist). Hebrew עמידה does not feature in these meanings in the current dictionaries. Nathan (a.l.) translates both Arab. منتهى and انتهاء as העמדה, and Arab. مكث as עכוב.

ענה = Arab. ناب 'to attack'; cf. 25.24: אמר משה: המובן ממאמרו הראשון הוא שהליחה המתעפשת תחלה תהיה בתוך העורקים. וזמן המנוחה הוא הזמן אשר בין עיפוש חלק מזה הדבר

321 הגדולה והמעלה וההקדם: الرئاسة والتقدّم a.

ובין עיפוש מה שסמוך לו כמו שהומשל באשפה ותהיה הקדחת תענה והליחה מתעפשת בתוך העורקים כמו שאמר (Says Moses: The gist of his first statement is that the humour that putrefies gradually is within the vessels, and the period of abatement is that period between the putrefaction of a part of that thing and of that [part] which lies next to it, as he illustrated with [the example of] the dunghill. The fever attacks and the humour putrefies within the vessels, as he said). Hebrew ענה does not feature in this sense in the current dictionaries. Nathan (a.l.) translates Arab. ناب as עשה עונות.

עצירה: עצירת הבטן = Arab. احتباس الطبع 'constipation'; cf. 8.27: ועצירת הבטן יעורר כל כאב מהליחות הגסות ויחליש כח הטבע ויפסיד הפעולות הנפשיות ויקרה ממנו התרדמה הכבדה והפסד הדעת (Constipation stirs up every [kind of] pain coming from thick humours; it weakens the powers of nature and corrupts the psychical activities. Sometimes it causes a heavy torpor and loss of reason). Hebrew עצירת הבטן does not feature in the current dictionaries. Nathan (a.l.) translates Arab. احتباس الطبع as העצר הטבע. See entry עצר: העצר הטבע below.

עֶצֶם: עצם העגבות = Arab. القطن 'loins'; cf. 16.5: העצר הוסת ברוב ירדפוהו מקרים רעים או כולם או קצתם ואילו הם כובד הגוף ונפילת תאות המזון ופלצות וכאב על עצם העגבות או הצואר או הקדקוד[322] או הראש או שרשי העינים וקדחות שורפות ושתן במראה מעורב משחרות ואודם ויצא החלב מהשדים (Retention of the menstruation is mostly followed by some or all of the [possible] bad afflictions, namely heaviness of the body, loss of appetite, shivering, pain in the loins, neck, forehead, head or roots of the eyes, ardent fevers, a dark, reddish urine, flow of milk from the breasts). Hebrew עצם העגבות does not feature in the current dictionaries. Nathan (a.l.) transcribes Arab. القطن as קטן. In addition to עצם העגבות Zeraḥyah translates Arab. القطن as העצם העומד למטה מכל השדרה (see next entry).

-: העצם העומד למטה מכל השדרה = Arab. القطن 'loins'; cf. 17.14: ואילו[323] לפי דעתי צריכים להיותם מונעים עצמם מכל דבר שהוא מוליד הזרע ויאכלו מזון ורפואה שתכבה הזרע ויטריחו עליון גופם בשישחקו לכדור הקטון או הגדול או להעתיק האבנים וימשה העצם העומד למטה מכל השדרה הנקרא קוטון אחר צאתו מבית המרחץ במשיחות מקררות (As to the regimen of these people my advice is that they abstain from anything producing sperm, consume foods and medications that suppress its formation and exercise the upper parts of their body by playing with a small or large

322 הקדקוד: اليافوخ a.

323 ואילו: وتدبير هؤلاء a.

ball or by lifting stones. After bathing he should anoint his loins with cooling oils). Hebrew העצם העומד למטה מכל השדרה does not feature in the current dictionaries. Nathan (a.l.) translates Arab. القطن as שפל השדרה. See also previous entry.

עַצְמוּת = Arab. قوام 'consistency'; cf. 2.14: ויהיה בעצמותו עובי והיא מתיילדת בגופות החולים לבד (Its consistency [i.e. that of black bile] is thick, and it originates especially in the bodies of ill people). Hebrew עצמות does not feature in this sense in the current dictionaries. Nathan (a.l.) translates Arab. قوام as עצמיות, and Moses Ibn Tibbon as תכונה.

עוצר הבטן: עֹצֶר = Arab. احتباس البطن 'constipation'; cf. 9.55: תקשה רפואת חולשת פי האסטומכה ומהירות הקרבונקלי עם עוצר הבטן כי מה[324] שיתיר הבטן יביא הקרבונקלי ויהפך הנפש ואשר יחזק פי האסטומכה יעצור הבטן (It is difficult to treat weakness of the cardia of the stomach and quick nausea associated with constipation because everything that relieves the bowels causes nausea and upsets the soul, while that which strengthens the cardia of the stomach causes constipation). Hebrew עוצר הבטן does not feature in the current dictionaries. Ben Yehuda (BM 4660) mentions עצר את הבטן (to cause constipation) as featuring in medieval literature. Nathan translates Arab. احتباس البطن just like Zeraḥyah as עוצר הבטן.

עוצר הניפוש : - = Arab. عسر النفس 'dyspnea'; cf. 23.79: החולי הנקרא צרות הניפוש ועוצר הניפוש בייחוד הוא החולי המתחדש מלחויות עבות דבקות עומדות בחלקי קנה הריאה וזה השם אמנם יפול על זה החולי ביחוד (The illness which is called 'orthopnea' and 'dyspnea' in particular is that originating from thick, viscous humours that are stuck in the [different] parts of the windpipe. This term is indeed used for this illness in particular). Hebrew עוצר הניפוש does not feature in the current dictionaries.

עצר = I. Arab. عسر 'to be difficult'; cf. 6.94: ועל כן תהיה חולי השיתוק החזק ממית בהכרח והחלוש יעצור רפואתו כמו שאמר בוקראט (Therefore, a severe stroke is necessarily fatal and a mild one is difficult to heal, as Hippocrates stated). Hebrew עצר does not feature in this sense in the current dictionaries; II. Arab. قبض 'to be astringent'; cf. 7.34: סבת שברון השיניים והתפוצצם הוא בעבור חלקותם ומפני זה ראוי שתקשה אותם ותחזקם ברפואה העוצרת (The reason for the breaking

324 מה: كل ما a.

and corrosion of teeth lies in their softness. Therefore, it is necessary to harden and strengthen them with astringent drugs). Hebrew עצר in the sense of 'to be astringent', a semantic borrowing from the Arabic قبض does not feature in this sense in the current dictionaries. Nathan (a.l.) translates Arab. عسر as קשה, and Arab. قبض as קובץ. See as well ZA 140.

עשה = Arab. استعمل 'to take, to consume' cf. 3.92: שים עינך והשגחתך שלא יתחדש בכבד ובטחול ובכליות קושי וברוב יקרו אילו המורסות הקשות למי שימצאנו מורסא חמה באחד מאילו השלשה אברים ואחר כן יעשה מאכלים שמולידים ליחות גסות או דבקות (Pay attention and be extremely careful that no hardness occurs in liver, spleen, or kidneys. Mostly, these hard conditions occur to somebody who suffers from a hot tumor in one of these three organs and then takes foods that produce coarse and viscous humours). Hebrew עשה does not feature in this sense in the current dictionaries. Nathan (a.l.) and Shem Tov (s.v. הרגיל) translate Arab. استعمل as הרגיל. The same term is used by Hillel for the Latin equivalent 'administrare'.

עששית = Arab. ثريّا 'Pleiades'; cf. 3.18: בעלות הכוכבים הנקראים עששית הוא תחלת הקיץ (The rising of the Pleiades [marks] the beginning of summer). Hebrew עששית (lantern) in the sense of 'Pleiades' is a non-attested semantic borrowing from Arab. ثريّا which means both 'Pleiades' and 'a cluster of lamps, generally resting in holes in the bottom of a lantern' (L336). Nathan (a.l.) transcribes Arab. ثريّا as תריא.

פּוֹשֶׁר: **היה פושר** = Arab. فتر 'to be weak'; cf. 1.32: פעולות המושקולי כולם בזמן השינה יהיו פושרים (All the activities of the muscles become weak during sleep). Hebrew פשר does not feature in this sense in the current dictionaries. Nathan (a.l.) translates Arab. فتر as שקע.

פחד = Arab. خطر 'danger'; cf. 12.38: וכשידוקר הגיד הדופק על רחבו בשני חצאיו אין בו פחד כי הוא יתקווץ כל אחד משני קצותיו אל הצד אשר הוא בו (When a pulsatile vessel is cut in its width, it is not dangerous because every part contracts to its own side). In addition to פחד Zeraḥyah has סכנה ופחד (cf. 15.13) and the standard סכנה (cf. 23.38) for Arab. خطر. Hebrew פחד does not feature in this sense in the current dictionaries. Nathan (a.l.) translates Arab. خطر with the standard Hebrew term סכנה.

נִפְסָק (פסק) = Arab. مفارق ‘intermittent’; cf. 25.23: כי הקדחות הנפסקות והם אשר הפסקם מבואר[325] מורגש אמנם יהיה זה בהיות הליחה המולידה לקדחת מתחרך[326] רץ בגוף כולו (Intermittent fevers, that is, those that have a sensible abatement, occur only when the humour that produces the fever moves and flows throughout the entire body). Hebrew נִפְסָק, Part. Nif‘al from פסק does not feature in this sense in the current dictionaries. Nathan (a.l.) translates Arab. مفارق ‘intermittent’ as נִפְסָק as well.

פרנס = Arab. غذا ‘to feed’; cf. entries מרקחת and פרנסה. Hebrew פרנס only features in the current dictionaries in the sense of ‘to sustain’ (BM 5193). Nathan translates Arab. غذا as הנהיג and זן respectively. Cf. ZA 141: ‘to maintain (Arabic: to feed)’. See as well entry מפרנס.

היה מתפרנס: התפרנס (פרנס) = Arab. اغتذى ‘to be nourished’ cf. 1.56: האסטומכא והמעים יהיו מתפרנסים בשני דברים: האחד מהם המזון אשר ילך בהם ויתעכל בהם והאחר מה שימשכו מן הכבד (The stomach and intestines are nourished by two things: the first thing is the food that passes through them and is digested in them; and the second thing is that which they attract from the liver). Hebrew התפרנס does not feature in this sense in the current dictionaries. This section has not been translated by Nathan. Cf. BA 181: ‘nutriri’.

פרנסה = Arab. غذاء ‘nourishment’; cf. 9.124: הנהגת שיברון העצם אחר מה שתצטרך ממלאכת היד הוא שתנהיג החולה בהנהגה מדקדקת בתכלית. והרבה פעמים תצטרך אל שלשול הבטן ברפואה ובהתחלה. אבל[327] אחר כן תפרנסהו במזון טוב הכימוס והרבה יהיה פרנסתו ושיהיה בו דבקות (The therapy for a bone fracture should, after necessary surgery, consist of an extremely thinning diet. It is often first of all necessary to purge the bowels with a remedy. While the fracture heals, one should feed the patient with food that has good chymes and that is nutritious and viscous. Hebrew פרנסה only features in the current dictionaries in the sense of ‘provision, maintenance, outfit’ (JD 1231), or ‘subsistence, livelihood’ (BM 5195–6). In addition to פרנסה for Arab. غذاء, Zeraḥyah uses the standard term מזון; cf. 9.127. Nathan translates Arab. غذاء both in 9.124 and 9.127 as מזון. Cf. BA 181: ‘nutrimentum’.

---

325 מבואר מורגש: محسوسا a.

326 מתחרך: متحرّكا a.

327 אבל אחר כן: فأمّا وقت تولّد الدشبد a.

פתח = I. Arab. بطّ 'to lance'; cf. 15.25: החולי שבעין הנקרא ברדה צריכה לחיתוך. וכן הטרי המקובץ בעין בחולי הנקרא אלכמנא ברוב תרופא ברפואה מתירה לא בדבר שמייבש יובש חזק כי הוא יריק הרוב ויקפיא הנשאר. ואנחנו הריקונו זה הטרי כשפתחנו הקרום הנקרא קרנית במקום האכליל (Hailstone in the eyelid requires excision. The same applies to the pus collected in the eye in the illness called 'kumna'.[328] However, in most cases it can be treated with dissolving medications that do not have a strong drying effect because these evacuate most of the pus and congeal the rest. I have evacuated this pus by lancing the horn-like tunic, in the rim); II. Arab. شقّ 'to incise'; cf. 15.48: כשתראה הרפואה לא תהיה לה יכולת להתיר הטרי כולו אבל יגבר עליה הטרי ונצח אותה ראוי שתפתח אותו הצמח ותפתחנו במקום העליון שבו והיותר דק ועשה שיהיה הטרי ניגר ושים מה שייבש מבלתי עקיצה (If you see that the medications are unable to dissolve the entire pus, but that the pus overpowers them and prevails over them, it is necessary to lance and incise the abscess at its highest and thinnest point. Let the pus flow out and then put drying [medicines] on it that do not have a biting effect). Hebrew פתח does not feature in these senses in the current dictionaries. Nathan (a.l.) translates Arab. بطّ as שטח and Arab. شقّ as שסע. See also entry קרע.

פתיחה = Arab. بطّ 'incision'; cf. 15.49: וכשליחות ישתעפו באבר בין האברים המתדמים חלקיהם ויתחייב שתריק מן האבר בעצמו ראוי שתשים על אותו האבר רפואה תדחה מה שירוץ לו. וההרקה תהיה עם הפתיחה ועם הרפואה המתירה וכל שכן אם תרגיש שיהיה בין האברים המתדמים החלקים דבר עצור וכלוא (When humours become entangled in a part of the body that is between the homoiomerous parts and have to be evacuated from that very part, one should [first] put medicines on that spot which repel that which streams to it, and then one should evacuate them through an incision and dissolving drugs, especially when you suspect that something [of those humours] is being retained in those spots which are between the homoiomerous parts). Hebrew פתיחה does not feature in these senses in the current dictionaries. Nathan (a.l.) translates Arab. بطّ as חתך.

צלע: מה שתחת הצלעות = Arab. ما دون الشراسيف 'hypochondria'; cf. 6.55: סימני המורסות החדות[329] בכבד שמונה סימנים והם הקדחת השורפת והצמא הגדולה וביטול התאוה בכליות[330] ואודם הלשון תחלה ואחר כך ישתחר ויקיא מרות דומות לאודם הביצה ובסוף הענין

328 I.e., 'hidden <matter>'; the formation of pus behind the cornea, cf. Galen, *De methodo medendi* XIV, 19 (KX, p. 1019).

329 החדות: الحارّة a.

330 בכליות (= بالكلى): بالكلّية a.

יהיה זנגארי הוא וירדידט וכאב בצד הימין עד הקטיולא ילך וכל שכן כשתמשוך מה שתחת הצלעות למעלה (There are eight symptoms of an inflammation in the liver: burning fever, severe thirst, a total lack of appetite, a tongue which becomes initially red and then black, vomiting of bile which initially has the colour of egg yolks and then turns verdigris green, a pain in the right side which extends to the collar bone, especially when the hypochondria is pulled upwards…). Hebrew מה שתחת הצלעות does not feature in the current dictionaries. Nathan (a.l.) translates Arab. ما دون الشراسيف as מה שלמטה מצדי הכסלים. In addition to מה שתחת הצלעות Zeraḥyah has מה שתחת החלצים (cf. entry חלצים).

צִפּוֹרֶן: ציפורן = Arab. ظفرة 'pterygium'; cf. 15.24: רפואת הציפורן אשר תהיה בעין בעודנו קטון יהיה בדברים מטהרים כרפואת הגרב כשתוסיף ותתקשה אז תרפא בברזל (As long as the pterygium[331] in the eye is small, it can be treated with cleansing medications similar to medications for trachoma. If it increases and hardens, it should be treated by surgery). The Hebrew term is defined by Ben Yehuda (BM 5609) as 'an eye disease, i.e. unguis' in attestations from Nathan ha-Me'ati's translation of Ibn Sīnā's *K. al-Qānūn* and from his translation of our text. Cf. Shem Tov, s.v. צפורן.

צָרוּת: צרות הניפוש = Arab. ضيق النفس 'orthopnea'; cf. entries חול and עוצר הניפוש. Hebrew צרות הניפוש does not feature in the current dictionaries. Nathan (a.l.) translates Arab. ضيق النفس as צרות הנשימה. See as well entry נִפּוּשׁ.

קִבּוּץ = Arab. قَبْض 'astringency'; cf. 13.45: מדבריו: כל המשלשלים כל אשר תרחצם יפחות פעולתם. וכן כשתרתיחם. וכל אשר תשחקם היטב יהיה[332] הזקם יותר מתועלתם בפעולת השלשול. ואם המשלשל יהיה בטוח ירבה השתן. וכל העוצרים יהיו הפך כי כל אשר תרחץ המשלשל והארכת בישולו תוסיף קיבוץ. וכן כל אשר תשחקנו יוסיף קביצה ועוצר לשתן כמו כן (He [Abū l-ʿAlā' ibn Zuhr] further said: The more one washes purgatives, the more one diminishes their purgative effect. The same applies if one boils them. The more one pulverizes them, the more likely they are to be lethal rather than purgative. When they are safe, they induce micturition. But all astringent things act conversely. The more one washes or boils them, the more astringent they become. Similarly, the more one pulverizes them,

331 'pterygium'; i.e., a winglike membrane growing over the eye from the inner corner; cf. Galen, *De methodo medendi* XIV, 19 (KX, p. 989).

332 יהיה הזקם יותר מתועלתם בפעולת השלשול: أولى بأن تقتل منها بأن تسهل منها a.

the more astringent they become and also hold back the urine. Hebrew קִבּוּץ does not feature in this sense in the current dictionaries (cf. BM 5675–7). Nathan (a.l.) translates the Arabic قَبْض as קביצות. Moses Ibn Tibbon translates Arab. قَبْض just like Zeraḥyah as קִבּוּץ.

קביצה = Arab. قَبْض 'astringency'; cf. previous entry. Hebrew קביצה does not feature in this sense in the current dictionaries. Nathan (a.l.) translates the Arabic قَبْض as קביצות.

קוֹבֵץ = Arab. قابض 'astringent'; cf. 8.63: האסטומכא והכבד יותר צריכים משאר האברים אל דברים קובצים (The stomach and liver need astringent substances [when superfluities stream into them] more than the other organs of the body). Hebrew קובץ does not feature in this sense in the current dictionaries. Nathan (a.l.) translates Arab. قابض as קובץ as well. Another term used by Zeraḥyah for 'astringent' is עוצר; see entry עצר. See as well ZA 143.

קדחת: הקדחת העונה בכל יום = Arab. الحمّى النائبة كلّ يوم 'quotidian fever'; cf. 8.65: אמנם הקדחת העונה בכל יום אי אפשר שתתחדש אלא עם חולי באסטומכא כמו שהרביעית אי אפשר שתתחדש אלא עם חולי הטחול (Quotidian fever hardly ever occurs without a stomach illness, just as quartan fever hardly ever occurs without an illness in the spleen). Hebrew הקדחת העונה בכל יום does not feature in the current dictionaries. Nathan (a.l.) translates the Arab. الحمّى النائبة كلّ يوم as הקדחת שעונתה בכל יום.

הקדים (קדם) = Arab. تقدّم 'to order'; cf. 9.48: ותעשה זה ביום השני ותקדים החולה בהכנסת המרחץ (Do the same on the second day and order the patient to go to the bathhouse…) In the sense of 'to order' Hebrew הקדים is a semantic borrowing from Arab. تقدّم that does not feature in the secondary literature. Nathan (a.l.) translates Arab. تقدّم as קירב.

קְלוּי = Arab. قلي 'frying'; cf. 20.64: ראוי שתתנהג[333] בכל המזונות בכלל כי מה שיהיה מהם חריף ומחודד או מר יהיה מזונו מעט. ומה שיהיה מהם אין טעם לו מה שהגיע ממזונו אל הגוף מרובה וברוב מה שיהיה מתוק וכל שכן אם יהיה גרם קשה בין שיהיה אילו הטעמים והמאכלים[334] בטבע או נקנים במלאכה כלומר בבישול ובצלי אש ובקלוי ובשרוי במים ודומה לאילו (One should bear in mind a factor common to all foods that whatever is sharp and spicy or bitter provides little nourishment, whilst whatever is

333 שתתנהג: أن تذكر a.

334 והמאכלים: om a.

tasteless provides the body with rich nourishment, even more so whatever is sweet and especially when its substance is firm. [This is the case] regardless whether these tastes are natural or acquired through [human] preparation, that is cooking, roasting, frying, macerating in water and the like). Hebrew קִלּוּי does not feature in the current dictionaries. Nathan (a.l.) translates Arab. قلي as קליה.

קלפה I. = Arab. طبقة 'tunic'; cf. 3.52: הלחות הכפורי והביציי הזכוכיי וכן הכת הקרניי אין בו גידים בשום פנים אבל תתפרנס הלחות הזכוכיי בהזיע הלחות הזכוכיי והזכוכיית במה שיגיע לה מן הקלפה השכבית אשר היא מרובה בגידים הדופקים ובלתי דופקים (The crystalline, vitreous, and albuminoid humours, and likewise the hornlike tunic, do not contain any vessels at all. The crystalline humour is nourished from the vitreous humour by transudation, and the vitreous [humour] is nourished from what reaches it from the netlike tunic, which has many arteries and veins). II. Plur. קליפות = Arab. صفاقات 'tunics' cf. 3.53: כמו שיכלול החוש לעור ... כן ירגשו כמו כן[335] הקרומות והקליפות והגידים הדופקים ובלתי דופקים והרחם והמיעים והשלפוחית והאסטומכא וכל הקרביים ואע"פ שיהיה בעצבים שני הכחות יחד וכלי התנועה היא המושקולי (Just as the skin has sensation...so, too the membranes, tunics, arteries, veins, uteri, intestines, urinary bladder, stomach, and all the viscera have sensation but no motion, although the nerves have both faculties, while the instrument of motion is the muscle). Hebrew קלפה does not feature in this sense in the current dictionaries. Nathan (a.l.) translates Arab. طبقة as עור and Arab. صفاقات as עורות. Hillel uses the term כתנות for Latin 'tunica', while Shem Tov (s.v. גלד) has הגלד הענבי for Arab. الطبقة العنبية. For the different terminology used in medieval literature for the tunics of the eye see Kaufmann, *Die Sinne*, p. 86; See as well the explicit statement of Zeraḥyah quoted in the introduction, above, about the difficulty involved in translating the Arabic terms for three different kinds of membranes, i.e. *aghshiyya*, *ṣifāqāt*, and *ṭabaqāt* into Hebrew, since Hebrew only has *qelippot* and *qerumot*, while *qelippot* is not all at applicable to any of these three [membranes], because it is mostly used for the peels of edible fruits.

קרא: קרא על = Arab. قرأ على 'to study under'; cf. 8.69: אמר משה וכן אני לא ראיתיהו במערב ולא אמר שום אחד מאותם הזקנים אשר קראתי עליהם שהוא ראם (Says Moses: I too have not seen it in the Maghreb, nor did any one of the elders under

335 כן: ولا تتحرّك add a.

whom I studied inform me that he had seen it). Hebrew קרא על in the sense of 'to study under' is a non-attested loan translation of the Arab. قرأ على. Nathan (a.l.) translates the Arabic as קרא לפני.

קרירות = Arab. نافض 'rigor'; cf. 7.23: יתקבץ בגוף ליחה פליאומטיקא זכוכיית ולא תתעפש ותחדש ריגור ימים רבים זו אחר זו וכל זמן היות האדם נח ולא יתנועע כלל וינוח הקרירות ההוא (Sometimes a vitreous phlegmatic humour collects in the body but does not putrefy and thus causes rigor lasting for many successive days. As long as that person is at rest and does not move at all, the rigor is also at rest). Hebrew קרירות does not feature in the sense 'rigor' in the current dictionaries. In addition to the Hebrew term קרירות Zeraḥyah (a.l.) uses a Hebrew transcription of Latin 'rigor', i.e. ריגור. Nathan (a.l.) translates Arab. نافض as רתת (trembling). Masie (MD 634) has for 'rigor': קפיאה and צפידה.

קרע = Arab. شقّ 'to dissect'; cf. 15.31: כשתהיה קורע הקרום הקרני יהיה תחלת מה שיפגושך הלחות הדק הדקיק ויהיה ניגר וזב והוא הלחות אשר הרבה פעמים אנו רואים שיגר ויצא מן הנקב אשר ינקב בעין אשר ימחט המים. ואחרי כן יתכווץ העין בעצמו[336] (If you dissect the hornlike tunic, the first thing you find is the fine and thin liquid streaming and pouring out. It is the moisture which you often see flowing out from the opening made in the eye that is being operated for a cataract. This is followed by the whole eye becoming shriveled, contracted, and hollow). Hebrew קרע features in the current dictionaries in the sense of 'to rend, tear' (BM 6202) or 'to tear, split; esp. to rend the garment in mourning' (JD 1424). In the Nifʿal it is attested in Rabbinical literature in the sense of 'to be torn; to be cut open, be operated upon by a section' (JD 1424). In the sense of 'to dissect' קרע is a semantic borrowing from the Arab. شقّ which features in the Arabic translation literature for Greek ἀναπτύσσω (to cut open) (cf. UW 107: 'aufschneiden').

Nathan (a.l.) translates Arab. شقّ as שסע. In addition to קרע for شقّ Zeraḥyah uses פתח (see entry פתח).

קִשּׁוּר = Arab. رباط 'ligament'; cf. 1.8: העצבים לא יהיה דבק שום דבר מהם בתנוך בלעז קרטילייני ולא בקישור ולא בשמן ולא בעצם אלא בשניים לבדם מן כל העצמות כי הם יתדבקו בשרשיהם עצבים חלקים (No part of a nerve is attached to cartilage, ligaments, fat, or bones. The only exceptions among all the bodily parts are the teeth,

336 בעצמו: بأسرها a وتقلّصها وغورانها a add.

for soft nerves are attached to their roots). Hebrew קִשּׁוּר in the sense of 'ligament' features in BM 6265 in an attestation from Nathan's translation of this term. Hebrew קִשּׁוּר indeed features in Nathan (a.l.) for Arab. رباط. Shem Tov (s.v. אסר) uses אסר and קשירה for the same Arabic term. See as well entries קשר and קשירה.

קוֹשִׁי: קוֹשִׁי = Arab. إنعاظ 'erection'; cf. 22.61: וכשתשחק זרע האורוגא והושמה בבצים שאינם מבושלים אלא מעט עם מעט מלח האשטינק ויעשה[337] מהם חסו יוסיף בזרע ויחזק הקושי מאד (If rocket [*Eruca sativa*] seed is pulverized and put into soft-boiled eggs with a little bit of salted skink and then sipped, it increases the sperm and greatly strengthens the erection). Hebrew קושי only features in a medical sense in Low LXXVI, namely as 'travail, the act of going through labor pains'. Nathan (a.l.) translates Arab. إنعاظ as קושי as well.

קשירה = Arab. رباط 'ligament'; cf. 15.29: רפואה הלחה הניגרת לא תעמוד אלא בקשר ועל כן תשים רפואת הגרב[338] יבישה כי הקשירה צריכה להיות על העין כולו (A moist liquid medicine only stays at its place when applied in a ligament. Therefore, medicines for lachrymal fistula should be dry, because the ligament has to cover the whole eye…). Hebrew קשירה does not feature in this sense in the current dictionaries. Nathan (a.l.) also uses קשירה, and Hillel (s.v. קשירה) has plur. קשירות for the Latin equivalent ligamenta 'ligaments'.

קֶשֶׁר = Arab. رباط 'ligament'; cf 1.7: הקשרים העגולים והיתרים יחשוב מי שאין לו עיון בניתוח שהן עצבים (Someone who is not knowledgeable in anatomy supposes the round ligaments and tendons to be nerves). Hebrew קֶשֶׁר does not feature in this sense in the current dictionaries. However, it also features in Moses Ibn Tibbon (s.v. קֶשֶׁר) as a translation of رباط, and in Hillel (s.v. קֶשֶׁר) to render Latin 'ligatura'. Nathan (a.l.) translates Arab. رباط as קִשּׁוּר.

ראוי: היה ראוי = Arab. لزم 'to remain'; cf. Introduction: כי אני אלו התרתיו[339] על אחד מאותן המקומות היתה ראויה אותה הקושיא בעצמה (for, if I were to refer [the reader] to one of these [other] places, the same objection would still apply). Hebrew היה ראוי in the sense of 'to remain' is a non-attested semantic borrowing from the Arab. لزم.

337 ויעשה מהם חסו: وتحسى a.

338 הגרב: الغرب a.

339 התרתיו על: أحلته على a.

רוֹאֶה: הרואה שלעין = Arab. حدقة 'pupil'; cf. 25.17: אמר משה זה תמה כי המים היורדים בעין וחבלת הקרנית העמוקה בהיותה נכח הרואה שלעין ואחר כן עלתה בשר תזיק בחוש הראות תחלה[340] ואי זו חולי שבא לעצב אשר יהיה בו חוש הראות באילו החליים ודומיהם (Says Moses: I wish I knew whether a cataract in the eye and a deep ulceration of the hornlike [tunic], if they are opposite the pupil and are joined together, are harmful for the sense of vision or not, and from what kind of damage the nerve through which the sense of vision is active suffers in these illnesses and similar ones). Hebrew הרואה שלעין does not feature in this sense in the current dictionaries. Nathan (a.l.) translates Arab. حدقة as אישון. In addition to הרואה שלעין, Zeraḥyah has שומר for Arab. ناظر which also means 'pupil' (see below).

רחיצה = Arab. غسالة 'extraction'; cf. 2.2: כמו שימצא בגוף[341] לחות מימיי כאלו הוא רחיצת החלק הגס אשר בו כן ימצא בכל הליחות לחות מימיי רקיק (Just as milk contains a watery fluid that is as it were, the extraction of the thick part, so, too, all humours contain a fine watery fluid). Hebrew רחיצה in the sense of 'extraction' is a semantic borrowing from Arab. غسالة which does not feature in the current dictionaries. Nathan (a.l.) translates Arab. غسالة just like Zeraḥyah as רחיצה.

רֵחַיִם = Arab. رحا 'lit. millstone, and then a hard formation in a woman's womb, after Greek μύλη'; cf. 23.97: הרחים הנולדים ברחמי הנשים הוא בשר יולידהו האשה אין צורה לו (The [illness called] 'millstone' which develops in the uteri of women is the formless flesh which a woman produces. Hebrew רֵחַיִם in the sense of 'a hard formation in a woman's womb' is a non-attested semantic borrowing from Arab. رحا. Nathan (a.l.) also translates Arab. رحا as רֵחַיִם.

רמז = Arab. أشار 'to advise'; cf. 3.85: ולא ארמוז בהזרתו לעולם אלא לעתים רחוקות שנזיר במעט הזרה כשלא יהיה שם כאב ויהיה הגוף נקי (I never advise application of a restraining treatment, except for a light one when there is no pain and when the body is clean). Hebrew רמז only features in the current dictionaries in the sense of 'to indicate' (BM 6610–11) or 'to gesticulate, hint' (JD 1481–2). Nathan (a.l.) translates Arab. أشار as יעץ.

340 תחלה: أو لا تضرّ a.

341 בגוף: في اللبن a.

רַעַם = Arab. قرقرة 'intestinal rumblings'; cf. 7.55: כשתאכל מזון ולא יקרה לך ממנו נפיחה[342] ולא רעם ולא רפפות ולא שונגלוצו...אין ספק שבזה האסטומכא נתקבצה על המזון על דרך הרעש (If you take food without suffering from intestinal rumblings or inflation or palpitation or hiccups…there is no doubt that the stomach has contracted over the food in a trembling way). Hebrew רַעַם does not feature in the sense of 'intestinal rumblings' in the current dictionaries. Nathan (a.l.) translates the Arab. قرقرة as קרקורים בבטן.

ריפא (רפא) = Arab. عالج 'to practise'; cf. 20.62: המזון שהוא קשה להתיר והוא מזון הדברים שהם עבים ודבקים כמו מזון בשר החזיר והלחם הטוב הנקי ושלא יתקרב בו שום טורח ויתמיד לעשות זה המזון ימהר לו החולי ממילוי כמו שמי שירפא הטורח ויתמיד להיות ניזון עם הירקות ומי השעורים יפסיד גופו וימהר אליו הטיצי (Food which is hard to dissolve is that consisting of thick, sticky things such as pork and pure bread. If someone who does not exercise would constantly take this food, he would soon suffer from the illness of overfilling, just as if someone who practises bodily exercise would constantly feed himself with vegetables and barley juice, his body would be destroyed and waste away quickly). Hebrew ריפא in the sense of 'to practise' is a non-attested semantic borrowing from the Arabic عالج. Nathan (a.l.) translates Arab. عالج as התעסק.

רפידה: רפידות = Arab. رفائد 'pads'; cf. 15.65: בהיות העצם נשבר תשים הרפידות טבולות ביין קובץ ושחור וכל שכן בקייץ. כי אתה אם תעשה בקיץ השמן או הקירוטי יתחדש באברים עיפוש (In the case of broken bones apply pads immersed in astringent dark wine, especially in the summer. For if you use olive oil or cerate, putrefaction develops in [those] parts). Hebrew רפידות in the sense of 'pads' is a semantic borrowing from Arab. رفائد. The Hebrew term features in Ben Yehuda (BM 6683), a.o., in an attestation from Nathan's translation of Maimonides' *Medical Aphorisms*. Ben Yehuda defines the term as תחבשת שעל אברים שבורים (A bandage on broken limbs). רפידות indeed features in Nathan's translation of Arab. رفائد in this aphorism.

רפפות = Arab. اختلاج 'palpitation'; cf. 7.40: הרפפות סבתו רוח עב כלוא במקום קשה[343] לא ימצא מקום שיצא ממנו (The cause of palpitation is a thick wind that is confined to a narrow spot from which it cannot escape). Hebrew רפפוּת only features in a variant reading, namely רפפה, Plur. רפפוֹת in the current

---

342 נפיחה ולא רעם: قرقرة و لا نفخة a.

343 קשה: متكاثف a.

dictionaries. Thus it is mentioned in JD 149 in the sense of a) 'loose lattice work; b) cases of levitical uncleanness arising from vibrations caused by unclean persons'. According to Ben Yehuda (BM 6689) Hebrew רפפה means 'convulsion' as it features, for instance, in *Sefer Refafot*. The term *refafot* as it features in this work actually means 'twitches', i.e. the involuntary twitches of different parts of the body, from which the future of that person is predicted. This kind of magic is also called palmomancy (cf. G. Bohak, *Fragments of Twitch Divination from the Cairo Genizah* (forthcoming). Cf. SG resh 12. Nathan (a.l.) translates Arab. اختلاج as רפרוף.

רצון קיא: רצון = Arab. تهوّع 'nausea'; cf. 6.34: ומי שיקרה לו השקוטומיאה מפני פי האסטומכא יקדים לו דפיקת הלב ורצון קיא (Is someone is affected by vertigo or dizziness that originates from the cardia of the stomach, it is preceded by palpitation of the heart and nausea). Hebrew רצון קיא does not feature in the current dictionaries. Nathan (a.l.) translates Arab. تهوّع as חפץ קיא. Synonyms of רצון קיא are בחילה and קבס (MD 494).

הרקיק (רקק) = Arab. روّق 'to purify'; cf. 7.15: והרוח החיונית בישרון האויר היוצא ולפתוח סתמי העור ולנקות כלי הניפוש מן העובי ומן הדבקות ולפתוח סתמיהם ושיכניס בגופו דברים שירקיקו דם הלב ויסירו העכירות מרוחו עם הרפואות (As for the animal pneuma [it should be balanced] through balancing the outside air, and through opening the pores of the skin, and through cleansing the respiratory organs from the thick and viscous [humours], and through opening the obstruction caused by them, and through the consumption of that which, in combination with drugs, has the property to purify the blood of the heart and to remove the turbidity from its air). Hebrew הרקיק does not feature in the sense of 'to purify' in the current dictionaries. Nathan (a.l.) translates Arab. روّق as זיכך.

שאף = Arab. استنشق 'to inhale through the nose'; cf. 9.6: בהיות המותרות הניגרים מן האף מימיות בלתי מבושלים היותינו מתקנים אותם יהיה בדברים אשר תטבול הראש כדי שיחמם המוח ועם הדברים אשר תשאף ואשר יריק באוזן (If the mucous discharge from the nose is watery and uncocted, we stop it with things with which we foment the head in order to heat the brain, and with those things that are inhaled through the nose, and with those things that are dripped into the ears). In the sense of 'to inhale through the nose' Hebrew שאף does not feature in the current literature. In Biblical literature שאף (absolute and in combination with רוח) is attested for in the sense of 'to gasp, to pant' (KB 1375). Nathan (a.l.) translates Arab. استنشق as שאף ריח.

שָׁדוּף = Arab. سقيم 'ill'; cf. 8.14: אבל כשיהיו אותם האברים שדופים החולי לקח חוקו מעצם הגוף והפחד עליו מרובה ואי אפשר שיתרפא החולה עד שתשוב אל האברים השרשיים כחם המיוחד בהם (But when these organs are ill, then the illness has taken possession of the very substance of the body, and the danger is great, and the patient cannot be cured unless the specific strength of these main organs returns to them). Hebrew שדוף occurs in the Bible (KB 1423, s.v. שדף), medieval and modern literature (EM 1781) in the sense of 'dried out' (especially of grain). It is not attested in a medical sense. Nathan (a.l.) translates Arab. سقيم as עלול.

השיב (שוב) = Arab. عوّد 'to accustom'; cf. 7.51: כשירצה האדם לרומם קולו ראוי לו שישיב רוחו ויפתח פיו מאד עד שיכנס בו אויר מרובה ירחיב הגרון ויהיה הקול גדול (If someone wishes to raise his voice, he should become accustomed to opening his mouth wide so that he lets in much air, which widens the larynx. Then the voice is loud). Hebrew השיב in the sense of 'to accustom' is a semantic borrowing from the Arab. عوّد which does not feature in the current dictionaries. Nathan (a.l.) translates Arab. عوّد as הרגיל.

שׁוֹכֵן = Arab. ساكن 'motionless'; cf. 1.15: ורוב אברי הפנים יתנועעו ברצון והעצמות שוכנות ואינם צריכים ליתרים (Most of the parts of the face move voluntarily, while the bones are motionless and do not need tendons). Hebrew שכן in the sense of 'to be motionless' is a non-attested semantic borrowing from Arabic سكن which can mean both 'to dwell' and 'to be still'. Nathan (a.l.) translates Arab. ساكن as נח.

שׁוֹמֵר = Arab. ناظر 'pupil'; cf. 15.30: המים אחר שירד ויפחות[344] מפני השומר ראוי שתחזיק אותו עם המחט שעה גדולה במקומות אשר ירצה שינוח בו כדי שיתאחז בו (When [in the case of a cataract operation] the moisture has descended from the surface of the pupil, the couching needle should be held for a long time in the place one wants the moisture to settle, so that it becomes firmly fixed there). Hebrew שומר does not feature in this sense in the current dictionaries. Nathan (a.l.) translates Arab. ناظر as רואה. See as well entry רואה.

344 ויפחות: وينحطّ a.

שׁוֹרֵץ: המורסא השורצת = Arab. الورم الساعي 'shingles'; cf. 2.25: מפני היות המזונות שהם רעים בכימוס שתי מינים דקים ועבים כי מה שהוא מן הכימוס הרע דק יחדש חליים חדים וקדחות פוראלינטי ואם יבוא אל אבר יחדש מורסת הריזיפילה בער' חמרה והמורסא השורצת כלומר המתפשטת הנה והנה וכאבים וחליים[345] אחרים (There are two kinds of foods with bad chymes: thin and thick. The bad chyme that is thin causes acute diseases and malignant fevers; and, when it reaches an organ, it causes erysipelas, shingles, and other pains). Hebrew המורסא השורצת, a semantic borrowing from Arab. الورم الساعي does not feature in the current dictionaries. Nathan (a.l.) translates Arab. الورم الساعي as המורסא המתרחבת.

שכינה = Arab. سكون 'rest'; cf. 1.27: אבל מי שהוא ישן ויש בו שכרות או טורח חזק או חולשה הוא ירפה כל אברי גופו בתכלית הרפיון וישיב המושקולי בצורה הממוצעת ויהיה שוכן שכינה שלמה בהיותו ישן (When someone is asleep while he is drunk or very tired or weak, he causes all the limbs of his body to be extremely relaxed; his muscles are in the intermediate position and are completely at rest during sleep). Hebrew שכינה does not feature in this sense in the current dictionaries. Nathan (a.l.) translates Arab. سكون as מנוחה.

שִׁלּוּחַ: שילוח הדם = Arab. انبعاث الدم 'haemorrhage'; cf. 15.41: יכריחנו העניין אל הכויה בהיות שילוח הדם בעבור חולי[346] שנפל באבר או בעבור עיפוש שקרהו (We are forced to cauterize if the haemorrhage is caused by corrosion or putrefaction affecting the organ). Hebrew שילוח הדם, a loan translation of the Arab. انبعاث الدم does not feature in the current dictionaries. Nathan (a.l.) translates Arab. انبعاث الدم as השתלח הדם.

שלם: שלם על = Arab. اشتمل على 'to contain'; cf. Introduction: המאמר הראשון ישלם על פרקים יהיו נתלים בהנחת המלאכה כלומר צורת אברי גוף האדם ופעולותיו וכוחותיו (The first treatise containing aphorisms which concern the subject of the [medical] art, by which I mean the form of the organs of the human body and their functions and faculties). Hebrew שלם על is not attested in this sense in the current dictionaries. Nathan a.l. translates Arab. اشتمل على as תלוי ב. Instead of שלם על Zeraḥyah has the common כלל ב for Arab. اشتمل على; cf. Introduction: השער השלישי יכלול בו שרשי המלאכה וסדרים כוללים (The third treatise contains aphorisms that concern the principles of the [medical] art and general rules).

---

345 וחליים: a om.

346 חולי: أكلة a.

שמירה = Arab. حمية 'diet'; cf. 13.38: ראוי שיהיה נזהר כל מה שאפשר בשאר מיני ההרקות במי שעניין גופו יהיה[347] חלק ורך ובעל בשר[348] ואספוגי ומהר ניתך. וכן מי שנתרבה בו השומן והרזון ויהיה הרקת אילו בשמירה הממוצעת והחפיפה והקרישטירי המחליקים והנטילות[349] והתחבושות ובעשיית השיאף[350] ובמרחץ ותקיז מי שעניינו כן לפי מה שיורוך בו ענייני החולה (One should be careful and considerate as much as possible concerning the other types of evacuation in the case of someone whose bodily condition is such that his flesh is soft and slack, lean and quick to dissolve. Similarly, in the case of someone who is extremely fat or lean. Such a person should be first of all evacuated by means of a moderate diet, massage, mild enemas, the application of fomentations and poultices and softening suppositories, and bathing. Be careful to apply these [means] according to the indications provided by the conditions of the patient). Hebrew שמירה is not attested in the sense of 'diet' in the current dictionaries. Nathan (a.l.) translates Arab. حمية as שמירה והנהגה. Hillel Ben Samuel (s.l. שמירה) uses Hebrew שמירה to translate the Latin parallel to حمية, i.e. dieta.

שינוי: שִׁנּוּי = Arab. اختلاف 'diarrhoea'; cf. 21.11: החלב היותר מעולה משאר החלבים מלבד חלב האשה הוא חלבי בעלי חיים שהם קרובים מטבע האדם כחזירות והצאן והעזים והסוסים. ואם יתקן כשיתחמם חלוקי[351] אבנים אחרי[352] שקדם ותכבס בחלב אחר[353] חממם לאש והתלבנם עד שיחסר מן החלב מימיותו ויותר לחותו ואחרי כן ירד מהאש וישתנה[354] ישכך התרת הבטן המרובה ויפסיק שינוי הדברים הנמצא בהם שמנות (The best [kind of] milk after women's milk is from animals whose nature is close to that of human beings, such as pigs, sheep, goats, and horses. When the milk is prepared by making solid smooth stones glowing hot once they has been washed and by extinguishing (cooling) them in the milk, then by boiling the milk so that most of the moist, watery part disappears, and it is then taken from the fire and drunk, it alleviates dysentery and stops the diarrhoea of oily things). In the sense of 'diarrhoea' Hebrew שִׁנּוּי is a non-attested semantic

347 יהיה: أن يكون لحمه add a.

348 ובעל בשר ואספוגי: سخيفا a.

349 והנטילות: والتنطيل a.

350 השיאף: الأشياف الملیّنة a.

351 חלוקי אבנים: حجارة صمّ ملص a.

352 אחרי שקדם ותכבס בחלב: بعد غسلها وتطفأ فيه a.

353 אחר חממם לאש והתלבנם: ثمّ يطبخ اللبن طبخا a.

354 וישתנה: ويستعمل a.

borrowing from the Arabic اختلاف. Nathan (a.l.) translates Arab. اختلاف as שלשול.

שעמום = Arab. وسواس '(melancholic) delusion'; cf. 2.16: החליים המתחדשים מהמרה השחורה הם הסרטן והצרעת והגרב והחולי אשר יתקלף בו העור וקדחת רביעית והוסוסא הוא השעמום ועובי הטחול. (Diseases caused by black bile are cancer, elephantiasis, mange, the disease in which the skin peels off, quartan fever, delusion, and thickness of the spleen). Hebrew שעמום is mentioned as featuring in Rabbinic literature in the sense of 'melancholy' in EM 1870, and in the sense of 'dullness, idiocy' in JD 1611. Ben Yehuda (BM 7355) refers to it in the sense of a 'mental disease'. Nathan (a.l.) translates Arab. وسواس as בלבול. See as well entry מְשֻׁעֲמָם.

שקיקה = Arab. شقيقة 'migraine'; cf. 6.35: בעלי השקיקה והוא חולי הנק' מיגרניאה קצתם ימצא מישוש הכאב יוצא מהגלגלת וקצתם ימצאנו יגיע אל עומק הראש והכאב יכלה במגרניאה אל הגבול המגיע בין שני צלעות הראש (Some of those who suffer from migraine feel the sensation of the pain on the outside of the skull, while others feel it deep inside the head. The pain of [those suffering from] migraine ends at the line that separates the two halves of the head). As a medical term Hebrew שקיקה does not feature in Ben Yehuda nor in Even Shoshan. It is mentioned, however, in Masie (MD 468), referring to Nathan's Hebrew translation of Ibn Sīnā's *K. al-Qānūn*. Nathan (a.l.) translates Arab. شقيقة as פלוח הראש.

שֵׁרוּי = Arab. نقيع 'macerating'; cf. entry קִלּוּי. Hebrew שֵׁרוּי does not feature in the current dictionaries. Nathan (a.l.) translates Arab. نقيع as שריה.

שָׂרִי = Arab. رئيس 'major'; cf. 25.70: ואמנם הקדמתי לך זאת ההקדמה להעירך מעניין גליאנוס זה החכם המשובח שידעת דעתו באברים השריים שהם שלשה והם הלב והמוח והכבד (I have only made this statement as an introduction to what I will remind you of concerning the matter of Galen, this learned and eminent man. You know that according to his opinion there are three major organs: the heart, the brain and the liver). Hebrew שָׂרִי, an adjective derived from שַׂר does not feature in the current dictionaries. Nathan (a.l.) translates Arab. رئيس as ראשי. Shem Tov (s.v. אבר) translates Arab. رئيس as מושל, and Moses Ibn Tibbon (BIZ 9:8) translates the plural الأعضاء الرئيسة as האברים הראשים.

שִׁתּוּק = Arab. سكتة ‘apoplexy, stroke’; cf. 6.1: יורה על השיתוק אם הוא חזק וימית על כל פנים או חלוש ואפשר שיתרפא וזה[355] קשה מענין הניפוש כי העדר תנועת הניפוש בכלל עד שלא יושג ויהיה זה יותר חזק ממה שיהיה מן השיתוק (One can predict whether an apoplexy will be severe and necessarily fatal or weak and curable — though it is difficult — from the condition of the respiration. For when the movement of respiration is totally missing, so that it can not be noticed, it is the fastest [killing] kind of apoplexy there is). Hebrew שִׁתּוּק features in Ben Yehuda (BM 7495) a.o. in a quotation from Nathan’s Hebrew translation of our passage. However, just as Even Shoshan, Ben Yehuda (ibid.) only explains the term as ‘paralysis’.

שָׁתוּק = Arab. مسكوت ‘suffering from a stroke’; cf. 1.38: ולא יקשה עליך היות השכור והשתוק כשלא יעורו בשום דבר מאלו כי אלו הם חולים לא בריאים (It is not difficult for you [to understand] that a drunk person or someone who suffered from a stroke does not notice any of these, because they are not healthy, but ill). Hebrew שָׁתוּק does not feature in this sense in the current dictionaries. Nathan (a.l.) translates Arab. مسكوت as בעל השתוק; cf. entry שִׁתּוּק.

שתיקה = Arab. سكتة ‘apoplexy, stroke’; cf. 9.12: אפשר שיזדמן שיהיה האדם שוכב על ערפו בלילה כלה ואז התקדם אליו חולי השתיקה[356] וויציאו בהתמלא בטני המוח מאותם המותרות (It sometimes happens to a person that he lies on his back the entire night and that [when he arises in the morning] he is overtaken by a stroke, torpor, or an epileptic fit, since the ventricles of his brain are filled with those superfluities). Hebrew שתיקה only features in the current dictionaries in the sense of ‘silence’ (BM 7498-7499). Nathan translates Arab. سكتة as שִׁתּוּק

תוספת: **תוספות** = Arab. زوائد ‘the lobes [of the liver]’; cf. 24.54: החבלה השוקעת אשר תהיה בתוספות הכבד אפשר שתתרפא (A deep wound that occurs in the lobes of the liver can be cured). Hebrew תוספת features in BM 7692 (referring to MD 56) in the medical sense of ‘appendix’ only. Nathan (a.l.) translates Arab. زوائد as יותרות.

תיק = Arab. قالب ‘cast’; cf. 15.68: שברי הרגל צריך אל תיק כדי שלא יסתער האבר בזמן התנועה וראוי שתעיין היטב בחולי המגיע[357] ללב כי אם יהיה ההזק המתחדש מהלב[358] יותר

355 וזה: وإن كان a.

356 השתיקה: والإغماء add a.

357 המגיע ללב (= الموجب القلب) : الموجب القالب a.

358 מהלב: من القالب a.

מתועלתו לא תעשנו (Fractures of the leg require a cast, so that the limb is not troubled during moving. You should carefully investigate the injuries which require a cast, for if the harm caused by the cast is greater than its benefit, do not apply it). Hebrew תיק does not feature in a medical sense in the current dictionaries; cf. JD 1665: 'casing, sheath'. Nathan translates Arab. قالب as דפוס. Shem Tov (SG Tav 16) uses Hebrew תיק to translate Arab. غلاف (a receptacle used as a repository; and a covering, or an envelope; scabbard, or sheath; a case, or covering, enclosing the scabbard; enclosing membrane; pellicle of the egg; the calyx of a flower; cf. L 2284).

תכלית = Arab. مبلغ 'extent'; cf. 8.8: והמזון לפי תכלית תוספתו בכח החולי ואיחורו בבישול יהיה תכלית חיזוקו ותטה לעולם לצד היותר צריך לעזור (And to the extent that food aggravates a disease and delays its coction, to that extent it strengthens [the patient]. Therefore, one should always turn to that [aspect] which is in most need of support). Hebrew תכלית does not feature in this sense in the current dictionaries; cf. BM 7749: 'end, extreme limit'; KT 4.197: 'Ende, Endlichkeit, Grenze, Extrem'. See as well EP 122: '1. final cause; 2. end'. Nathan (a.l.) translates Arab. مبلغ as המרצה.

תחת: תחת השחי = Arab. الإبطان 'the armpits'; cf. 7.71: אמנם השחוק אשר יהיה במישוש הנראה שלתחת השחי ותחת כפות הרגלים וכן השחוק אשר אנו עושים בראותינו הדברים שאדם שוחק עליהם או שישמע אותם אין לי בידיעת הסבה בזה דרך כלל (As for laughter occurring through tickling the armpits [on the outside] and the footsoles, as well as laughter which occurs when seeing or hearing comical things, it is absolutely impossible to find out its cause). Hebrew תחת השחי does not feature in secondary literature. Nathan (a.l.) translates Arab. الإبطان as אצילים, while Hillel uses the same Hebrew term as Zeraḥyah, i.e. תחת השחי to translate the Latin parallel subascellas.

Abbreviations

AD = The Academy of the Hebrew Language. *Dictionary of Medical Terms*. English-Hebrew. Hebrew-English. (Jerusalem 1999).

AL = André, J., *Les noms des plantes dans la Rome antique*. (Paris 1985).

BA = Bos, G., *Aristotle's De Anima*. Translated into Hebrew by Zeraḥyah ben Isaac ben She'altiel Ḥen. A Critical Edition with an Introduction and Index. (Leiden 1994).

BDB = Brown, F. with the cooperation of S.R. Driver and Ch.A. Briggs, *A Hebrew and English Lexicon of the Old Testament with an appendix containing the Biblical Aramaic based on the Lexicon of William Gesenius as translated by E. Robinson* (Oxford 1907. Repr. 1978).

BIR = Bar Ilan Responsa Project.

BIZ = Bos, G., Ibn *al-Jazzār on Skin Diseases and Other Afflictions of the Outer Part of the Body*. Critical edition, English translation and introduction of Bk. 7 chs. 7–30 of *Zād al-musāfir wa-qūt al-ḥāḍir* (Provisions for the Traveller and the Nourishment of the Settled). With a study of the Romance terminology by Guido Mensching and Julia Zwink (forthcoming).

BL = Barkaï, Ron, *Les infortunes de Dinah ou la gynécologie juive au Moyen-Age*. (Paris 1991).

BLS = Brockelmann, C., *Lexicon Syriacum*, Editio secunda aucta et emendata. (Halle 1928).

BM = Ben Yehuda, Eliezer, *Millon ha-Lashon ha-Ivrit. Thesaurus Totius Hebraitatis et Veteris et Recentioris*. 17 vols. (Berlin-Tel Aviv 1910–59. Repr. Tel Aviv 1948–59).

BMH = Bos, G., *Maimonides, On Hemorrhoids*, Critical edition of the Arabic text and Hebrew translations (forthcoming).

BMP = Maimonides, *On Poisons and the Protection against Lethal Drugs*. A New Parallel Arabic-English Translation by Gerrit Bos with Critical Editions of medieval Hebrew translations by Gerrit Bos and medieval Latin translations by Michael R. McVaugh. (Provo 2009).

BMR = Maimonides, *On the Regimen of Health*. A New Parallel Arabic-English Translation by Gerrit Bos with Critical Editions of medieval Hebrew translations by Gerrit Bos and Latin translations by Michael R. McVaugh (forthcoming).

BP = Biville, F., 'Pathologie de la voix', in A. Debru et G. Sabbah (eds), *Nommer la maladie. Recherches sur la lexique gréco-latin de la pathologie*. (Saint-Étienne 1998), 63–81.

BZ = Bos, G., *Ibn al-Jazzār on Sexual Diseases*: A critical edition, English translation and introduction of Bk. 6 of *Zād al-musāfir wa-qūt al-ḥāḍir* (Provisions for the Traveller and the Nourishment of the Settled). (London 1997).

CN = Caballero-Navas, C., *The Book of Women's Love. Sefer Ahavat Nashim*. (London 2004).

D = Dozy, R.P.A., *Supplément aux Dictionnaires arabes*. 2 vols. (Leiden-Paris 1927).

DA = Dalman, G., *Aramäisch-Neuhebräisches Handwörterbuch zu Targum, Talmud und Midrasch*. (2nd rev. and enl. ed. Frankfurt a. Main 1922).

DAS = Dalman, G., *Arbeit und Sitte in Palästina*, 8 vols. (Repr. Hildesheim 1964–87, Berlin 2001).

DKT= De Koning, Pieter, *Trois traités d'anatomie arabes*. Nachdruck der Ausgabe Leiden 1903, hrsg. von Fuat Sezgin, Frankfurt am Main, Institut für Geschichte der Arabisch-Islamischen Wissenschaften an der Johann Wolfgang Goethe-Universität. (1986).

DT = *Dioscurides Triumphans. Ein anonymer arabischer Kommentar (Ende 12. Jahr. n. Chr.) zur Materia medica*. Arabischer Text nebst kommentierter deutscher Übersetzung hrsg. von Albert Dietrich (Abh. der Akad. der Wiss. in Göttingen, Phil. Hist. Klasse, Dritte Folge, Nr. 172). I–II. (Göttingen 1988).

EM = Abraham Even-Shoshan, *Ha-Millon he-Ḥadash*, repr. in 5 vols. (Jerusalem 2000).

EP = Efros, I., *Philosophical Terms in the Moreh Nebukim*. (New York 1924).

FA = Fonahn, A., *Arabic and Latin Anatomical Terminology. Chiefly from the Middle Ages*, (Kristiania 1922).

FEW = Wartburg, W. von, *Französisches Etymologisches Wörterbuch*, (Bonn, Leipzig, Tübingen, Basilea 1922 seqq).

GA = García González, A., *Alphita. Edición crítica y comentario*. (Firenze 2007).

GS = Goltz, D., *Studien zur Geschichte der Mineralnamen in Pharmazie, Chemie und Medizin von den Anfängen bis Paracelsus*. (Wiesbaden 1972).

H = Hall, Susan P., *The Cyrurgia Magna of Brunus Longoburgensis*. A Critical Edition. Ph.D. (Oxford 1957).

HA = Hyrtl, J., *Das arabische und hebräische in der Anatomie*. (Wien 1879, repr. Schaan, Liechtenstein 1981).

Hillel = Bos, G., 'Medical terminology in the Hebrew tradition: Hillel Ben Samuel of Verona, Sefer Keritut'.

JD = Jastrow, M., *A dictionary of the Targumim, the Talmud Bavli and Yerushalmi, and the midrashic literature*, repr. 2 vols. (New York 1950).

JNK = Judah Ben Solomon Natan, *Kelal Qaẓar mi ha-Sammim ha-Nifradim* (= Hebrew translation of Abū Ṣalt's *K. al-Adwiya al-mufrada (On Simple Medicines)*, in M. Steinschneider, 'Abu's'Salt (gest. 1134) und seine Simplicia, ein Beitrag zur Heilmittellehre der Araber', *Archiv für pathologische Anatomie und Physiologie und für klinische Medicin*. Hrsg. von R. Virchow. Vierundneunzigster Band. Neunte Folge. Vierter Band. (Berlin 1883, 28–65).

KA = Kohut, A., *Arukh shalem. Aruch Completum*, and Krauss, *Tosefet he-Arukh*. Additamenta. Repr. in 9 vols. (Tel Aviv 1970).

KB = Koehler, L. and W. Baumgartner, *The Hebrew and Aramaic Lexicon of the Old Testament*. Subsequently revised by W. Baumgartner and J.J. Stamm. With assistance from B. Hartmann, Z. Ben-Hayyim, E.Y. Kutscher, Ph. Reymond. Translated and edited under the supervision of M.E.J. Richardson. 5 vols. (Leiden 1994–2000).

KG = Krauss, S., *Griechische und Lateinische Lehnwörter im Talmud, Midrasch und Targum*. Mit Bemerkungen von Immanuel Löw, 2 vols. (Berlin 1898–9).

KS = David Kaufmann, *Die Sinne: Beiträge zur Geschichte der Physiologie und Psychologie im Mittelalter aus hebräischen und arabischen Quellen* (Budapest 1884).

KT = Klatzkin, J., *Thesaurus Philosophicus linguae hebraicae et veteris et recentioris* (Repr. 4 parts in 2 vols. New York 1968).

KZ = Kroner, H., *Zur Terminologie der arabischen Medizin und zu ihrem zeitgenössischen hebräischen Ausdrucke*. An der Hand dreier medizinischer Abhandlungen des Maimonides. (Berlin 1921).

L = Lane, E.W., *Arabic-English Lexicon*, I, 1–8. (London 1863–79).

LC = Levy, J., *Chaldäisches Wörterbuch über die Targumim und einen grossen Theil des rabbinischen Schriftthums*. 2 parts. in 1 vol. (Köln 1959).

LF = Löw, I., *Die Flora der Juden*, 4 vols. (Vienna/Leipzig 1928–34, repr. Hildesheim 1967).

Low = Lowinger, A., 'Register of Hebrew and Aramaic terms', translated and edited by S. Paley, in J. Preuss, *Biblisch-talmudische Medizin. Beiträge zur Geschichte der Heilkunde und der Kultur überhaupt*. (Repr. New York 1971).

LS = Liddell, H.G. and R. Scott, *A Greek English Lexicon*. Revised and augmented throughout by H.S. Jones a.o. (With a supplement 1968, repr. Oxford 1989).

LSD = Lewis, Charlton T. and Charles Short, *A Latin Dictionary. Founded on Andrew's Edition of Freund's Latin Dictionary*. Revised, enlarged, and in great part rewritten. (Oxford 1966).

LW = Levy, Jacob, *Wörterbuch über die Talmudim und Midraschim. Nebst Beiträgen von H. Leberecht Fleischer*. Zweite Aufl. mit Nachträgen und Berichtigungen von L. Goldschmidt. I-IV. (Berlin-Vienna 1924).

M = Moses Ibn Tibbon.

MA = Maimonides, *Medical Aphorisms*, see N and Z.

Ma'agarim =Mif'al ha-Millon ha-Histori la-Lashon ha-Ivrit: http://hebrew-treasures.huji.ac.il/

MD = Masie, A.M., *Dictionary of Medicine and Allied Sciences. Latin-English-Hebrew*. Edited by S. Tchernichowsky. (Jerusalem 1934).

MH = Meyerhof, M., *The Book of the Ten Treatises on the Eye ascribed to Hunain Ibn Ishâq (809 - 877 A.D.)*. (Cairo 1928).

Moses Ibn Tibbon = Bos, G., *Medical terminology in the Hebrew tradition: Moses Ben Samuel Ibn Tibbon*.

MZ = Moses Ibn Tibbon, *Ẓedat ha-Derakhim* (translation of Ibn al-Jazzār, *Zād al-musāfir*), bk. 6, Bayerische Staatsbibliothek 19. (Munich).

N(athan) = Maimonides, *Medical Aphorisms*. Critical Edition of the Hebrew translation by Nathan ha-Me'ati (forthcoming).

R = Rosner, F., *Moses Maimonides' Glossary of Drug Names. Translated and annotated from Max Meyerhof's French edition* (Maimonides' Medical Writings 7, Haifa 1995).

S(hem Tov Ben Isaac) = Bos, G., 'Medical terminology in the Hebrew tradition: Shem Tov Ben Isaac, *Sefer ha-Shimmush*, book 30'.

SDA = Sokoloff, M., *A Dictionary of Jewish Babylonian Aramaic of the Talmudic and Geonic Periods*. (Ramat Gan 2002).

SG = *Sefer ha-Šimmuš*, bk. 29, Shem Tov Ben Isaac medical synonyms (list 1), ed. by G. Bos and G. Mensching in collaboration with F. Savelsberg and M. Hussein (forthcoming).

Shem Tov: see S(hem Tov Ben Isaac).

SIN = Mensching, Guido, *La Sinonima delos nonbres delas medeçinas griegos e latynos e arauigos*. (Madrid 1994).

SL = Albucasis. *On Surgery and Instruments*. A definitive edition of the Arabic text with English translation and commentary by M.S. Spink and G.L. Lewis. (London 1973).

SN = Sontheimer, D., 'Nachricht von einer arabisch-medicinischen Handschrift, vermutlich des Ibn-Dschezla', *Janus* 2 (1847), 246–72 (repr. in *Beiträge zur Geschichte der arabisch-Islamischen Medizin*). Aufsätze I (1819–69), hrsg. von F. Sezgin, in Zusammenarbeit mit M. Amawi, D. Bischoff, E. Neubauer. (Frankfurt am Main 1987), 92–128.

SP = Shem Tov Ben Isaac, *Sefer ha-Shimmush*, MS Paris, BN héb. 1163.

SR = Charles Singer and C. Rabin, *Prelude to Modern Science: Being a Discussion of the History Sources and Circumstances of the 'Tabulae Anatomicae Sex' of Vesalius*. (Cambridge 1946).

SSH = Sermoneta, J., *Hillel Ben Shemu'el of Verona. Sefer Tagmulé ha-Nefesh (Book of the Rewards of the Soul)*. Critical Edition with Introduction and Commentary. (Jerusalem 1981).

UW = Ullmann, M., *Wörterbuch zu den griechisch-arabischen Übersetzungen des neunten Jahrhunderts*. (Wiesbaden 2002).

VL = Vullers, I.A., *Lexicon Persico-Latinum Etymologicum*, 2 vols. (Bonn 1855–64, repr. Graz 1962).

WKAS = *Wörterbuch der klassischen arabischen Sprache*. Hrsg. durch die Deutsche Morgenländische Gesellschaft. In Verbindung mit A. Spitaler bearb. v. Jörg Krämer u. Helmut Gätje (ab Lief. 3 bearb. von M. Ullmann). (Wiesbaden 1957ff.).

Z = Zeraḥyah ben Isaac ben She'altiel Ḥen, Hebrew translation of Maimonides' *Medical Aphorisms* (see N).

ZA = Zonta, M., 'A Hebrew Translation of Hippocrates' De superfoetatione: Historical Introduction and Critical Edition', *Aleph* 3 (2003), 100–43.

Index

אבה 128
אבנט 16
אֵבֶר ← תרדמה
האבר המושל 76
אבר שיש לו מתרים רבים 60
האיברים המיוחסים 17
האיברים המעולים 128
אֲגֻדָּה: אגודות 76
אגודות הבשר 77
אָדָם ← זיו
אֹדֶם: אודם הביצה 128
אדרופיקי 43
אורובי ← קמח
אח ← דם
אִכּוּל: איכול 77, 128
אכילה 129
(אכל) אוכלת 129
אליה 77
אִמּוּן 17
(אמן) אימן 17
אֹמֶץ: אומץ המעים 77
אמצעי ← גיד
אספוגות 129
אִסֹּר / אֱסָר 77
אף ← הגרה
אֹפֶל: אופל 130
אֹפֶן :אופן העצירה 35
אפר: אפר העינים 78
אצבע: אצבע קטנה 78
אצילה 78
אצילי 79
אריגה: אריגת העכביש 17
אריה ← חֳלִי
ארכובה ← פלך
אשה ← נֶקֶב, קבה
אשך: האשך הבשרי 79
האשך הזמורי 79
האשך המימי 79
האשך המעיי 79
האשך הרוחיי 79
אתרוג ← חִמּוּץ
בֵּאוּר: ביאור 130
(באר) מבואר 160
בגד: בגדים 17
(בדל) מַבְדִּיל ← כסה
(בדק) בדק עצמו 79
בחינה 18
בִּטּוּל 130
(בטח) הבטיח 131
(בטל) ביטל 131
התבטל 131
בֶּטֶן 131 ← התרה, חלק, כסה, עצירה, עֹצֶר, שִׁפּוּל
(בטן) מובטן 132
ביצה ← אֹדֶם, מֹחַ
בית: בית הפרשות 79
בלבול: בלבול הדעת 132
בליטה 80
בלל 53
(בעבע) נתבעבע הצמח 80
בקיעה 132
ברזל 54 ← כלי, נְסֹרֶת
בַּשָּׁמוּת 132
בשר ← אֲגֻדָּה, כיס
בשרי ← אשך
בֶּתֶק 80
גְּזֵרָה 81
גחלת 133
גיד 18, 81
הגיד האמצעי 54
הגיד המדני 82
גיד הדופק 134
גיד הראש 82
גידים 133
גלב ← תער
גלגל 82
גלד: הגלד הענבי 82
גלידה 82
(גלל) מגולל 99
גְּמָמוּת 18
גְּמָמִי ← חבלה
גְּנוּחַ 83
גפן: גפנים 134
גפרית: גפרית חי 19
גרב 83
גרגור: גרגורים 83

גרגתני 84
גרד 84, 134
גרה 84
גרון ← נחרה
גרידה 19
גרידת המעים 134
גריקא ← זפת
גרירה 84
גֶּרַע 85 ←מסמר
גרעין :גרעינים 135
גרר: גרר במגרה 85
(גרש) גירש 19
דִּבּוּק ← פרוד
(דבק) נדבק 135
דִּבֵּק 135
מדביק 59
מְדֻבָּקִים 28
דֶּבֶק: דבק היד 20
דבקים 20
דבקה: דבקות 135
דְּבֵקוּת 136 ← הפרדה, התרה
דבקות הזהב 136
דבר: דברים מחליקים 26
דבש ← יערה
דבש מְקֻצָּף 20
דבשת 85
דופק ← דפק
דחיקה 20
דָּחַק 21
דֹּחַק: בדֹחַק 21
דליות 85
דם ← הגרה, הטפה, רעיפה
דם שני האחים 71
דעת ← בלבול
(דפק) דופק ← גיד
דק ← שחין
דקירה 137
דקר 137
דרדני 85
הבטחה 137
הברה 86
הגלדה 86
הגרה: הגרת הדם 138
הגרת הדם מהאף 138
הדבקה 21
הִדּוּק 86
הזלה: הזלות הראש 86
הזרה 21, 87, 138

הטפה: הטפת דם מהנחירים 138
הטפות 87
הטפחה 87
הידרוקן 139
הכרה ← הקדמה
המעדה 88
המעדת המעים 139
הנהגה: הנהגת השמירה 40
הנחה 139
העדפה: העדפות 22, 88
(הפך) הפך ל- 139
התהפך 22, 23
הפרדה: הפרדת הדבקות 140
הפשטה 22
הקדמה: הקדמת ההכרה 140
הקעה 55
הקפאה 140
הרגל: הרגלים 140
הרגשה 140
הריון 141
השבה 22
השבת השברים 88
השבון 22
הַשְׁוָיוֹת 141
השמטה 141
השמטות 23
הַשְׁמָעוּת 23
השקעה 141
השתדלות: השתדלות הרפואה 142
התחכחות 23
התיתרות 142
התכה 142
התכי 143
התלבדות 88
התלהבות 55, 89
התפוצצות 89
התרה 55
התרת הבטן 143
התרת הדבקות 24
התרת השתן 143
ווירוס 43
וינטוסי 43
ויתן: ויתנים 24
וריד 89
זאב ← מות
זהב ← דְּבֵקוּת
(זור) הזיר 143
המזירים 24

Index

זיו: זיו האדם 143
זיכום 89
זינה 25
זיפק 43
זירבו 43
זַכּוּת 144
זמורה 89
זמורי ← אשך
זמן 25
זנב ← חָלָל
זנב העין 90
זפת: זפת גריקא 45
זקן ← שִׁבֹּלֶת
הזקן התחתון 90
זרוע 144 ← חֶבֶל, פרק
זרעון 71
(חבא) נֶחְבָּא 169
חִבּוּש: חיבוש 90, 144
(חבל)[1]: חיבל 145
התחבל 145
(חבל)[2]: התחבל 145
חֶבֶל: חבל הזרוע 90
חֵבֶל/חֶבֶל: חבלים 145
חֲבָלָה: חבלות 25, 146
החבלות הגממיות 19
(חבר) מחברת ← רפואה
מחובר 161
(חבש) נחבש 91
חִבֵּש 91
מְחַבֵּש 101
התחבש 91
מְחֻדָּד: מחודד 161
חוט 146
החוטים הנתלים 91
חוֹל 147
חזירי ← צמח
(חזק) חיזק 147
מוחזק 161
חָח 92
חטה: שני החטים 92
חֹטֶם: חוטם ← עֹקֶץ
חי ← גפרית, יין, סיד
חיק: חיק העין 92
(חכם) מחוכם 59
חלאה: חלאת הים 25
חָלָב ← מיץ
חֵלֶב 147 ← כיס
החלב אשר על הקרב 92
החלב המכסה (את) הקרב 92, 147
חלול: חלולים 148
חלוקה 92
(חלחל) מתחלחל 93
חֳלִי 148
חולי האריה 56
חולי הנחש 56
חולי הפיל 56
חולי הצד 148
חולי השועל 56
חָלָל 148
חלל הזנב 93
חלל העורף 93
חללות 94
חלצים: (מ)תחת החלצים 93, 149
(חלק) להחליק הבטן 149
החליק הטבע 150
מחליק ← דבר, רפואה
חָלָק 149
חלקות/ חֲלָקוּת / חַלְקוּת 26, 150
חלקות המיעים 150
חַם ← צבות, צמח
חִמּוּץ: חימוץ האתרוגים 150
חמרמרות 56
חֹמֶש: חומש 91
חניקה 94
חֶנֶק 151
חספניתא 57
חפז 151
חפיפה 57, 151
(חפש) מחפש 101
חֲרִיכוּת 94
חשב 151
חתום ← חתם
חִתּוּם 57
(חתך) נחתך 152
חתם 152
חתום ← טירה
התחתם 58
החתים 57
מחתימים 59
טִבּוּל: טיבולים 153
טבל 153
טבע ← חלק
טָחוּל 154
טיחה 85, 95
טיסיס 43
טירה: טירה חתומה 45

טנטא 44
(טפח) הטפיח 95
טָרַח 154
טֹרַח: טורח 154
בטֹרַח 26
טרפשה 95
טשטי 44
יד ← דֶּבֶק, מסרק, משמוש, פרק
יום ← קדחת
יוצא ← יצא
(יחס) מְיֻחָס: מיוחסים ← אֵבָר
יין: יין חי 55
ים ← חלאה, קֶצֶף
יערה: יערת הדבש 155
(יצא) יוצא 155
הוציא 155
יציאה: יציאות 58
יציקה 26
ירידה: ירידת המים בעין 155
ירך ← כף, עקר, ראש
ירקנות 156
(ישן) התישן 96
יָשָׁר 156
(יתר) מיותר 162
התיתר 156
יֶתֶר: יתרים 157
כד 96
כִּוּץ 96, 157
כוליא 96
כורת ← כרת
כותח 157
כח: כח המפרנס 164
כיס 158
כיס הבשר 158
כיס החלב 159
כיס המים 159
כיס המעים 159
כיס מקוה המים 97
כיסים 97
כלב: כלב שוטה 59
כלונס: כלונסות 97
כלי: כלי נוקב 98
כלי ברזל 97
כלי הממשש 27
כמהים/ כמהין 27
(כנס) נכנס 159
(כסה) הַמְכַסֶּה הַמַּבְדִּיל 29
מכסה הבטן 102
כף 27
כף הירך 98
כָּפוּל 159
כפל 160
נכפל 160
הכפיל 160
כריתות 27
כרכשה 98
(כרת) כורת: כורתים 26
כשיל 98
כת: הכת הקרניי 160
כתות 160
כֻּתֹּנֶת: כתנות 27
(לבד) מתלבד 98
לוח: לוחות 28
לופיני ← קמח
לחות: לחויות ממעידות 104
לטש 98
לכלך 99
לעוסה: לעוסות 99
לצרטי 44
לקה 160
מְבֹאָר ← באר
מַבְדִּיל ← בדל
מֻבְטָן ← בטן
מגולל ← גלל
מגופה 99
מַגְזֵר 100
מַגְזֵרָה: מגזרות 100
מֻגְלִי: מוגלי 160
מגרה ← גרר
מדביק ← דבק
מֻדְבָּק ← דבק
מדחה 100
מדני ← גיד
מוסקולו 44
מוצא 28
מורסא :המורסא השורצת 191
(מות) ממית הזאב 163
מזון ← מיץ
מזיר ← זור
מזלג 29, 100
מזלגי ← מסמר
מֹחַ: מוח הביצים 161
מחבוא 101
מְחֻבָּר: מחובר ← חבר

מחברת ← חבר
מְחַבֵּשׁ ← חבש
מְחֻדָּד: מחודד ← חדד
מְחֻזָּק: מוחזק ← חזק
מְחֻכָּם: מחוכם ← חכם
מְחִלָּה 29
מחליק ← חלק
מחפש ← חפש
מחשבה 162
מחתים: מחתימים ← חתם
מְיַחֵס ← אֵבֶר
מים ← ירידה, כיס, עדשה, עשן
  לעשות מי רגלים 101
מימי ← אשך
מימיות 101
מיץ: מיץ חלב 71
  מיץ המזון 162
מירק 44
מְיֻתָּר: מיותר ← יתר
מֵיתָר: מתרים ← אבר
מכה: מכות 29
מכוה 101
  מכוה סכיני 102
מִכְחֹל: מכחול 102
מכסה ← חֵלֶב, כסה, קרום
(מלא) ממולא 163
  התמלא 162
מִלּוּי: מילוי 163
מלקחים 30,102
מלתעה/ מלתעת ← מתלעת
ממית ← מות
מְמֻלָּא: ממולא ← מלא
מְמֹרְסָם: ממורסם ← מרסם
ממשש ← משש
מנגע: מנגעים ← נגע
מנע 163
מָסָך 164
מסמר 103
  מסמר מזלגי 103
  מסמר הגרע 103
מסרק: מסרק היד 103
  מסרק הרגל 103
מעבר: מעבר השתן 103
מעי ← אֹמֶץ, גרידה, המעדה, חֲלָקוֹת, כיס, מעידה
  המעי התחתון 30
מעידה ← לחה
  מעידת המעים 164
מעיי ← אשך
מַעֲלֶה ← אֵבֶר
מְעֻנָּג: מעונג ← ענג
מעצור ← עצר
מפרנס ← פרנס
מְפֻשָּׁט ← פשט
מצב 165
מצנפת: מצנפות 60
מצעת 165
מקבת 104
מקוה ← כיס
מקום 165 ← נֶקֶב
מקומי 166
מָקוֹר: מקורים 166
מַקּוֹר 104
מקורי 166
מְקֻצָּף ← קצף
מַרְאֶה 61, 167
מְרֻבָּע: מרובע 105
מרוצה 167
מרחץ ← רגל
מֹרֶךְ: מורך 167
מרכב: מירכב 167
(מרסם) ממורסם 163
  התמרסם 168
מרפק ← פרק
מרקחת 168
מְשִׁיחוּת 31
(משך) נמשך זו אחר זו 168
מְשֻׁכָּךְ ← שכך
(משל) מושל ← אֵבֶר
משלחת 31
משמוש: המישמוש בידים 168
משמרת ← קנה
משמש 169
מְשֻׁעֲמָם ← שעמם
מַשְׂרֵט: משרטים 105
(משש) ממשש 30 ← כלי
מתאים ← תאם
מתחלחל ← חלחל
מתלעת/ מלתעה/ מלתעת 31
(מתן) המתין על 169
מתנגע ← נגע
נאדי ← שקוי
(נגע) מנגעים ← סם
  מתנגע 62
נֶגַע 31, 62 ← עשה
  הנגעים הנוקבים 33
נהג 32

(נוח) הֵנִּיחַ מן 169
נוקב ← נָקַב
נֶחְבָּא ← חבא
נחיר ← הטפה
נחרה: נחרת הגרון 105
נחש ← חֳלִי
נחשת ← פרח, קל(י)פה
נטייה: נטיית הפה 105
נִיּוּת 170
נִכְאוּת 170
(נכה) הכה 170
(נכר) הכיר על 170
נמלה 32, 170
נסירה 32
נְסֹרֶת: נסורת ברזל 32
נער 106
נִפּוּשׁ 171 ← עֹצֶר, צָרוּת
(נָקַב) נוקב ← כלי, נֶגַע
נֶקֶב: נקב אותו מקום של אשה 33
הנקב התחתון 33
(נקה) לְהִנָּקוֹת 33
נְקָה 33
נקיון 43, 62
נקיות 34
נקירה 171
(נשג) השיג 171
נשך 172
(נתר) נִתַּר 173
התיר 172
סִבּוּב 63
סוף: סוף הפרשות 106
סור 34
סיד: הסיד החי 34
סכיני ← מכוה
סם: סמים מנגעים 60
סַמּוּת 173
סמרות 173
(סנן) סינן 34
סְנַפִּיר: סנפירות 63
סַעַר 173
סערה 174
(ספג) הספיג 174
ספוגי ← עֶצֶם
ספרד ← עפר
(עבה) עיבה 175
עגבה: עגבות ← עֶצֶם
עִגּוּל 63
עגול העין 106
(עדף) עוֹדֵף 175
עדשה: עדשי המים 71
עוגה 63
עוֹדֵף ← עדף
עונה 175 ← קדחת
עופרת ← קל(י)פה
עוֹתֵק ← עתק
עַיִן ← אפר, זנב, חיק, ירידה, עִגּוּל, ראה, ראש
עַיִן: עין בעין 176
עכביש ← אריגה
עֲלִיָּה 176
עלילה 34
עמידה 176
ענבי ← גלד
(ענג) מעונג 30
ענה 176
עפר: עפר ספרד 72
עֵצָה 106
עִצּוּם: עיצום 107
עִצּוּר 64
עצירה ← אֹפֶן
עצירת הבטן 177
עצלה 64
(עצם) התעצם 107
עֶצֶם: העצם העומד למטה מכל השדרה 177
עצם העגבות 177
העצמים הספוגיים 107
עַצְמוּת 178
עצר 35, 178
לעצור עצמו מן 35
מעצור 30, 60
עֹצֶר: עוצר הבטן 178
עוצר הניפוש 178
עֹקֶץ: עוקץ החוטם 107
עקר: עיקרי הירכים 107
ערבוב: ערבוב שכל 65
עֹרֶף ← חָלָל
ערקה 108
עשה 65, 179
עשה הנגע 65
עִשּׁוּן 35
עשן: עישן במים 35
עששית 179
(עתק) עוֹתֵק 175
פדלקון 108
פדלקן: לפדלקן 108
פה ← נטייה

Index

פּוֹשֵׁר ← פשר
פחד 179
(פטר) הפטיר 108
פיל ← חֲלִי
פישטולא 45
פיתקא 109
פֶּלַח 109
פלחי השפתים 109
פלך: פלך הארכובה 109
(פסק) נִפְסָק 180
הפסיק 65
פרוד: פרוד (ה)דבוק 66
פרונקא: פרונקות 110
פרח: פרח הנחשת 36
פרנס 180
מפרנס ← כח
היה מתפרנס 180
פרנסה 180
פרק: פרק היד 36, 110
פרק המרפק 110
פרק קנה הזרוע הסמוך ליד 110
פרשה: פרשות ← בית, סוף
(פשט) נפשט 36
פִּשֵּׁט המעים 36
מְפֻשָּׁט 31
(פשר) היה פושר 179
פתח 181
פתיחה 181
צבות: צבות חמה 110
צד ← חֲלִי
צילחתא 111
צֶלַע: מה שתחת הצלעות 181
צלעות 111
צמח 36, 111 ← בעבע
צמח חזירי 111
צמח חם 111
צִפּוֹרֶן: צ(י)פורן 111, 182
צָרוּת: צרות הניפוש 182
קֵבָה: קיבת האשה 112
קִבּוּץ 66, 182
קביצה 183
(קבס) נִקְבָּס 112
קבסא 66
(קבץ) קוֹבֵץ 183
קדחת: הקדחת העונה בכל יום 183
(קדם) הקדים 183
קִוּוּץ 37, 66
קטן ← אצבע
קיא ← רצון
קילור: קילורים 112
קלוח: קלוחים 67
קִלּוּי 183
קליבוסתא 37
קל(י)פה 184
קלפת נחשת 72
קלפת עופרת 37
קליפות 67, 112
קמח: קמח אורובי 45
קמח לופיני 46
קנה ← פרק
קנה משמרת 38
(קצף) מְקֻצָּף ← דבש
קֶצֶף: קצף הים 72
קרא: קרא על 184
קרב ← חֵלֶב
קרום: קרום מכסה 38
קרירות 185
קרן: קרנים 113
קרני הראש 113
קרני הרחם 113
קרניי ← כת
קרע 185
קִשּׁוּר 185
קֹשִׁי: קושי 186
קשירה 186
קשירות 38
קשיש: קשישים 113
קשקש 113
קֶשֶׁר 38, 186
קשרים 68
(ראה) הרואה שלעין 187
ראוי: היה ראוי 186
ראות 113
ראש ← גיד, הזלה, קרן, רִבּוּעַ
ראש העין 114
ראשי הירכים 114
רִבּוּעַ: רבוע הראש 39
רבידא 114
רגיל 114
היה רגיל 39
(רגל) הרגיל 39, 114
הרגיל במרחץ 39
רֶגֶל ← מים, רגל
רוֹאֶה ← ראה
רוחיי ← אשך
רַחַיִם 187

רחיצה 187
רחם ← קרן
ריאומה 45
ריקות 115
ריר 68
רמז 187
רִסּוּק / ריסוק 68, 115
רעיפה: רעיפת הדם 115
רַעַם 188
(רפא) ריפא 188
רפואה ← השתדלות
רפואה מחברת 25
רפואה מחליקה 26
רפואה מתאימה 41
הרפואות אשר יודעו במשככות 61
רפידה: רפידות 188
רפפות 188
רצון: רצון קיא 189
רִקּוּחַ 68
(רקק) הרקיק 189
(רתע) הרתיע לאחור 116
שאף 189
שבב: שבבים 116
שִׁבֹּלֶת: שבולת הזקן 116
שבר ← השבה
(שדף) שָׁדוּף 190
השתדף 116
שדרה ← עֶצֶם
(שוב) השיב 190
שוטה ← שטה
שׁוֹכֵן ← שכן
שׁוֹמֵר ← שמר
שועל ← חֳלִי
שׁוֹרֵץ ← שרץ
שחי: תחת השחי 42, 195
שחין: השחין הדק 116
שחפת 117
(שטה) שוטה ← כלב
שטות 69, 117
(שטח) השטיח 117
שיבא 118
שכיבה 40
שכינה 191
(שכך) משככות ← רפואה
שכל ← ערבוב
(שכן) שׁוֹכֵן 190
שלהבת 69
שִׁלּוּחַ: שילוח הדם 19
שלם: שלם על 191
שמיטה 118
שמיר 118
שמירה 69, 192 ← הנהגה
(שמר) שׁוֹמֵר 190
שִׁנּוּי: שינוי 192
שעיעות 40
שעיר 40
שעירות 40
שעמום 193
(שעמם) מְשֻׁעֲמָם 169
(שעע) שְׁעַשַׁע 41
שפה ← פֶּלַח
שִׁפּוּל: שפולי הבטן 41
שקוי: השקוי הנאדי 118
שקיעה 119
שקיקה 193
שקע: השקיע 119
שֵׁרוּי 193
שָׂרִי 193
(שרץ) שׁוֹרֵץ 191 ← מורסא
שִׁתּוּק 194
שָׁתוּק ← שתק
שתיקה 194
שתן ← התרה, מעבר
(שתק) שָׁתוּק 194
(תאם) מתאים ← רפואה
תונבא 120
תוספת: תוספות 194
תוצאה :תוצאות 41
תַּחְבֹּשֶׁת: תחבושת 42
תחתון ← זקן, נֶקֶב
תיק 194
תכונה 69
תכלית 70, 195
(תלה) נתלים ← חוט
תלולית: תלוליות של בשר 120
(תמד) התמיד 70
תער 42
תער הגלבים 120
תפירה 42
תפירות 120
תרדמה 70
תרדמת האברים 70